Core Curriculum for Nephrology Nursing

Sixth Edition

Editor: Caroline S. Counts, MSN, RN, CNN

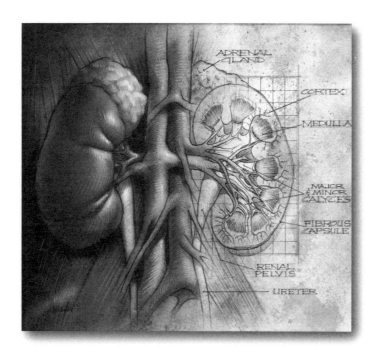

MODULE 6

The APRN's Approaches to Care in Nephrology

ANNA American Nephrology Nurses' Association
www.annanurse.org

Core Curriculum for Nephrology Nursing, 6th Edition

Editor and Project Director
Caroline S. Counts, MSN, RN, CNN

MODULE 6 • The APRN's Approaches to Care in Nephrology
Module Editors: Kim Alleman, Katherine Houle

Publication Management
Anthony J. Jannetti, Inc.
East Holly Avenue/Box 56
Pitman, New Jersey 08071-0056

Managing Editor: Claudia Cuddy
Editorial Coordinator: Joseph Tonzelli
Layout Design and Production: Claudia Cuddy
Layout Assistants: Kaytlyn Mroz, Katerina DeFelice, Casey Shea, Courtney Klauber
Design Consultants: Darin Peters, Jack M. Bryant
Proofreaders: Joseph Tonzelli, Evelyn Haney, Alex Grover, Nicole Ward
Cover Design: Darin Peters
Cover Illustration: Scott M. Holladay © 2006
Photography: Kim Counts and Marty Morganello (*unless otherwise credited*)

MODULE 6. The APRN's Approaches to Care in Nephrology
Copyright © 2015 American Nephrology Nurses' Association
ISBN 978-1-940325-11-8

American Nephrology Nurses' Association, East Holly Avenue/Box 56, Pitman, New Jersey 08071-0056
www.annanurse.org ■ Email: anna@annanurse.org ■ Phone: 888-600-2662

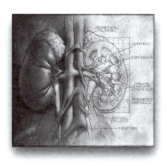

Foreword

The American Nephrology Nurses' Association has had a long-standing commitment to providing the tools and resources needed for individuals to be successful in their professional nephrology roles. With that commitment, we proudly present the sixth edition of the *Core Curriculum for Nephrology Nursing*.

This edition has a new concept and look that we hope you find valuable. Offered in six separate modules, each one will focus on a different component of our specialty and provide essential, updated, high-quality information. Since our last publication of the *Core Curriculum* in 2008, our practice has evolved, and our publication has been transformed to keep pace with those changes.

Under the expert guidance of Editor and Project Director Caroline S. Counts, MSN, RN, CNN (who was also the editor for the 2008 *Core Curriculum*!), this sixth edition continues to build on our fundamental principles and standards of practice. From the basics of each modality to our roles in advocacy, patient engagement, evidence-based practice, and more, you will find crucial information to facilitate the important work you do on a daily basis.

The ANNA Board of Directors and I extend our sincerest gratitude to Caroline and commend her for the stellar work that she and all of the section editors, authors, and reviewers have put forth in developing this new edition of the *Core Curriculum for Nephrology Nursing*. These individuals have spent many hours working to provide you with this important nephrology nursing publication. We hope you enjoy this exemplary professional resource.

Sharon Longton, BSN, RN, CNN, CCTC
ANNA President, 2014-2015

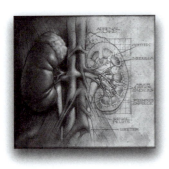

What's new in the sixth edition?

The 2015 edition of the *Core Curriculum for Nephrology Nursing* reflects several changes in format and content. These changes have been made to make life easier for the reader and to improve the scientific value of the *Core*.

1. The *Core Curriculum* is divided into six separate modules that can be purchased as a set or as individual texts. Keep in mind there is likely additional relevant information in more than one module. For example, in Module 2 there is a specific chapter for nutrition, but the topic of nutrition is also addressed in several chapters in other modules.

2. The *Core* is available in both print and electronic formats. The electronic format contains links to other websites with additional helpful information that can be reached with a simple click. With this useful feature comes a potential issue: when an organization changes its website and reroutes its links, the URLs that are provided may not connect. When at the organization's website, use their search feature to easily find your topic. The links in the *Core* were updated as of March 2015.

3. As with the last edition of the *Core*, the pictures on chapter covers depict actual nephrology staff members and patients with kidney disease. Their willingness to participate is greatly appreciated.

4. Self-assessment questions are included at the end of each module for self-testing. Completion of these exercises is not required to obtain CNE. CNE credit can be obtained by accessing the Evaluation Forms on the ANNA website.

5. References are cited in the text and listed at the end of each chapter.

6. We've provided examples of references in APA format at the beginning of each chapter, as well as on the last page of this front matter, to help the readers know how to properly format references if they use citations from the *Core*. The guesswork has been eliminated!

7. The information contained in the *Core* has been expanded, and new topics have been included. For example, there is information on leadership and management, material on caring for Veterans, more emphasis on patient and staff safety, and more.

8. Many individuals assisted in making the *Core* come to fruition; they brought with them their own experience, knowledge, and literature search. As a result, a topic can be addressed from different perspectives, which in turn gives the reader a more global view of nephrology nursing.

9. This edition employs usage of the latest terminology in nephrology patterned after the National Kidney Foundation.

10. The *Core Curriculum for Nephrology Nursing*, 6th edition contains 233 figures, 234 tables, and 29 appendices. These add valuable tools in delivering the contents of the text.

Thanks to B. Braun Medical Inc. for its grant in support of ANNA's *Core Curriculum*.

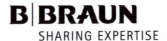

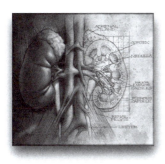

Preface

The sixth edition of the *Core Curriculum for Nephrology Nursing* has been written and published due to the efforts of many individuals. Thank you to the editors, authors, reviewers, and everyone who helped pull the *Core* together to make it the publication it became. A special thank you to Claudia Cuddy and Joe Tonzelli, who were involved from the beginning to the end — I could not have done my job without them!

The overall achievement is the result of the unselfish contributions of each and every individual team member. At times it was a daunting, challenging task, but the work is done, and all members of the "Core-team" should feel proud of the end product.

Now, the work is turned over to you — the reader and learner. I hope you learn at least half as much as I did as pieces of the *Core* were submitted, edited, and refined. Considering the changes that have taken place since the first edition of the *Core* in 1987 (322 pages!), one could say it is a whole new world! Even since the fifth edition in 2008, many changes in nephrology have transpired. This, the 2015 edition, is filled with the latest information regarding kidney disease, its treatment, and the nursing care involved.

But, buyer, beware! Evolution continues, and what is said today can be better said tomorrow. Information continues to change and did so even as the chapters were being written; yet, change reflects progress. Our collective challenge is to learn from the *Core*, be flexible, keep an open mind, and question what could be different or how nephrology nursing practice could be improved.

Nephrology nursing will always be stimulating, learning will never end, and progress will continue! So, the *Core* not only represents what we know now, but also serves as a springboard for what the learner can become and what nephrology nursing can be. A Chinese proverb says this: "Learning is like rowing upstream; not to advance is to drop back."

A final thank-you to the Core-team and a very special note of appreciation to those I love the most. (Those I love the most have also grown since the last edition!) For their love, support, and encouragement, I especially thank my husband, Henry, who thought I had retired; my son and daughter-in law, Chris and Christina, and our two amazing grandchildren, Cate and Olin; and my son-in-law, Marty Morganello, and our daughter, Kim, who provided many of the photographs used in this version of the *Core*. It has been a family project!

Last, but certainly not least, I thank the readers and learners. It is your charge to use the *Core* to grow your minds. Minds can grow as long as we live — don't drop back!

Caroline S. Counts
Editor, Sixth Edition

Module 6

Module 6 was designed and written for Advance Practice Registered Nurses (APRNs) under the guidance of the module's editors, Katherine Houle and Kim Alleman. Its topics are meant for the APRN new to nephrology practice as well as for those with experience. The module is divided into 5 chapters. The first addresses professional issues related to the APRN and end-of-life issues. In the next chapter, chronic kidney disease stages 1 through 5 are presented. Chapter 3 offers an overview of treatment options for kidney replacement therapy. It includes transplant, hemodialysis, the vascular access, peritoneal dialysis, and home dialysis. The next chapter covers acute kidney injury (AKI) and presents useful information pertaining to AKI, its causes, and its treatments. Chapter 5 discusses care of the pediatric patient by the APRN.

Additional information on almost all of these topics can be found in the other modules of the *Core Curriculum for Nephrology Nursing*. The APRN will find this information useful as well.

Special thanks go to Robin Davis, Child Life Specialist at Texas Children's Hospital, for providing photos of real patients and staff.

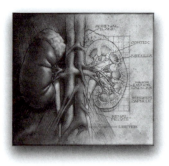

Chapter Editors and Authors

Lisa Ales, MSN, NP-C, FNP-BC, CNN
Clinical Educator, Renal
Baxter Healthcare Corporation
Deerfield, IL
Author: Module 3, Chapter 4

Kim Alleman, MS, APRN, FNP-BC, CNN-NP
Nurse Practitioner
Hartford Hospital Transplant Program
Hartford, CT
Editor: Module 6

Billie Axley, MSN, RN, CNN
Director, Innovations Group
FMS Medical Office
Franklin, TN
Author: Module 4, Chapter 3

**Donna Bednarski, MSN, RN, ANP-BC,
  CNN, CNP**
Nurse Practitioner, Dialysis Access Center
Harper University Hospital
Detroit, MI
Editor & Author: Module 1, Chapter 3
Editor & Author: Module 2, Chapter 3
Author: Module 6, Chapter 3

Brandy Begin, BSN, RN, CNN
Pediatric Dialysis Coordinator
Lucile Packard Children's Hospital at Stanford
Palo Alto, CA
Author: Module 5, Chapter 1

Deborah Brommage, MS, RDN, CSR, CDN
Program Director
National Kidney Foundation
New York, NY
Editor & Author: Module 2, Chapter 4
Editor: Module 4, Chapter 3

**Deborah H. Brooks, MSN, ANP-BC, CNN,
  CNN-NP**
Nurse Practitioner
Medical University of South Carolina
Charleston, SC
Author: Module 6, Chapter 1

Colleen M. Brown, MSN, APRN, ANP-BC
Transplant Nurse Practitioner
Hartford Hospital
Hartford, CT
Author: Module 6, Chapter 3

Loretta Jackson Brown, PhD, RN, CNN
Health Communication Specialist
Centers for Disease Control and Prevention
Atlanta, GA
Author: Module 2, Chapter 3

**Molly Cahill, MSN, RN, APRN, BC,
  ANP-C, CNN**
Nurse Practitioner
KC Kidney Consultants
Kansas City, MO
Author: Module 2, Chapter 3

Sally F. Campoy, DNP, ANP-BC, CNN-NP
Nurse Practitioner, Renal Section
Department of Veterans Affairs
Eastern Colorado Health System
Denver VA Medical Center, Denver, CO
Author: Module 6, Chapter 2

Laurie Carlson, MSN, RN
Transplant Coordinator
University of California –
  San Francisco Medical Center
San Francisco, CA
Author: Module 3, Chapter 1

Deb Castner, MSN, APRN, ACNP, CNN
Nurse Practitioner
Jersey Coast Nephrology & Hypertension
  Associates
Brick, NJ
Author: Module 2, Chapter 3
Author: Module 3, Chapter 2

Louise Clement, MS, RDN, CSR, LD
Renal Dietitian
Fresenius Medical Care
Lubbock, TX
Author: Module 2, Chapter 4

Jean Colaneri, ACNP-BC, CNN
Clinical Nurse Specialist and Nurse
  Practitioner, Dialysis Apheresis
Albany Medical Center Hospital, Albany, NY
Editor & Author: Module 3, Chapter 1

Ann Beemer Cotton, MS, RDN, CNSC
Clinical Dietitian Specialist in Critical Care
IV Health/Methodist Campus
Indianapolis, IN
Author: Module 2, Chapter 4
Author: Module 4, Chapter 2

Caroline S. Counts, MSN, RN, CNN
Research Coordinator, Retired
Division of Nephrology
Medical Unversity of South Carolina
Charleston, SC
Editor: Core Curriculum for Nephrology Nursing
Author: Module 1, Chapter 2
Author: Module 2, Chapter 6
Author: Module 3, Chapter 3

Helen Currier, BSN, RN, CNN, CENP
Director, Renal Services, Dialysis/Pheresis,
  Vascular Access/Wound, Ostomy,
  Continence, & Palliative Care Services
Texas Children's Hospital, Houston, TX
Author: Module 6, Chapter 5

Kim Deaver, MSN, RN, CNN
Program Manager
University of Virginia
Charlottesville, VA
Editor & Author: Module 3, Chapter 3

Anne Diroll, MA, BSN, BS, RN, CNN
Consultant
Volume Management
Rocklin, CA
Author: Module 5, Chapter 1

Daniel Diroll, MA, BSN, BS, RN
Education Coordinator
Fresenius Medical Care North America
Rocklin, CA
Author: Module 2, Chapter 3

**Sheila J. Doss-McQuitty, MBA, BSN, RN,
  CNN, CCRA**
Director, Clinical Programs and Research
Satellite Healthcare, Inc., San Jose, CA
Author: Module 2, Chapter 1

Paula Dutka, MSN, RN, CNN
Director, Education and Research
Nephrology Network
Winthrop University Hospital, Mineola, NY
Author: Module 2, Chapter 1

**Andrea Easom, MA, MNSc, APRN,
  FNP-BC, CNN-NP**
Instructor, College of Medicine
Nephrology Division
University of Arkansas for Medical Sciences
Little Rock, AR
Author: Module 6, Chapter 2

Rowena W. Elliott, PhD, RN, CNN, CNE, AGNP-C, FAAN
Associate Professor and Chairperson
Department of Advanced Practice
College of Nursing
University of Southern Mississippi
Hattiesburg, MS
Editor & Author: Module 5, Chapter 2

Susan Fallone, MS, RN, CNN
Clinical Nurse Specialist, Retired
Adult and Pediatric Dialysis
Albany Medical Center, Albany, NY
Author: Module 4, Chapter 2

Jessica J. Geer, MSN, C-PNP, CNN-NP
Pediatric Nurse Practitioner
Texas Children's Hospital, Houston, TX
Instructor, Renal Services, Dept. of Pediatrics
Baylor College of Medicine, Houston, TX
Author: Module 6, Chapter 5

Silvia German, RN, CNN
Clinical Writer, CE Coordinator
Manager, DaVita HealthCare Partners Inc.
Denver, CO
Author: Module 2, Chapter 6

Elaine Go, MSN, NP, CNN-NP
Nurse Practitioner
St. Joseph Hospital Renal Center
Orange, CA
Author: Module 6, Chapter 3

Norma Gomez, MSN, MBA, RN, CNN
Nephrology Nurse Consultant
Russellville, TN
Editor & Author: Module 1, Chapter 4

Janelle Gonyea, RDN, LD
Clinical Dietitian
Mayo Clinic
Rochester, MN
Author: Module 2, Chapter 4

Karen Greco, PhD, RN, ANP-BC, FAAN
Nurse Practitioner
Independent Contractor/Consultant
West Linn, OR
Author: Module 2, Chapter 1

Bonnie Bacon Greenspan, MBA, BSN, RN
Consultant, BBG Consulting, LLC
Alexandria, VA
Author: Module 1, Chapter 1

Cheryl L. Groenhoff, MSN, MBA, RN, CNN
Clinical Educator, Baxter Healthcare
Plantation, FL
Author: Module 2, Chapter 3
Author: Module 3, Chapter 4

Debra J. Hain, PhD, ARNP, ANP-BC, GNP-BC, FAANP
Assistant Professor/Lead AGNP Faculty
Florida Atlantic University
Christine E. Lynn College of Nursing
Boca Raton, FL
Nurse Practitioner, Cleveland Clinic Florida
Department of Nephrology, Weston, FL
Editor & Author: Module 2, Chapter 2

Lisa Hall, MSSW, LICSW
Patient Services Director
Northwest Renal Network (ESRD Network 16)
Seattle, WA
Author: Module 2, Chapter 3

Mary S. Haras, PhD, MS, MBA, APN, NP-C, CNN
Assistant Professor and Interim Associate
  Dean of Graduate Nursing
Saint Xavier University School of Nursing
Chicago, IL
Author: Module 2, Chapter 2

Carol Motes Headley, DNSc, ACNP-BC, RN, CNN
Nephrology Nurse Practitioner
Veterans Affairs Medical Center
Memphis, TN
Editor & Author: Module 2, Chapter 1

Mary Kay Hensley, MS, RDN, CSR
Chair/Immediate Past Chair
Renal Dietitians Dietetic Practice Group
Renal Dietitian, Retired
DaVita HealthCare Partners Inc.
Gary, IN
Author: Module 2, Chapter 4

Kerri Holloway, RN, CNN
Clinical Quality Manager
Corporate Infection Control Specialist
Fresenius Medical Services, Waltham, MA
Author: Module 2, Chapter 6

Alicia M. Horkan, MSN, RN, CNN
Assistant Director, Dialysis Services
Dialysis Center at Colquitt Regional
  Medical Center
Moultrie, GA
Author: Module 1, Chapter 2

Katherine Houle, MSN, APRN, CFNP, CNN-NP
Nephrology Nurse Practitioner
Marquette General Hospital
Marquette, MI
Editor: Module 6
Author: Module 6, Chapter 3

Liz Howard, RN, CNN
Director
DaVita HealthCare Partners Inc.
Oldsmar, FL
Author: Module 2, Chapter 6

Darlene Jalbert, BSN, RN, CNN
HHD Education Manager
DaVita University School of Clinical
  Education Wisdom Team
DaVita HealthCare Partners Inc., Denver, CO
Author: Module 3, Chapter 2

Judy Kauffman, MSN, RN, CNN
Manager, Acute Dialysis and Apheresis Unit
University of Virginia Health Systems
Charlottesville, VA
Author: Module 3, Chapter 2

Tamara Kear, PhD, RN, CNS, CNN
Assistant Professor of Nursing
Villanova University, Villanova, PA
Nephrology Nurse, Fresenius Medical Care
Philadelphia, PA
Editor & Author: Module 1, Chapter 2

Lois Kelley, MSW, LSW, ACSW, NSW-C
Master Social Worker
DaVita HealthCare Partners Inc.
Harrisonburg Dialysis
Harrisonburg, VA
Author: Module 2, Chapter 3

Pamela S. Kent, MS, RDN, CSR, LD
Patient Education Coordinator
Centers for Dialysis Care
Cleveland, OH
Author: Module 2, Chapter 4

Carol L. Kinzner, MSN, ARNP, GNP-BC, CNN-NP
Nurse Practitioner
Pacific Nephrology Associates
Tacoma, WA
Author: Module 6, Chapter 3

Kim Lambertson, MSN, RN, CNN
Clinical Educator
Baxter Healthcare
Deerfield, IL
Author: Module 3, Chapter 4

Sharon Longton, BSN, RN, CNN, CCTC
Transplant Coordinator/Educator
Harper University Hospital
Detroit, MI
Author: Module 2, Chapter 3

Maria Luongo, MSN, RN
CAPD Nurse Manager
Massachusetts General Hospital
Boston, MA
Author: Module 3, Chapter 5

Suzanne M. Mahon, DNSc, RN, AOCN, APNG
Professor, Internal Medicine
Division of Hematology/Oncology
Professor, Adult Nursing, School of Nursing
St. Louis University, St. Louis, MO
Author: Module 2, Chapter 1

Nancy McAfee, MN, RN, CNN
CNS – Pediatric Dialysis and Vascular Access
Seattle Children's Hospital
Seattle, WA
Editor & Author: Module 5, Chapter 1

Maureen P. McCarthy, MPH, RDN, CSR, LD
Assistant Professor/Transplant Dietitian
Oregon Health & Science University
Portland, OR
Author: Module 2, Chapter 4

M. Sue McManus, PhD, APRN, FNP-BC, CNN
Nephrology Nurse Practitioner
Kidney Transplant Nurse Practitioner
Richard L. Roudebush VA Medical Center
Indianapolis, IN
Author: Module 1, Chapter 2

Lisa Micklos, BSN, RN
Clinical Educator
NxStage Medical, Inc.
Los Angeles, CA
Author: Module 1, Chapter 2

Michele Mills, MS, RN, CPNP
Pediatric Nurse Practitioner
Pediatric Nephrology
University of Michigan
C.S. Mott Children's Hospital, Ann Arbor, MI
Author: Module 5, Chapter 1

Geraldine F. Morrison, BSHSA, RN
Clinical Director, Home Programs & CKD
Northwest Kidney Center
Seattle, WA
Author: Module 3, Chapter 5

Theresa Mottes, RN, CDN
Pediatric Research Nurse
Cincinnati Children's Hospital & Medical Center
Center for Acute Care Nephrology
Cincinnati, OH
Author: Module 5, Chapter 1

Linda L. Myers, BS, RN, CNN, HP
RN Administrative Coordinator, Retired
Home Dialysis Therapies
University of Virginia Health System
Charlottesville, VA
Author: Module 4, Chapter 5

Clara Neyhart, BSN, RN, CNN
Nephrology Nurse Clinician
UNC Chapel Hill
Chapel Hill, NC
Editor & Author: Module 3, Chapter 1

Mary Alice Norton, BSN, FNP-C
Senior Heart Failure/LVAD/Transplant
  Coordinator
Albany Medical Center Hospital
Albany, NY
Author: Module 4, Chapter 6

Jessie M. Pavlinac, MS, RDN, CSR, LD
Director, Clinical Nutrition
Oregon Health and Science University
Portland, OR
Author: Module 2, Chapter 4

Glenda M. Payne, MS, RN, CNN
Director of Clinical Services
Nephrology Clinical Solutions
Duncanville, TX
Editor & Author: Module 1, Chapter 1
Author: Module 3, Chapter 2
Author: Module 4, Chapter 4

**Eileen J. Peacock, MSN, RN, CNN,
  CIC, CPHQ, CLNC**
Infection Control and Surveillance
  Management Specialist
DaVita HealthCare Partners Inc.
Maple Glen, PA
Editor & Author: Module 2, Chapter 6

Mary Perrecone, MS, RN, CNN, CCRN
Clinical Manager
Fresenius Medical Care
Charleston, SC
Author: Module 4, Chapter 1

Susan A. Pfettscher, PhD, RN
California State University Bakersfield
  Department of Nursing, Retired
Satellite Health Care, San Jose, CA, Retired
Bakersfield, CA
Author: Module 1, Chapter 1

Nancy B. Pierce, BSN, RN, CNN
Dialysis Director
St. Peter's Hospital
Helena, MT
Author: Module 1, Chapter 1

Leonor P. Ponferrada, BSN, RN, CNN
Education Coordinator
University of Missouri School of Medicine –
  Columbia
Columbia, MO
Author: Module 3, Chapter 4

Lillian A. Pryor, MSN, RN, CNN
Clinical Manager
FMC Loganville, LLC
Loganville, GA
Author: Module 1, Chapter 1

Timothy Ray, DNP, CNP, CNN-NP
Nurse Practitioner
Cleveland Kidney & Hypertension Consultants
Euclid, OH
Author: Module 6, Chapter 4

Cindy Richards, BSN, RN, CNN
Transplant Coordinator
Children's of Alabama
Birmingham, AL
Author: Module 5, Chapter 1

Karen C. Robbins, MS, RN, CNN
Nephrology Nurse Consultant
Associate Editor, *Nephrology Nursing Journal*
Past President, American Nephrology Nurses'
  Association
West Hartford, CT
Editor: Module 3, Chapter 2

Regina Rohe, BS, RN, HP(ASCP)
Regional Vice President, Inpatient Services
Fresenius Medical Care, North America
San Francisco, CA
Author: Module 4, Chapter 8

Francine D. Salinitri, PharmD
Associate (Clinical) Professor of
  Pharmacy Practice
Wayne State University, Applebaum College of
  Pharmacy and Health Sciences, Detroit, MI
Clinical Pharmacy Specialist, Nephrology
Oakwood Hospital and Medical Center
Dearborn, MI
Author: Module 2, Chapter 5

Karen E. Schardin, BSN, RN, CNN
Clinical Director, National Accounts
NxStage Medical, Inc.
Lawrence, MA
Editor & Author: Module 3, Chapter 5

Mary Schira, PhD, RN, ACNP-BC
Associate Professor
Univ. of Texas at Arlington – College of Nursing
Arlington, TX
Author: Module 6, Chapter 1

Deidra Schmidt, PharmD
Clinical Pharmacy Specialist
Pediatric Renal Transplantation
Children's of Alabama
Birmingham, AL
Author: Module 5, Chapter 1

Joan E. Speranza-Reid, BSHM, RN, CNN
Clinic Manager
ARA/Miami Regional Dialysis Center
North Miami Beach, FL
Author: Module 3, Chapter 2

Jean Stover, RDN, CSR, LDN
Renal Dietitian
DaVita HealthCare Partners Inc.
Philadelphia, PA
Author: Module 2, Chapter 4

Charlotte Szromba, MSN, APRN, CNNe
Nurse Consultant, Retired
Department Editor, Nephrology Nursing
  Journal
Naperville, IL
Author: Module 2, Chapter 1

Kirsten L. Thompson, MPH, RDN, CSR
Clinical Dietitian
Seattle Children's Hospital, Seattle, WA
Author: Module 5, Chapter 1

Lucy B. Todd, MSN, ACNP-BC, CNN
Medical Science Liaison
Baxter Healthcare
Asheville, NC
Editor & Author: Module 3, Chapter 4

Susan C. Vogel, MHA, RN, CNN
Clinical Manager, National Accounts
NxStage Medical, Inc.
Los Angeles, CA
Author: Module 3, Chapter 5

Joni Walton, PhD, RN, ACNS-BC, NPc
Family Nurse Practitioner
Marias HealthCare
Shelby, MT
Author: Module 2, Chapter 1

Gail S. Wick, MHSA, BSN, RN, CNNe
Consultant
Atlanta, GA
Author: Module 1, Chapter 2

Helen F. Williams, MSN, BSN, RN, CNN
Special Projects – Acute Dialysis Team
Fresenius Medical Care
Denver, CO
Editor: Module 4
Editor & Author: Module 4, Chapter 7

Elizabeth Wilpula, PharmD, BCPS
Clinical Pharmacy Specialist
Nephrology/Transplant
Harper University Hospital, Detroit, MI
Editor & Author: Module 2, Chapter 5

Karen Wiseman, MSN, RN, CNN
Manager, Regulatory Affairs
Fresenius Medical Services
Waltham, MA
Author: Module 2, Chapter 6

Linda S. Wright, DrNP, RN, CNN, CCTC
Lead Kidney and Pancreas Transplant
  Coordinator
Thomas Jefferson University Hospital
Philadelphia, PA
Author: Module 1, Chapter 2

Mary M. Zorzanello, MSN, APRN
Nurse Practitioner, Section of Nephrology
Yale University School of Medicine
New Haven, CT
Author: Module 6, Chapter 3

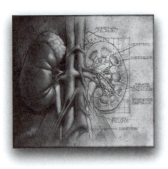

Reviewers

The Blind Review Process

The contents of the *Core Curriculum* underwent a "blind" review process by qualified individuals. One or more chapters were sent to chosen people for critical evaluation. The reviewer did not know the author's identity at the time of the review.

The work could be accepted (1) as originally submitted without revisions, (2) with minor revisons, or (3) with major revisions. The reviewers offered tremendous insight and suggestions; some even submitted additional references they thought might be useful. The results of the review were then sent back to the chapter/module editors to incorporate the suggestions and make revisions.

The reviewers will discover who the authors are now that the *Core* is published. However, while there is this published list of reviewers, no one will know who reviewed which part of the *Core*. That part of the process remains blind.

Because of the efforts of individuals listed below, value was added to the sixth edition. Their hard work is greatly appreciated.

Caroline S. Counts, Editor

Marilyn R. Bartucci, MSN, RN, ACNS-BC, CCTC
Case Manager
Kidney Foundation of Ohio
Cleveland, OH

Christina M. Beale, RN, CNN
Director, Outreach and Education
Lifeline Vascular Access
Vernon Hills, IL

Jenny Bell, BSN, RN, CNN
Clinical Transplant Coordinator
Banner Good Samaritan Transplant Center
Phoenix, AZ

M. Geraldine Biddle, RN, CNN, CPHQ
President, Nephrology Nurse Consultants
Pittsford, NY

Randee Breiterman White, MS, RN
Nurse Case Manager Nephrology
Vanderbilt University Hospital
Nashville, TN

Jerrilynn D. Burrowes, PhD, RDN, CDN
Professor and Chair
Director, Graduate Programs in Nutrition
Department of Nutrition
Long Island University (LIU) Post
Brookville, NY

Sally Burrows-Hudson, MSN, RN, CNN
Deceased 2014
Director, Nephrology Clinical Solutions
Lisle, IL

LaVonne Burrows, APRN, BC, CNN
Advanced Practice Registered Nurse
Springfield Nephrology Associates
Springfield, MO

Karen T. Burwell, BSN, RN, CNN
Acute Dialysis Nurse
DaVita HealthCare Partners Inc.
Phoenix, AZ

Laura D. Byham-Gray, PhD, RDN
Associate Professor and Director
Graduate Programs in Clinical Nutrition
Department of Nutritional Sciences
School of Health Related Professions
Rutgers University
Stratford, NJ

Theresa J. Campbell, DNP, APRN, FNP-BC
Doctor of Nursing Practice
Family Nurse Practitioner
Carolina Kidney Care
Adjunct Professor of Nursing
University of North Caroline at Pembroke
Fayetteville, NC

Monet Carnahan, BSN, RN, CDN
Renal Care Coordinator Program Manager
Fresenius Medical Care
Nashville, TN

Jacke L. Corbett, DNP, FNP-BC, CCTC
Nurse Practitioner
Kidney/Pancreas Transplant Program
University of Utah Health Care
Salt Lake City, UT

Christine Corbett, MSN, APRN, FNP-BC, CNN-NP
Nephrology Nurse Practitioner
Truman Medical Centers
Kansas City, MO

Sandra Corrigan, FNP-BC, CNN
Nurse Practitioner
California Kidney Medical Group
Thousand Oaks, CA

Maureen Craig, MSN, RN, CNN
Clinical Nurse Specialist – Nephrology
University of California Davis Medical Center
Sacramento, CA

Diane M. Derkowski, MA, RN, CNN, CCTC
Kidney Transplant Coordinator
Carolinas Medical Center
Charlotte, NC

Linda Duval, BSN, RN
Executive Director, FMQAI: ESRD Network 13
ESRD Network
Oklahoma City, OK

Damian Eker, DNP, GNP-C
ARNP, Geriatrics & Adult Health
Adult & Geriatric Health Center
Ft. Lauderdale, FL

Elizabeth Evans, DNP
Nephrology Nurse Practitioner
Renal Medicine Associates
Albuquerque, NM

Susan Fallone, MS, RN, CNN
Clinical Nurse Specialist, Retired
Adult and Pediatric Dialysis
Albany Medical Center
Albany, NY

Karen Joann Gaietto, MSN, BSN, RN, CNN
Acute Clinical Service Specialist
DaVita HealthCare Partners Inc.
Tiffin, OH

Deborah Glidden, MSN, ARNP, BC, CNN
Nurse Practitioner
Nephrology Associates of Central Florida
Orlando, FL

**David Jeremiah Grubbs, RN, CDN,
    Paramedic, ACLS, PALS, BCLS,
    TNCC, NIH**
Clinical Nurse Manager
Crestwood, KY

**Debra J. Hain, PhD, ARNP, ANP-BC,
    GNP-BC, FAANP**
Associate Professor/Lead Faculty AGNP Track
Florida Atlantic University
Christine E. Lynn College of Nursing
Boca Raton, FL
Nurse Practitioner, Cleveland Clinic Florida
Department of Nephrology
Weston, FL

Brenda C. Halstead, MSN, RN, AcNP, CNN
Nurse Practitioner
Mid-Atlantic Kidney Center
Richmond and Petersburg, VA

Emel Hamilton, RN, CNN
Director of Clinical Technology
Fresenius Medical Care
Waltham, MA

Mary S. Haras, PhD, MBA, APN, NP-C, CNN
Associate Dean, Graduate Nursing Programs
Saint Xavier University School of Nursing
Chicago, IL

**Malinda C. Harrington, MSN, RN,
    FNP-BC, ANCC**
Pediatric Nephrology Nurse Practitioner
Vidant Medical Center
Greenville, NC

Diana Hlebovy, BSN, RN, CHN, CNN
Nephrology Nurse Consultant
Elyria, OH

Sara K. Kennedy, BSN, RN, CNN
UAB Medicine, Kirklin Clinic
Diabetes Care Coordinator
Birmingham, AL

Nadine "Niki" Kobes, BSN, RN
Manager Staff Education/Quality
Fresenius Medical Care – Alaska JV Clinics
Anchorage, AK

Deuzimar Kulawik, MSN, RN
Director of Clinical Quality
DaVita HealthCare Partners Inc.
Westlake Village, CA

Kristin Larson, RN, ANP, GNP, CNN
Clinical Instructor
College of Nursing
Family Nurse Practitioner Program
University of North Dakota
Grand Forks, ND

Deborah Leggett, BSN, RN, CNN
Director, Acute Dialysis
Jackson Madison County General Hospital
Jackson, TN

Charla Litton, MSN, APRN, FNP-BC, CNN
Nurse Practitioner
UHG/Optum
East Texas, TX

Greg Lopez, BSN, RN, CNN
IMPAQ Business Process Manager
Fresenius Medical Care
New Orleans, LA

Terri (Theresa) Luckino, BSN, RN, CCRN
President, Acute Services
RPNT Acute Services, Inc.
Irving, TX

Alice Luehr, BA, RN, CNN
Home Therapy RN
St. Peter's Hospital
Helena, MT

Maryam W. Lyon, MSN, RN, CNN
Education Coordinator
Fresenius Medical Care
Dayton, OH

**Christine Mudge, MS, RN, PNP/CNS,
    CNN, FAAN**
Mill Valley, CA

Mary Lee Neuberger, MSN, APRN, RN, CNN
Pediatric Nephrology
University of Iowa Children's Hospital
Iowa City, IA

Jennifer Payton, MHCA, BSN, RN, CNN
Clinical Support Specialist
HealthStar CES
Goose Creek, SC

April Peters, MSN, RN, CNN
Clinical Informatics Specialist
Brookhaven Memorial Hospital Medical Center
Patchogue, NY

David J. Quan, PharmD, BCPS
Health Sciences Clinical Professor of Pharmacy
Clinical Pharmacist, Liver Transplant Services
UCSF Medical Center
San Francisco, CA

Kristi Robertson, CFNP
Nephrology Nurse Practitioner
Nephrology Associates
Columbus, MS

E. James Ryan, BSN, RN, CDN
Hemodialysis Clinical Services Coordinator
Lakeland Regional Medical Center
Lakeland, FL

June Shi, BSN, RN
Vascular Access Coordinator
Transplant Surgery
Medical University of South Carolina
Charleston, SC

Elizabeth St. John, MSN, RN, CNN
Education Coordinator, UMW Region
Fresenius Medical Care
Milwaukee, WI

Sharon Swofford, MA, RN, CNN, CCTC
Transplant Case Manager
OptumHealth
The Villages, FL

Beth Ulrich, EdD, RN, FACHE, FAAN
Senior Partner, Innovative Health Resources
Editor, *Nephrology Nursing Journal*
Pearland, TX

David F. Walz, MBA, BSN, RN, CNN
Program Director
CentraCare Kidney Program
St. Cloud, MN

Gail S. Wick, MHSA, BSN, RN, CNNe
Consultant
Atlanta, GA

Phyllis D. Wille, MS, RN, FNP-C, CNN, CNE
Nursing Faculty
Danville Area Community College
Danville, Il

Donna L. Willingham, RN, CPNP
Pediatric Nephrology Nurse Practitioner
Washington University St. Louis
St. Louis, MO

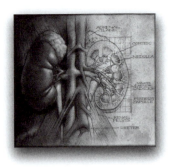

Contents at a Glance

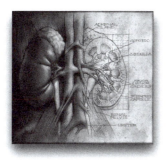

Expanded Contents

The table of contents contains chapters and sections with editors and authors for all six modules. The contents section of this specific module is highlighted in a blue background.

Module 1   Foundations for Practice in Nephrology Nursing

Module 2 Physiologic and Psychosocial Basis for Nephrology Nursing Practice

Module 3   Treatment Options for Patients with Chronic Kidney Failure

Module 4   Acute Kidney Injury

Module 5 Kidney Disease in Patient Populations Across the Life Span

Module 6 The APRN's Approaches to Care in Nephrology

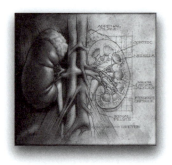

Examples of APA-formatted references

A guide for citing material from Module 6 of the *Core Curriculum for Nephrology Nursing, 6th edition.*

Module 6, Chapter 1

Example of reference for Chapter 1 in APA format. Use author of the section being cited. This example is based on Section B – End-of-Life and Palliative Care.

Brooks, D. (2015). Professional issues for the APRN in nephrology: End-of-life and palliative care. In C.S. Counts (Ed.), *Core curriculum for nephrology nursing: Module 6. The APRN's approaches to care in nephrology* (6th ed., pp. 1-18). Pitman, NJ: American Nephrology Nurses' Association.

Interpreted: Section author. (Date). Title of chapter: Title of section written by that author. In ...

For citation in text: (Brooks, 2015) (Use the author of the section you are citing.)

Module 6, Chapter 2

Example of reference for Chapter 2 in APA format. Use author of the section being cited. This example is based on Section B – APRN Role in CKD, Stages 4 to 5, Not on Dialysis.

Easom, A. (2015). Overview of CKD for the APRN: APRN role in CKD, stages 4 to 5, not on dialysis. In C.S. Counts (Ed.), *Core curriculum for nephrology nursing: Module 6. The APRN's approaches to care in nephrology* (6th ed., pp. 19-52). Pitman, NJ: American Nephrology Nurses' Association.

Interpreted: Section author. (Date). Title of chapter: Title of section written by that author. In ...

For citation in text: (Easom, 2015) (Use the author of the section you are citing.)

Module 6, Chapter 3

Example of reference for Chapter 3 in APA format. Use author of the section being cited. This example is based on Section D – Approaches to Care by the APRN in Peritoneal Dialysis.

Zorzanello, M.M. (2015). Overview of treatment options for CKD for the APRN: Approaches to care by the APRN in peritoneal dialysis. In C.S. Counts (Ed.), *Core curriculum for nephrology nursing: Module 6. The APRN's approaches to care in nephrology* (6th ed., pp. 53-110). Pitman, NJ: American Nephrology Nurses' Association.

Interpreted: Section author. (Date). Title of chapter: Title of section written by that author. In ...

For citation in text: (Zorzanello, 2015) (Use the author of the section you are citing.)

Module 6, Chapter 4

Example of reference for Chapter 4 in APA format. One author for entire chapter.

Ray, T. (2015). Overview of acute care for the APRN. In C.S. Counts (Ed.), *Core curriculum for nephrology nursing: Module 6. The APRN's approaches to care in nephrology* (6th ed., pp. 111-152). Pitman, NJ: American Nephrology Nurses' Association.

Interpreted: Chapter author. (Date). Title of chapter. In ...

For citation in text: (Ray, 2015)

Module 6, Chapter 5

Example of reference for Chapter 5 in APA format. Both authors for entire chapter.

Currier, H., & Geer, J. (2015). Overview of pediatric nephrology for the APRN. In C.S. Counts (Ed.), *Core curriculum for nephrology nursing: Module 6. The APRN's approaches to care in nephrology* (6th ed., pp. 153-200). Pitman, NJ: American Nephrology Nurses' Association.

Interpreted: Chapter authors. (Date). Title of chapter. In ...

For citation in text: (Currier & Geer, 2015)

CHAPTER **1**

Professional Issues for the APRN in Nephrology

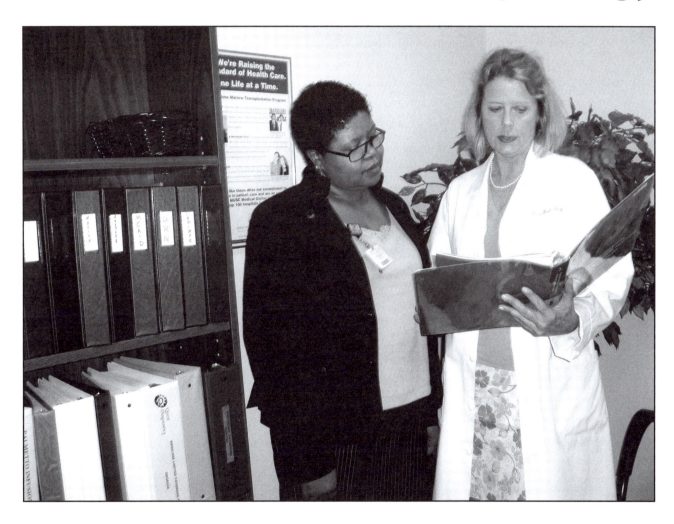

Chapter Editors
Kim Alleman, MS, APRN, FNP-BC, CNN-NP
Katherine Houle, MSN, APRN, CFNP, CNN-NP

Authors
Deborah Brooks, MSN, ANP-BC, CNN, CNN-NP
Mary Schira, PhD, RN, ACNP-BC

CHAPTER **1**

Professional Issues for the APRN in Nephrology

This offering for **1.3 contact hours** is provided by the American Nephrology Nurses' Association (ANNA).

American Nephrology Nurses' Association is accredited as a provider of continuing nursing education by the American Nurses Credentialing Center Commission on Accreditation.

ANNA is a provider approved by the California Board of Registered Nursing, provider number CEP 00910.

This CNE offering meets the continuing nursing education requirements for certification and recertification by the Nephrology Nursing Certification Commission (NNCC).

To be awarded contact hours for this activity, read this chapter in its entirety. Then complete the CNE evaluation found at **www.annanurse.org/corecne** and submit it; or print it, complete it, and mail it in. Contact hours are not awarded until the evaluation for the activity is complete.

Example of reference for Chapter 1 in APA format. Use author of the section being cited. This example is based on Section B – End-of-Life and Palliative Care.

Brooks, D. (2015). Professional issues for the APRN in nephrology: End-of-life and palliative care. In C.S. Counts (Ed.), *Core curriculum for nephrology nursing: Module 6. The APRN's approaches to care in nephrology* (6th ed., pp. 1-18). Pitman, NJ: American Nephrology Nurses' Association.

Interpreted: Section author. (Date). Title of chapter: Title of section written by that author. In ...

Cover photo by Sandra Cook.

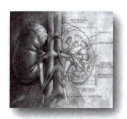

Professional Issues for the APRN in Nephrology

Purpose

The purpose of this chapter is to present an overview of advanced practice nursing and the professional issues related to advanced practice. Information related to the roles and practice of advanced practice nurses, regulation, and licensure will be addressed.

Objectives

Upon completion of this chapter, the learner will be able to:
1. Describe the advanced practice nursing roles with specific relevance to nephrology nursing.
2. Summarize the essential elements and issues regarding scope of practice and regulation of advanced practice registered nurses.
3. Determine current professional issues in advanced practice nursing.
4. Discuss end-of-life and palliative care as it pertains to nephrology nursing.
5. Outline how advanced practice nurses can identify, assess, evaluate, and manage patients and families who could benefit from end-of-life and palliative care services.
6. Identify available resources for managing end-of-life and palliative care for patients with kidney disease.

SECTION A
Professional Issues in Advanced Practice Nursing
Mary Schira

I. Introduction to advanced practice registered nursing.

A. Advanced practice registered nurse (APRN) roles.
   1. An advanced practice registered nurse is a registered nurse (RN) with graduate (master's or doctoral) level education prepared to provide direct patient care within four defined roles. APRN roles that are recognized in the United States are the clinical nurse specialist, nurse anesthetist, nurse practitioner, and nurse midwife.
   2. The four APRN roles have legal authority and title protection in individual state practice acts.
   3. For the purposes of advanced practice nursing in nephrology, the clinical nurse specialist and nurse practitioner roles are most relevant.
   4. For all advanced practice roles, graduate level education is currently (in most states) required for licensure and practice as an APRN. RNs previously prepared as nurse practitioners and nurse-midwives without graduate education continue to practice, but all education programs are now at the graduate level.
   5. The specific scope of practice for each APRN is governed by the individual state, and thus is state-specific.

B. Clinical nurse specialist (CNS).
   1. A clinical nurse specialist is a registered nurse with graduate preparation (master's or doctorate) with expertise in a specific area of nursing practice (National Association of Clinical Nurse Specialists, 2014).
   2. Practice focus.
      a. A clinical nurse specialist has a practice focus that may be based on a setting, disease process, specialty, or healthcare problem.
      b. Nephrology is an example of a specific practice focus and expertise of a CNS. The CNS in nephrology may have a strong focus in kidney replacement therapies, chronic kidney disease, transplantation, or any area of care needed by individuals with chronic (or acute) kidney disease.

3. Practice sites.
   a. Practice sites for the CNS are across the continuum of healthcare delivery settings.
   b. Many hospital systems employ CNSs as on-unit consultants and leaders to improve the care provided by the nursing staff and serve as resources for the staff and patients.
4. Additional information regarding the role, educational preparation, and practice sites for the CNS is available from the National Association of Clinical Nurse Specialists (http://www.nacns.org).

C. Nurse practitioner (NP).
   1. A nurse practitioner is a registered nurse with graduate level education with expertise in diagnosing and treating health conditions, disease prevention, and managing the health of individuals, families, and groups (American Association of Nurse Practitioners, 2013).
   2. Practice focus.
      a. There are two major methods to determine the practice focus of the NP – primary versus high acuity care, and life span vs. age-specific care.
      b. The overall goal of a primary care NP is to provide health promotion and health protection services to individuals in their care. In addition, primary care NPs manage the episodic and chronic healthcare needs of individuals who are physiologically stable. The primary care NP may provide care across the life span (e.g., family NP) or be limited to a more narrow age range (e.g., primary care pediatric NP).
      c. The overall goal of an acute care NP is to provide care for individuals who are experiencing physiologic instability or who require a high degree of healthcare technology (e.g., ventilator support) to restore health (American Association of Critical Care Nurses, 2012). Unlike primary care NPs, acute care NPs provide care to a more narrow age range (e.g., adult gerontology acute care NP, or neonatal NP).
      d. The practice focus of the NP is not related to a specific site or setting where the care is delivered, but rather the needs of the individual for whom the NP is providing care.
      e. In nephrology, depending on the needs of the individual with CKD, both primary and acute care NPs provide care. It is the responsibility of the individual NP to assure that they have achieved the necessary education to support their practice and that their education and practice is consistent with the scope of practice defined in their state practice act.
   3. Practice/employment sites.
      a. Practice sites for the NP are in any area of health care, consistent with the NP's educational preparation, certification, and licensure.
      b. In nephrology, NPs practice in a variety of settings, including CKD clinics, outpatient dialysis units, in-patient dialysis units, and hospitals (including general medical-surgical and intensive care units).
   4. Additional information regarding the role, educational preparation, and practice sites for the nurse practitioner is available from the American Association of Nurse Practitioners (http://www.aanp.org).

II. Scope of practice.

A. Advanced practice registered nursing regulation.
   1. In 2008, the Consensus Model for APRN Regulation: Licensure, Accreditation, Certification & Education (APRN Consensus Work Group) was adopted with the intent to develop standards for the education and licensure of APRNs.
   2. The model represents the combined work of multiple organizations, groups, and stakeholders and has become the accepted standard by which APRN practice is currently being addressed in education and licensure.
   3. The title "APRN" is legally protected in state laws, and the licensure and scope of practice of an APRN is determined by the education and national certification examination completed by the APRN.
   4. As per Consensus Model, APRNs are educated and licensed in one of four roles.
      a. Certified registered nurse anesthetist (CRNA).
      b. Certified nurse midwife (CNM).
      c. Clinical nurse specialist (CNS).
      d. Certified nurse practitioner (CNP).
   5. APRNs are educated in at least one of six population foci.
      a. Family and individual across the life span.
      b. Adult-gerontology.
      c. Pediatrics.
      d. Neonatal.
      e. Women's health/gender-related.
      f. Psychiatry and mental health.
   6. LACE elements of APRN regulatory model.
      a. Licensure.
      b. Accreditation.
      c. Certification.
      d. Education.
   7. Specific guidelines are provided as a reference and guide for state licensing, national certification, accreditation bodies, and educational programs.
   8. Additional information regarding the practice of clinical nurse specialists is available through the

National Association of Clinical Nurse Specialists (http://www.nacns.org/).

9. Additional information regarding the practice of nurse practitioners is available through the American Association of Nurse Practitioners (http://www.aanp.org/).

B. APRN specialty practice – nephrology.
1. In the regulatory model, specialty practice builds on the role and population-focused competencies. As a result, specialties are not included in the licensure requirement.
2. Advanced practice nursing in nephrology is an example of a recognized APRN specialty. For licensure, an APRN in nephrology must have a recognized role and population focus (e.g., family nurse practitioner).
3. The specialty practice and competencies of the APRN in nephrology are described and recognized by the specialty nursing organization, the American Nephrology Nurses' Association (ANNA).
4. The standards of nephrology nursing practice and standards of professional performance for advanced practice nurses in nephrology are available in Nephrology Nursing Scope and Standards of Practice (Gomez, 2011). This resource identifies the standards for all nephrology nurses, with additional competencies expected of the advanced practice registered nurse.
5. ANNA developed two position statements, Advanced Practice in Nephrology Nursing (ANNA, 2013) and ANNA, ASN, and RPA Joint Position Paper on Collaboration Between Nephrologists and Advanced Practice Registered Nurses (ANNA, 2012) These statements provide additional information and guidance regarding the role of advanced practice nurses in nephrology care. Both documents serve as resources for the important role of APRNs in the care of individuals with kidney disease.
6. National certification in specialty practice is not required but is encouraged. Specialty certification is available in nephrology: the certified nephrology nurse–nurse practitioner. Information regarding specialty certification for the nurse practitioner in nephrology is available from the Nephrology Nursing Certification Commission (https://www.nncc-exam.org/).

III. Professional issues.

A. Independence in practice.
1. An important aspect of the Consensus Model described previously is that all APRNs will be licensed independent providers.
2. There is wide variety among states related to the level of independence with which an APRN may

practice. Depending on the individual state, APRNs may be fully independent in practice or may be required to collaborate with or be supervised by a physician provider.
3. The greatest area of variability across states is in the area of prescriptive authority. Each state has specific rules and guidelines related to APRNs: who may write prescriptions, level of autonomy in writing prescriptions, and schedule drug prescriptive authority.
4. The variability of independence in practice is often confusing. The APRN is responsible for complying with the individual state law in which the care is provided. An ongoing resource of state practice laws and regulations is available from the American Association of Nurse Practitioners (http://www.aanp.org) and the National Association of Clinical Nurse Specialists (http://www.nacns.org).
5. The Nurse Licensure Compact (available in 24 states for registered nurse licensure) is not yet well developed for Advanced Practice Registered Nursing licensure. The goal of the APRN licensure compact is to allow the recognition of APRN licenses and practice authority across state lines. The targeted implementation date is 2016 (Nurse Licensure Compact Administrators, 2012).
6. In 2010, the Institute of Medicine released *The Future of Nursing: Leading Change, Advancing Health*. The first recommendation of this report called for the removal of barriers that limit the scope of practice for APRNs. The intent is that all APRNs could provide healthcare services to the extent of their education. The report provided specific suggestions for legislation and licensure reform to address removal of the barriers.

B. Education for the advanced practice nurse.
1. Master's degree education.
a. Currently, the majority of APRNs are prepared at the master's degree level of education. Curriculum requirements for APRN education programs are addressed in most state nurse practice acts.
b. Clinical nurse specialist core competencies and education program evaluation criteria are available from the National Association of Clinical Nurse Specialists (http://nacns.org).
c. Nurse practitioner curriculum guidelines, competencies, and education program evaluation criteria are available from the National Organization of Nurse Practitioner Faculties (NONPF) (http://nonpf.org). Competencies for NPs include core competencies expected of all nurse practitioners and additional population-

specific competencies that are consistent with the population foci identified in the Consensus Model previously discussed.

2. Doctor of nursing practice (DNP).
   a. In 2004, members of the American Association of Colleges of Nursing (AACN) endorsed a decision advocating a move of the entry level of preparation for advanced nursing practice to the doctoral level.
   b. Following a consensus building process, in 2006 the AACN published *The Essentials of Doctoral Education for Advanced Nursing Practice*. The document defines curriculum elements and competencies for the practice doctorate in nursing.
   c. The DNP has been endorsed by numerous nursing organizations, and development of programs and student enrollment in the degree has been strong. According to the AACN, there were 241 DNP programs with an enrollment of over 14,500 students in 2013 (AACN, 2014).
   d. At this time, the DNP is not required for entry-level education preparation for clinical nurse specialists or nurse practitioners. As the degree gains momentum, the DNP will replace master's level entry preparation for APRNs in the future (AACN, 2006).
   e. In some cases, there is confusion regarding the difference between a DNP and a PhD (Chism, 2009).
      (1) The DNP degree is practice focused, with emphasis on translation of evidence to practice.
      (2) The PhD degree is research focused, with emphasis on generating research and new knowledge.

C. Employment.
   1. Contracts and negotiation.
      a. The majority of APRNs are employed by others rather than self-employed. If an APRN is employed by others, job duties, reimbursement for services, and job benefits may be identified or delineated via an employment contract or a job description. Most APRNs have previously worked in positions with job descriptions but have not had employment contracts.
      b. An employment contract is a written agreement in which the employer and employee agree on terms of the working relationship (Buppert, 2015).
      c. Contracts may be complex and should be reviewed carefully prior to signing.
      d. Most contracts cover common issues of interest to the employer and employee.
         (1) The services to be performed, including on-call and/or weekend responsibilities.

         (2) Payment for services including productivity expectations and bonuses.
         (3) Duration of employment.
         (4) Benefits (sick and vacation time allowances, health insurance, malpractice insurance, phone allowance, car/mileage reimbursement if driving between clinic sites).
         (5) Continuing education funds and allowances (and whether time at continuing education conferences is included in vacation time).
         (6) Reasons for termination of employment.
         (7) Required time frame for resignation or termination notice.
         (8) "Non-compete" clauses, which may be time or geographic location limited.
      e. Contract items and issues are generally negotiated shortly after a job has been offered. The APRN should not sign a contract until comfortable that all issues have been addressed and satisfactorily negotiated.
      f. When negotiating a contract, the APRN should consider retaining an attorney to review the contract, especially when there are questions or concerns about any clauses (Buppert, 2015).
      g. The advantage of a contract is that the APRN has a written agreement for employment during the duration of the contract (unless otherwise noted in the contact). As a result, the contract provides some degree of employment security.
      h. A written contract also provides a mechanism through which the employee and employer can discuss issues that arise. As a result, a contract is protective to the employee and the employer.
      i. The American Association of Nurse Practitioners provides business and practice management resources related to employment negotiations and key items to consider in negotiating employment (http://www.aanp.org).
   2. Malpractice insurance.
      a. Although APRNs, and specifically NPs, are not frequently sued, most APRNs carry malpractice insurance.
      b. The purpose of malpractice insurance is the same as any type of insurance – to mitigate the financial impact of a malpractice or negligence lawsuit.
      c. The APRN should carry individual malpractice insurance even if covered under a hospital, dialysis clinic, or nephrology practice policy.
      d. Insurance has two general types – claims made and occurrence (Buppert, 2015).
         (1) With claims made coverage, the APRN is covered only when the policy is active and does not relate to when the incident actually occurred. As a result, if the APRN

retires, the APRN needs to keep the insurance active in case an incident that happened previously results in a lawsuit. Claims made coverage can be extended through purchasing a "tail" policy (Buppert, 2015).

    (2) Occurrence coverage extends to any event that occurred while the APRN was insured. As a result, occurrence coverage is generally considered stronger than claims made coverage.

D. Advanced practice nurse-sensitive outcomes.
1. Advanced practice nurses.
   a. APRNs contribute to the health and wellness outcomes of individuals across the life span and healthcare settings in which care is provided.
   b. Measuring outcomes in advanced practice nursing is a key element in supporting the role, practice, and value of the APRN (Kleinpell, 2013).
   c. A systematic review by Newhouse and colleagues (2011) indicated that APRNs provide high-quality, safe, and cost-effective care to a variety of populations in numerous types of healthcare settings.
2. Advanced practice nurses in nephrology.
   a. Consistent with all APRNs, those practicing in nephrology are expected to contribute to positive patient, family, and practice outcomes.
   b. Specific outcomes that are sensitive to measurement in advanced practice nursing in nephrology have not been identified and are an important area of ongoing work.

IV. Summary.

A. Advanced practice registered nurses.
1. Regulation and scope of practice of APRNs are evolving and changing.
2. Outcome data support the APRN as a positive provider in the healthcare delivery system.

B. Advanced practice registered nurses in nephrology.
1. APRNs in nephrology work with patients across the full continuum of CKD.
2. Position statements from the American Nephrology Nurses' Association are available to provide information and guidance for APRNs in nephrology.
3. Continued work needs to be accomplished to identify patient and practice-appropriate outcomes in nephrology.

I. Palliative care and hospice definitions and guidelines.

A. Definition of palliative care: an approach that improves the quality of life of patients and their families facing the problems associated with life-threatening illness, through the prevention and relief of suffering by means of early identification and impeccable assessment and treatment of pain and other problems, physical, psychosocial, and spiritual. (World Health Organization (WHO), http://www.who.int/cancer/palliative/definition).
1. Applies to adults and children and includes support to families.
2. Recognizes death as a normal process; does not attempt to hasten or postpone death.
3. Palliative care begins early in the illness and is in conjunction with other forms of therapy. Therefore, in caring for persons with any degree of kidney disease, palliative care begins at the time of diagnosis and becomes more prominent as the kidney disease progresses.

B. Goals of palliative care (Palliative Doctors, http://www.palliativedoctors.org/about/index.html; WHO, http://www.who.int/cancer/palliative/definition).
1. Work with patients of curable, chronic, and life threatening illnesses to help achieve best quality of life as defined by patient and family.
2. Assist patients to live as active and full lives as possible.
3. Provide relief of symptoms such as pain, shortness of breath, nausea, anxiety, constipation, or fatigue.
4. Offer assistance in planning advance directives.
5. Coordinate care with other healthcare teams.
6. Assist with emotional and spiritual needs.
7. Transition into hospice care for terminally ill patients.

C. Definition of hospice according to the National Hospice and Palliative Care Organization (NHPCO, n.d., http://www.nhpco.org).
1. Care for terminally ill persons.
2. Focus and goal is on caring rather than curing.
3. Care involves patient and family.
4. Goal is compassionate, pain free death.
5. Can be facilitated in home, hospital, skilled nursing facility, or hospice center.

D. Hospice guidelines (Tamura & Cohen, 2010; NHPCO, n.d., http://www.nhpco.org).
   1. Referral can be made by anyone.
   2. Patient's physician and the medical director of the hospice must certify patient's eligibility.
   3. Life expectancy is 6 months or less but this can be reevaluated.
   4. Hospice is not intended for patients who are benefiting from treatment and when cure is intended and expected. However, palliative care may be very appropriate: http://palliativedoctors.org/faq
   5. Cost is covered by Medicare, most Medicaid, most private insurers, HMOs, and other managed-care organizations. Hospice will provide current details.
   6. Medicare coverage.
      a. Hospice is Medicare approved under the Medicare Hospice Benefit (MHB). Covers:
         (1) Medical, nursing (RN and aide), social work, spiritual, nutritional, physical therapy/occupational therapy (PT/OT), volunteers, and bereavement support for family.
         (2) 95% of drugs for pain and other symptoms.
         (3) Inpatient respite care for caregiver responsibilities.
      Not covered:
         (4) 24-hour care except during a medical crisis when continuous nursing and short-term inpatient hospice care are available.
         (5) Personal services.
      b. Covered by Part A (Hospital insurance).
      c. Signed statement that hospice covers illness-related care.
   7. Dialysis and hospice Medicare guidelines.
      a. If terminal illness is not due to end-stage renal disease (ESRD), then Medicare will provide benefits for both hospice and dialysis.
      b. If terminal illness is due to ESRD, then Medicare requires hospice provider to pay for dialysis and supplies or patient chooses to withdraw from dialysis.
   8. The Institute of Medicine's (IOM) Committee on Approaching Death: Addressing Key End of Life Issues met in July 2013. The Coalition of Supportive Care of Kidney Patients spoke about the current availability of and barriers to services and has sent a letter of support with recommendations on changing funding regulations for palliative care and hospice for patients with kidney failure (http://www.kidneysupportivecare.org/Files/IOM Letter08232013.aspx).

II. Legal considerations of palliative care.

A. Patient has the right to refuse care even if it means death occurs.
   1. U.S. Supreme Court: a competent, nonterminally ill person has a liberty interest under the Due Process Clause of the 14th Amendment in refusing unwanted medical treatment including food and water – even if it means the person will die as a result (Cruzan v. Director, MDH, 1990; Saylor, 2012, Slide 108).
   2. Healthcare staff has an ethical and legal responsibility to honor a competent patient's decision (Saylor, 2012, slide 110).
   3. Questions to consider if the patient refuses dialysis (Saylor, 2012, slide 109).
      a. Are they terminal?
      b. Is there a state interest in keeping them alive?
      c. Would their death impact others?
      d. Would innocent parties such as minor children be impacted?

B. CPR: survival is not very high or the person may die within days to weeks after resuscitation. When discussing end-of-life options, does the person really understand and want this? (Saylor, 2012, slides 117/118).

C. More patients with kidney failure die in the hospital than at home or with hospice. Patients may not be aware of possible options for end-of-life care.

D. The Conditions for Coverage (CMS, 2008): http://www.cms.gov/Medicare/Provider-Enrollment-and-Certification/GuidanceforLawsAndRegulations/Dialysis.html
   1. Do not require advance directives be a part of the assessment for patients on dialysis.
   2. State that patients are entitled to be "informed about the right to have advance directives."
   3. State that facility's policies and procedures address advance directives and to inform patients of the policy.
   4. If a facility's policy does not intend to honor properly executed advance directives, arrangements should be made to transfer patient to another facility (V457).
   5. Advance directives should be recorded in the medical record (V730).
   6. The physician, nurse practitioner, clinical nurse specialist, or physician's assistant treating the patient with kidney failure can inform the patient of his or her medical condition and document it in the medical record (V461).
   7. The conditions suggest that patients look to social workers for guidance in pursuing advance directives.

E. Respect patient's goals, preferences, and choices, within the confines of state and federal law, for advance care planning (Mid-Atlantic Renal Coalition, http://www.esrdnet5.org).

F. Ethical practice standards include beneficence, justice, nonmaleficence, confidentiality, informed consent, and avoidance of conflict of interest (Mid-Atlantic Renal Coalition. www.esrdnet5.org).

III. Advance directives
(http://www.palliativedoctors.org/resources/directives.html).

A. Advance directives require the person to be 18 years or older. Mental illness may require additional physician and attorney input. Pregnancy may preclude honoring an advance directive (Caring Connections, http://www.caringinfo.org).

B. Living will (also known as a "declaration of a desire for a natural death") describes the type of treatment the patient wants in the event of terminal illness or vegetative state.

C. Medical power of attorney (also known as health care proxy [agent] or durable power of attorney for health care) names the person, chosen by the patient, who will make medical decisions on the patient's behalf if the patient is not able to make reasoned decisions. The patient does not need to be at the end of life for the agent to have authority to speak for the patient.

D. Physician orders for life-sustaining treatment (POLST) are orders written and signed by physician, nurse practitioner, or physician's assistant outlining what interventions and treatments are to be conducted. Areas include cardiopulmonary resuscitation, medical interventions (e.g., IV and intubation, antibiotics, artificially administered nutrition, and medical condition/goals). If a section is not completed, then full treatment is expected of that component. Form is HIPPA compliant and is to be transferred with patient (faxes and photocopies are valid). Update form with changes in health. Form can be voided by patient or designated surrogate (Coalition for Supportive Care of Kidney Patients, http://www.kidneysupportivecare.org/Files/POLST_Form.aspx).

IV. Patients to consider for palliative care.

A. Patients at increased risk for complications and death (USRDS, 2014, at http://www.usrds.org/adr.aspx). USRDS data for dialysis patients starts at day 1 of treatment, rather than 90 days.
  1. Elderly. Adjusted mortality increases with patient complexity in older patients.
  2. More hospitalizations and deaths for patients > 65 years old with CKD.
  3. Other comorbidities if the patient is > 66 years old. In patients with CKD, the mortality risk is twice as high if diabetes and cardiovascular disease are also present. When comparing patients with diabetes and cardiovascular disease, those with CKD have a nearly 50% higher mortality rate than those without CKD (USRDS, Vol. 1, Fig. 3.4).
  4. Decreased kidney function – 51% higher hospitalization rate in stage 4 or 5 than stage 1 or 2 for all causes of hospitalization including CVD and infection (USRDS, Vol. 1, Figure 3.5).
  5. Higher death rate in men than women with any stage of CKD including dialysis but very similar rates for all races. Mortality is 36% higher in patients with CKD vs non CKD (USRDS, Vol. 1, Table 3.1).
  6. Mortality in the dialysis population is 6 times greater than among Medicare patients of similar age without kidney disease (USRDS, Vol. 2, Figure 5.4).
  7. When compared with the same age group (patients on dialysis vs the general population), mortality in the dialysis group is 2 to 4 times higher than those with a diagnosis of diabetes, cancer, CHF, CVA, or MI (USRDS, Vol. 2, Table 5.3).
  8. Although patients with transplants fare the best with expected remaining lifetimes being 83% to 87% as long as their age-matched counterparts (USRDS, Vol. 2, Table 5.2), they should be assessed for end-of-life care issues.
  9. Patients at highest risk for death, and those suffering physical, mental, and spiritual pain (Davison, 2012).

B. Reassessment of patients who experience major changes in health or decision-making capabilities (RPA, 2010).

C. Considerations in the elderly (Berger & Hedayati, 2012).
  1. Frailty.
     a. Criteria include unintentional weight loss, slow walking, weakness, exhaustion, and low physical activity.
     b. Associated with increased risk of falls, disability, hospitalization, and death.
     c. In the general population, 7% of people over 65 years old and 40% over 80 years old met frailty criteria.
     d. Frailty increases with age but is a factor in CKD regardless of age.
     e. Twice as great a risk with mild CKD and 6 times the risk if eGFR < 45 mL/min.
     f. All patients with CKD need assessment for

physical and functional impairment with restorative action.

2. Falls.
   a. More frequent in patients over 65 years old on dialysis.
   b. Orthostatic blood pressure changes not necessarily greater in fall vs. nonfall patients on dialysis.
   c. Increased risk of mortality if on dialysis, over 75 years old, and have had one fall.

3. Functional impairment.
   a. Decreased ability to perform activities of daily living (ADLs) or instrumental activities of daily living (IADLs) such as management of medications, personal finances, cooking, driving, telephone use, or pet care.
   b. Initiation of dialysis does not appear to reverse functional impairment.
   c. Rehabilitation at the start of dialysis may maintain current function.

4. Cognitive impairment.
   a. Association between kidney failure and cognitive impairment including dementia.
   b. Risk increases with decline in kidney function.
   c. Causality has not been established.
   d. Initiation of dialysis in the elderly. Assess the patient's level of understanding regarding initiation of dialysis.

5. Nonmedical barriers.
   a. Transportation.
   b. Family support.
   c. Income.

6. Medical comorbidities.
   a. Reduced life expectancy due to age.
   b. Early initiation of dialysis may be harmful due to possible loss of residual function.
   c. Symptoms of frailty may be mistaken for symptoms of uremia (Swidler, 2013).
   d. Life expectancy on dialysis decreases with age compared to age-matched general population.

7. Hemodialysis vs. peritoneal dialysis.
   a. Choice of treatment needs to be individualized.
   b. Vascular access and fluid shifts may be difficult with HD.
   c. Functional impairment and limited social support may be difficult with PD.
   d. Studies have shown equivalent survival.

8. Conservative nondialytic therapy.
   a. Use multidisciplinary team approach to maximize care.
   b. Individualize patient and family goals for quality of life.
   c. May have lower rate of deaths occurring in hospital vs. home/hospice.
   d. May have lower hospitalization rate.

9. Transplantation. Better survival with less than a year of dialysis.

10. Swidler (2012) describes an approach to geriatric renal palliative care (GRPC) that divides the older adults (> 80 years old) into 3 categories or phenotypes. Although no standard geriatric assessment model exists, the available data suggests tailoring care to match group characteristics may help with improved planning and individualized care including starting or withdrawing dialysis. The phenotypes are as follows.
    a. Healthy/usual: better dialysis candidates with life expectancy averaging about 3 years, may be transplant candidates, fewer hospitalizations, and better quality of life scores.
    b. Vulnerable: typical dialysis patient, not a transplant candidate, increased hospitalizations and unpredictable events and outcomes.
    c. Frail: likely to die in less than a year, high risk for comorbidities and frequent hospitalizations. They are more likely to live in a nursing home.

V. Preparation of healthcare providers to address patient and family questions about end of life (Davison, 2010).

A. Traditionally not much formal training in discussing end-of-life issues.
   1. A survey of over 500 patients revealed that patients rely on their nephrologist and family doctor for information regarding overall health, yet over 90% of this same group stated their physicians had not discussed their overall longevity prognosis.
   2. These patients were strong proponents of being better informed and prepared for changes in their health, and most respondents relied on their physician and nurses for support during illness and treatments.
   3. This deficit is being recognized, and more educational energy is being directed toward this need.
   4. Online courses and webinars are available (see website list on page 14).

B. Communication skills can be learned and improved. Schell and colleagues (2013) report outcomes of a half-day workshop, NephroTalk, aimed at increasing skill and comfort of nephrology fellows discussing dialysis initiation or withdrawal of treatment. Two of the communication techniques can be incorporated into almost any patient and family discussions.
   1. Ask–tell–ask. This provides a focused point of discussion.
      a. Ask permission to discuss a topic such as: "I'd like to talk with you about advance care planning. Is this a convenient time for you?"
      b. Tell the intended information.

c. Ask the patient and family to provide feedback on what they heard. For example, "I want to be sure you don't have any questions. Can you please tell me your understanding of the information?"
2. NURSE acronym. This provides a framework for ensuring that emotional issues are acknowledged and addressed. Example below applies to an advance care planning discussion.
   a. **N**ame: "You look distressed."
   b. **U**nderstand: "Talking about serious illness can be distressing."
   c. **R**espect: "Your beliefs and values are very important to us."
   d. **S**upport: "We're here to help you and your family work through these decisions."
   e. **E**xplore: "What other information would be helpful?"

VI. Patient and family understanding of palliative care and information about the end-of-life process.

A. Patient survey (Davison, 2010) revealed the following information.
1. Many patients were not familiar with the term palliative care and less than half of those surveyed had completed any type of advance directive.
2. A desire for patient and family education with more involvement of families in end-of-life discussions and care.
3. More emphasis on pain and symptom management as disease progresses.
4. More education for healthcare staff in end-of-life issues.
5. Discussions with physicians about prognosis and care.
6. Routine discussions about end-of-life preferences including resuscitation.
7. Involvement of the entire team, including nursing and social work, in discussion.
8. Knowledge of and availability of resources such as support and counseling, hospice, palliative care team, social and spiritual care, and financial support.

B. Communication (Parry et al., 2013).
1. Families remembered small gestures a year later.
   a. Positive: private space.
   b. Negative: lack of communication with healthcare team.
2. Families reported less anxiety and more satisfaction when they had more information and participation in care.
3. Addressing emotions, end-of-life concerns, and quality-of-life concerns increased the communication with families and helped them participate in decisions.

4. Healthcare providers tended to underestimate patients' need for information and overestimate their understanding of provided information.

VII. Patient assessment.

A. Expanding and individualizing palliative care to meet the needs of patients (RPA, 2010; Tamura & Cohen, 2010).
1. Look at stage of CKD.
2. Screen for other comorbidities (e.g., depression).
3. Examine patient preferences, needs, and values (Saylor, 2012, slide 100).
   a. Qualitative goals may bring longer survival with potentially decreased quality of life. ("I want to live as long as possible and to have full treatment options.")
   b. Quantitative goals may improve quality but shorten survival time. ("It's important to me to be independent to the end.")
   c. Consider family dynamics, including family burden, care load, cost, role, and source of income.
   d. Expectations of treatment vs. reality of disease (Saylor, 2012, slide 111).
4. Estimate prognosis (see predictor model).
5. Explain and explore treatment options (Swidler, 2013).
   a. Include both the benefits and negative consequences.
   b. Patients' preferences may change as clinical situations change.
6. Implement advance care planning, which can include advance directives.
7. Assess and manage symptoms, especially if dialysis is not initiated or is stopped.
8. Refer for hospice as appropriate.

VIII. Screening for depression, pain, and distress.

A. Kidney Disease Quality of Life Short Form (KDQOL-SF) rates health in patients with kidney disease. The short form was developed from the original 1994 full-length form. Categories of items include symptoms, effect and burden of disease, social interaction and support, and physical and mental health status. The form is available in many languages. (See website list for information).

B. Patient Health Questionnaire-9 (PHQ-9) is a self-administered form to determine depression and monitor it over time. Can be used to monitor depression and treatment. (See website list for information).

C. Beck Depression Inventory (BDI) is a self-report inventory developed in 1961. It is used worldwide, available in different languages and in paper and computer format, used in psychiatric and nonpsychiatric populations, and has long and short forms. (See website list on page 14 for information.)

D. The McGill Pain Questionnaire (Melzack, 2005) has been validated and used in a wide variety of pain assessment settings including kidney disease. It is available in several languages and has been validated to be effective in both paper and electronic form (Cook et al., 2004). The higher the score (0–78), the greater the pain. Measurement and evaluation tools can be found at: http://www.npcrc.org/content/25/Measurement-and-Evaluation-Tools.aspx

E. Beck Anxiety Inventory (BAI) measures the amount of anxiety experienced over the past month and can be used for monitoring over time. This site includes the form and the scoring. http://dih.wiki.otago.ac.nz/images/8/80/Beck.pdf

F. McGill Quality of Life (QoL) questionnaire measures physical, psychological, existential, and support realms but also has a one-item question for patient to rate overall quality of life from 0 "very bad" to 10 "excellent." This was the first use of the item in patients with kidney failure. Patients with two or more symptoms reported lower QoL. Pain (extremities and cramps) was the most common symptom followed by sleep disturbance, tiredness, and shortness of breath (Kimmel et al., 2003).

G. Edmonton Symptom Assessment System (ESAS) has been used in palliative care to assess physical and psychological symptom distress. The authors added pruritus to the cancer version and validated the form with patients on hemodialysis and peritoneal dialysis. Symptoms reported as most severe were tiredness, decreased well-being, poor appetite, and pain with itching (Davison et al., 2006; http://meds.queensu.ca/assets/palliative-care/ppcip_esas.pdf (add "pruritus" in place of "other problem." Scoring is between 0 and 100).

IX. Predictions of mortality.

A. Use of the "surprise question" (SQ) with patients on dialysis (Moss et al., 2008): "Would I be surprised if this patient died in the next year?"
1. A "No" response was identified with older patients and the odds of dying within a year were 3.5 times higher in the No group vs. the Yes group.
2. In addition, the No group was older with more comorbidities, lower functional status, and lower albumin levels.
3. This is the first studied use of the SQ with dialysis

patients, and the clinicians were nurse practitioners.
4. In addition to helping clinicians consider the prognosis in a different way, the surprise question could help identify patients who might benefit from palliative care services.
5. The surprise question prognostic tool is at http://touchcalc.com/calculators/sq.

B. Predictive models for mortality (O'Connor & Corcoran, 2012).
1. Identification of factors that could predict the increased risk of short-term mortality would allow patients and families an opportunity to make informed decisions.
2. These are uncorrectable factors rather than modifiable risks. They followed 514 HD patients for 24 months. Five variables were identified that were independently associated with early mortality:
   a. Older age
   b. Dementia
   c. Peripheral vascular disease.
   d. Decreased albumin.
   e. "No" response to the surprise question.
3. Other variables that showed a relationship to poor survival were (Cohen et al., 2010):
   a. History of congestive heart disease.
   b. Chronic obstructive pulmonary disease.
   c. Cerebrovascular disease.
   d. Myocardial infarction.
   e. Diabetes.
   f. Cancer.

X. Advance care planning: guidance for patients.

A. Become familiar with or consider development of advance care planning guidelines for healthcare facility. Provide guidance and a timeline for addressing advance care planning with all patients. The Kidney End-of-Life Coalition (now Coalition for Supportive Care of Kidney Patients) developed guidelines for dialysis facilities (2006) (http://www.kidneysupportivecare.org/Advance-Care-Planning/For-Professionals.aspx).

B. Help patients and families make a plan (Caring Connections, http://www.caringinfo.org; Aging with Dignity, www.agingwithdignity.org; ANNA End-of-Life Modules).
1. Recognize that end-of-life discussions and decisions are personal and closely tied to individual values and beliefs. It is helpful to begin planning before a crisis occurs.
2. Become familiar with different types of advance directives.
3. Talk with the patient's family about end-of-life

wishes. Share specifics, as appropriate, preferred treatments and comfort level, how death would impact others, preferred place to die, service, burial or cremation plans, etc. Not all families are ready for this discussion, so written advance directives are helpful.

4. Appoint a health agent, in event of not being able to voice own choices, and put in writing for family and healthcare team. Agent or surrogate is person of patient's choosing, who will follow instructions of patient even if these differ from family wishes.

5. It is helpful to explain why this person is the health agent. If family difficulties are anticipated, may need to put in writing that the agent has full authority to carry out patient wishes.

6. Discuss advance directives with healthcare team and make a copy available for all medical records. Health team needs name and contact information of health agent. If advance directives cannot be honored by medical team for moral, ethical, or legal reasons, patient may need assistance finding a different healthcare site or dialysis facility.

XI. Initiate an end-of-life discussion with a patient
(Mid-Atlantic Renal Coalition, http://www.esrdnet5.org).

A. Have the conversation in a private setting such as a separate clinic room or conference room, at a separately scheduled appointment.

B. Patient needs to decide who else, if anyone, is present (family, friends, etc.) for the discussion.

C. Ask permission to discuss the topic. "I'd like to talk with you about the kind of care you would want if you became very sick. Could we talk about that? I'd feel better if I understood what is important to you."

D. If this type of conversation is a standard part of practice, inform the patient of this. "We have this conversation with everyone who starts dialysis. It's important to us to understand your healthcare wishes."

E. Be sensitive to patients' cultural beliefs, spiritual beliefs, and values. This includes a vast array of factors with a few being eye contact, touch, conversational style, decision making, level of comfort with discussing death, and family involvement.

F. Be encouraging and let the patient talk. Try to clarify the wants and wishes. Be attuned to how patient and medical goals mesh or conflict and how misunderstanding can be avoided. "You would be willing to try dialysis for a time but if you did not feel better you would want to discuss other options."

G. Ask about discussions with family and friends and if there is someone who could make health decisions if the patient were unable to do so. "I've noticed two daughters come to clinic with you. You would want Jeanne to be the final decision maker if you could not speak for yourself. Is your family aware of this choice?"

H. Be accepting of the patient's right to make decisions even if they do not match the family or healthcare team choices. "I understand you do not want dialysis under any circumstance. Can we talk about possible alternatives such as palliative care and hospice?"

I. Recognize that patients may not be amenable to discussions the first time.
1. Respect that and leave the door open for further discussions. "I understand you do not want to discuss this at this time. I'd like to leave some information for you."
2. This could be written, video, phone numbers, website, etc. For example: *Are you traveling without a map? A layperson's guide to advance care planning*, http://www.caringinfo.org/files/ public/brochures/Are_you_traveling_without_a_ map.pdf (Brandt, 2013).

XII. Resources for patients, families, and staff for end-of-life decisions.

A. *Advance Care Planning: For Dialysis Patients and Their Families* (2005), Mid-Atlantic Renal Coalition & the Academy for Educational Development, is a pamphlet for patients with suggestions on how to start conversations with family, friends and healthcare team about personal choices for illness and dying (http://www.kidneysupportivecare .org/Files/ACPBrochure-E.aspx).

B. *Advanced Chronic Kidney Disease – Care for the Dying Patient* (2010), Liverpool Care Pathway, is a patient and family booklet describing end-of-life symptoms and care for patients with kidney disease (http://www.sii-mcpcil.org.uk/publications/ publication-flip-book-viewer.aspx?publication=1400).

C. *Advance Chronic Kidney Disease – Care for the Dying Patient: A Guide for Health Professionals* (2010), Liverpool Care Pathway, is a guide for managing care in the final stages of life. It includes suggestions for medication management of common problems including pain, fluid status, gastrointestinal issues, electrolyte imbalance, and itching (http://www .sii-mcpcil.org.uk/publications/publication-flip- book-viewer.aspx?publication=1401).

D. *If You Choose Not to Start Dialysis Treatment* (2008) is a question and answer booklet for patients (http://www.kidney.org/atoz/pdf/IfYouChoose.pdf).

E. *When Stopping Dialysis Treatment is your Choice: A Guide for Patients and Families* (2006), is a question and answer booklet by the National Kidney Foundation, http://www.kidney.org/atoz/pdf/stopdialysis.pdf

XIII. Pain.

A. Pain assessment (WHO, 2008; http://www.kidneysupportivecare.org).
   1. World Health Organization (WHO) assessment guidelines for chronic nonmalignant pain in adolescents and adults include psychological, emotional, cultural, and social aspects. Classification of pain, cause, evaluation, management, and control are included (WHO, 2008).
   2. Patients may be reluctant to report pain (fear, finances, religion, cultural, belief that no relief is possible).
   3. Healthcare team may under-recognize and undertreat patient's pain.
   4. "Clinical algorithm and preferred medications to treat pain in dialysis patients" (2009). Describes pain scale, pain medication management, and adjuvant and side effect therapy. Developed by the Mid-Atlantic Renal Coalition and the Kidney End-of-Life Coalition, http://www.kidneysupportivecare.org/Files/PainBrochure9-09.aspx
   5. Edmonton Symptom Assessment System – 11 categories with 1–10 ranking scale and body diagram for making sites of symptoms, http://www.kidneysupportivecare.org/Files/EdmontonAssessment.aspx.
   6. Chronic pain assessment, http://www.liv.ac.uk/mcpcil/liverpool-care-pathway/

B. Types of pain.
   1. Nociceptive.
      a. Somatic, visceral, musculoskeletal.
      b. Pain receptors are intact.
      c. Described as aching, dull, throbbing, cramping, pressure.
   2. Neuropathic.
      a. Injury to pain receptors.
      b. Described as sharp, tingling, burning, stabbing, numb.
   3. Episodic or continuous.
   4. Mixed pain – both nociceptive and neuropathic.

Educational and Informational Websites

Aging with Dignity. Includes five wishes for end-of-life care planning. Form is recognized in 42 states and Washington, DC. Available in 27 languages. http://www.agingwithdignity.org

American Kidney Fund. Includes online course for ethics and end-of-life considerations for ESRD. http://www.kidneyfund.org

American Nephrology Nurses' Association. 4-part module series on end-of-life decision making and the role of the nephrology nurse. Available under professional development ANNA education modules. http://www.annanurse.org

American Hospice Foundation. Includes one-page fact sheet written for laypersons. http://www.americanhospice.org

Beck Depression Inventory (BDI). The form is copyrighted but available. http://www.apa.org/pi/about/publications/caregivers/practice-settings/assessment/tools/beck-depression.aspx

Caring Connections. Online state-specific advance directive forms and resources. http://www.caringinfo.org

Coalition for Supportive Care of Kidney Patients. Includes links to regulatory/legal documents and numerous end-of-life resources. http://www.kidneysupportivecare.org/For-Professionals/Palliative-Care-Hospice-Care.aspx

Hemodialysis mortality predictor. Downloadable app for iPhone. http://Touchcalc.com/calculators/sq

Johns Hopkins Opioid Conversion. Registration is free. Enter current medication and dose, then new regimen. Converted dose and appropriate warnings are displayed. iPhone version is available. http://www.hopweb.org

Kidney Disease Quality of Life Short Form (KDQOL-SF). (Manual for use and scoring). http://www.rand.org/content/dam/rand/pubs/papers/2006/P7994.pdf

Mid-Atlantic Renal Coalition, ESRD Network 5. Contains "Recommendations for addressing end-of-life care in ESRD." http://www.esrdnet5.org

National Kidney Foundation. http://www.kidney.org.

National Palliative Care Research Center. http://www.npcrc.org/content/25/Measurement-and-Evaluation-Tools.aspx

Palliative Doctors: Compassionate care at any stage of an illness. American Academy of Hospice and Palliative Medicine. Includes explanations of palliative care/hospice, patient stories, and resource guide. http://www.palliativedoctors.org/

Patient Health Questionnaire-9 (PHQ-9). http://www.cqaimh.org/pdf/tool_phq9.pdf. More questionnaires at http://www.cqaimh.org

This site includes reference, scoring, and validity data: http://www.phqscreeners.com

Physician Orders for Life-Sustaining Treatment (POLST) http://www.kidneysupportivecare.org/Files/POLST_Form.aspx

C. Pain medication management (consult current medication guide for doses and side effects).
  1. Educate patient and family on pain assessment, goals, management, and possible complications. Chronic pain often requires 24-hour medical management with additional medication for "breakthrough" pain.
  2. Work to control pain to a level acceptable to the patient. Total elimination may not be possible.
  3. Pain is a common symptom and includes musculoskeletal, dialysis associated, peripheral neuropathy, and peripheral vascular disease.
  4. Consider collaboration with pain management specialist.
  5. Analgesic pain ladder – 3 steps from mild to severe pain.
    a. Nonnarcotics – Step 1.
      (1) Nociceptive pain.
        (a) Acetaminophen – hepatically metabolized and does not require dose adjustment. Exceeding daily recommendation can lead to hepatotoxicity.
        (b) Nonsteroidal analgesics (NSAIDS) are generally not recommended because of platelet dysfunction with possible risk of gastrointestinal bleeding. They can also decrease residual kidney function.
        (c) Tramadol (Ultram®) – Step 2; for nociceptive pain; has some mu opioid activity. Titrate slowly (25–100 mg/day) and monitor for serotonin syndrome with SSRIs. Do not use extended release if CrCl < 30 mL/min.
      (2) Neuropathic pain (begin nociceptive meds if these are not effective):
        (a) Gabapentin (Neurontin®) (titrate from 10 to 100 mg/day) – needs to be adjusted based on level of kidney function; if ineffective, discontinue and use the following.
        (b) Pregabalin (Lyrica®) (titrate from 25 to 100 mg/day) – needs to be adjusted based on kidney function; if ineffective, discontinue and use the following.
        (c) Desipramine (titrate from 10 to 150 mg) needs to be adjusted based on kidney function.
    b. Opioids – Steps 2 and 3 for nociceptive and neuropathic pain. Safer to use with patients on dialysis.
      (1) Hydrocodone and oxycodone (OxyContin®) – Step 2 and hydromorphone (Dilaudid®) – Step 3; mostly metabolized in liver but active metabolite can accumulate in kidney failure.
      (2) Fentanyl – Step 3 if hydromorphone not strong enough. Good for chronic stable pain. Has no active metabolites and is well tolerated. Do not start dose higher than 12 mcg/hr in opioid naïve patient.
      (3) Methadone – step 3 if hydromorphone and fentanyl patch are ineffective; use by knowledgeable practitioner; prolonged QT interval possible in higher doses; does not accumulate in kidney failure and appears to be safe choice.
      (4) Caution: fentanyl, tramadol, and methadone are not dialyzable so titration needs to be done slowly.
  6. Do not use with patients on dialysis.
    a. Metabolites are excreted by the kidney, and the accumulation can cause neurotoxicity.
    b. Codeine and morphine are most likely to cause side effects including hypotension and respiratory depression.
    c. Morphine is often used in final stages for tachypnea.
    d. Meperidine (Demerol®) accumulation can cause seizures.
  7. Opioid toxicity can mimic uremia with sedation, hallucinations, asterixis, and myoclonus.

D. Management of opioid side effects and other symptoms.
  1. Sedation (acute event).
    a. Naloxone (Narcan®) 0.4–2 mg IV.
    b. Half-life of naloxone is shorter than opioid so repeat dose may be needed.
  2. Nausea/vomiting.
    a. Prochlorperazine (Compazine®) 2.5–10 mg PO, SC, PR prn. Use with caution in elderly.
    b. Haloperidol (Haldol®) 0.5–1 mg PO, SL, SC, IV bid-tid prn. No kidney adjustment needed. Use with caution in elderly.
    c. Metoclopramide (Reglan®) 5–10 mg PO, SC, IV qid prn. Decreased dose in kidney failure. Monitor for tardive dyskinesia, especially in elderly or long-term use.
    d. Dimenhydrinate (Dramamine®) 25–50 mg PO, SC, IV. Helps reduce opioid pruritus. No kidney adjustment needed.
    e. Ondansetron (Zofran®) 4–8 mg PO, IV tid prn. No kidney adjustment needed.
  3. Constipation.
    a. Start therapy when opioid therapy is begun.
    b. Stool softener (docusate sodium) and stimulant laxative (senna or bisacodyl).
  4. Cognitive changes. Lower dose or change to different pain medication.

E. Nonmedication pain management.
  1. Physical therapy – muscle cramps, spasms.
  2. Peripheral stimulation therapy (transdermal electronic nerve stimulation, acupuncture).

3. Nerve blocks.
4. Guided imagery.
5. Supportive care – treatment of comorbid conditions such as depression and anxiety.
6. Comfort measures – mouth care, lip moisturizer, skin care, light muscle massage, fans, cool compresses, etc.

F. Palliative care and hospice (Berger & Hedayati, 2012; Swidler, 2012).
   1. Address other symptoms (may have been present) – pain, muscle cramps, hunger, thirst, dyspnea.
   2. Distress may be proportional to frequency and management of symptoms.
   3. Increase use of hospice in earlier stages.

XIV. Ongoing areas of interest.

A. Validating and promoting palliative care. Moss and Armistead (2013) provided a synopsis of additional areas of needed research as identified by the Coalition for Supportive Care of Kidney Patients, led by the Mid-Atlantic Renal Coalition (MARC). Some of these of particular interest to nursing include the following.
   1. Communication between primary care and nephrology as it pertains to end of life.
   2. Regional variations in the use of hospice and withdrawal from dialysis.
   3. Better understanding of the needs and goals of patients at the end of life
   4. Actualizing the supportive care philosophy that makes the patient and family the true center of care.
   5. Understanding what patients really hear and understand from discussions about prognosis and treatment options.
      a. Do patients equate palliative care with hospice and death?
      b. Does literacy level influence decisions about end-of-life care?

B. Restructuring care of patients with kidney failure to include palliative care as a standard of care. Tamura and Meier (2013) propose five policies that could potentially increase availability and use of palliative care in this patient population. They acknowledge these would require changes in current regulations, funding, and more evidence-based research.
   1. Development of universal screening to assess for palliative care needs for all patients with kidney failure.
      a. Most dialysis care occurs outside of primary care, hospital, and specialist care settings – healthcare information is not easily shared and transferred.
      b. Consider initial screening as already discussed

in this chapter for the highest risk patients – Surprise Question, dementia, older age, peripheral vascular disease, and decreased albumin.
   c. Benefits could include more uniform screening regardless of location of patients (urban, rural, or region of the country).
   2. Modifications to the current Medicare ESRD Quality Incentive Program (QIP) to incorporate aspects of palliative care.
      a. All QIP standards already have to be endorsed by the National Quality Forum (NQF) (http://www.qualityforum.org). Palliative care already has approved QIP standards some of which could be adapted for the ESRD QIP.
      b. An example includes documentation of advance care planning and name of a healthcare agent (surrogate) with all patients > 65 years of age, or documentation that a discussion was held and patient does not wish to participate. Rationale includes findings that about one third of patients need a surrogate at the end of life and are more apt to receive their preferred treatment if this has been done.
      c. Evidence supports that less acute care is needed or used if palliative care is active.
      d. QIP would need to be adjusted to reflect patients who are actively followed by hospice.
      e. Collected data including admission rates, acuity scores, and use of palliative care services could all be analyzed for trends and outcomes.
   3. Increased and modified training for the multidisciplinary teams already providing care to the CKD/ESRD population, rather than dependence on specialty palliative care teams.
      a. Greater number of patients will need palliative care services, and most of these services are located in acute care settings, larger medical centers, and hospice settings.
      b. Increased availability and use of palliative care services would require changes in current regulations and reimbursements. As noted earlier, symptoms of pain, itching, gastrointestinal distress, sleep disturbances, and family support are all encompassed in palliative care.
      c. Increased training for all staff to screen, manage, and incorporate palliative care into CKD/ESRD care.
   4. Examination of current reimbursement.
      a. Consider use of Medicare Part B CKD stage 4 education to expand advance planning services.
      b. Examine current restrictions on use of hospice (see earlier section) in CKD population.
   5. Ongoing research to bolster evidence-based practice for palliative care methods.

a. Relatively little funding has been directed toward ESRD and palliative care research.
b. Development of demonstration projects could include other chronic illnesses such as heart disease, pulmonary disease, dementia, and frailty, all of which are present in the ESRD population.

References

American Association of Colleges of Nursing (AACN). (2006). *The essentials of doctoral education for advanced nursing practice.* Retrieved from http://www.aacn.nche.edu/publications/position/DNPEssentials.pdf.

American Association of Colleges of Nursing (AACN). (2014). *DNP fact sheet.* Retrieved from http://www.aacn.nche.edu/media-relations/fact-sheets/dnp.

American Association of Critical Care Nurses (AACCN). (2012). *Scope and standards of practice for the acute care nurse practitioner* (2nd ed.). Aliso Viejo, CA: Author.

American Association of Nurse Practitioners (AANP). (2013). *What's an NP?* Retrieved from http://www.aanp.org/all-about-nps/what-is-an-np.

American Nephrology Nurses' Association (ANNA). (2013). *Advanced practice in nephrology nursing.* Retrieved from http://www.annanurse.org/download/reference/health/position/advPractice.pdf

American Nephrology Nurses' Association (ANNA). (2012). *ANNA, ASN and RPA joint position paper on collaboration between nephrologists and advanced practice registered nurses.* Retrieved from http://www.annanurse.org/download/reference/health/position/nephCollaboration.pdf

APRN Consensus Work Group (2008). *Consensus model for APRN regulation: Licensure, accreditation, certification & education.* Retrieved from https://www.ncsbn.org/aprn.htm

Berger, J.R., & Hedayati, S.S. (2012). Renal replacement therapy in the elderly population. *Clinical Journal of the American Society of Nephrology, 7,* 1039-1046. doi:10:2215/CJN.10411011

Brandt, K. (2013). *Are you traveling without a map? A layperson's guide to advance care planning.* Caring Connections: National Hospice and Palliative Care Organization. http://www.caringinfo.org/files/public/brochures/Are_you_traveling_without_a_map.pdf

Buppert, C. (2015). *Nurse practitioner's business practice and legal guide* (5th ed.). Burlington: Jones & Bartlett.

Chism, L. (2009). Toward clarification of the doctor of nursing practice degree. *Advanced Emergency Nursing Journal, 31,* 287-297.

Cohen, L.M., Ruthazer, R., Moss, A.H., & Germain, M.J. (2010). Predicting six-month mortality for patients who are on maintenance hemodialysis. *Clinical Journal of the American Society of Nephrology, 5,* 72-79. doi:10.2215/CJN.03860609

Centers for Medicare and Medicaid Services (CMS). (2008, April 15). *Conditions for coverage for end-stage renal disease facilities,* Part II Federal Register. Department of Health and Human Services, 42 CFR Parts 405, 410, 413, et al. http://www.cms.gov/Regulations-and-Guidance/Legislation/CFCsAndCoPs/Downloads/ESRDfinalrule0415.pdf

Cook, A.J., Roberts, D.A., Henderson, M.D., VanWinkle, L.C., Chastain, D.C., & Hamill-Ruth, R.J. (2004). Electronic pain questionnaires: A randomized, crossover comparison with paper questionnaires for chronic pain assessment. *Pain, 110,* 310-317.

Cruzan v. Director, Missouri Department of Health, 497 U.S. 261, 264, 1990.

Davison, S.N. (2010). End-of-life care preferences and needs: Perceptions of patients with chronic kidney disease. *Clinical Journal of the American Society of Nephrology, 5*(2), 195-204. doi:10.2215/CJN.05960809 PMCID: MCC2827591

Davison, S.N. (2012). The ethics of end-of-life care for patients with ESRD. *Clinical Journal of the American Society of Nephrology, 7,* 2049-2057. doi:10.2215/CJN.03900412

Davison, S.N., Jhangri, G.S., & Johnson, J.A. (2006). Cross-sectional validity of modified Edmonton symptom assessment system in dialysis patients: a simple assessment of symptom burden. *Kidney International, 69,* 1621-1625. doi:10.1038/sj.ki.5000184

Gomez, N. (2011). *Nephrology nursing scope and standards of practice* (7th ed.). Pitman, NJ: American Nephrology Nurses' Association.

Institute of Medicine (IOM). (2010). *The future of nursing: Leading change, advancing health.* Retrieved from http://www.iom.edu/reports/2010/the-future-of-nursing-leading-change-advancing-health.aspx

Kimmel, P. L., Emont, S.L, Newmann, J. M., Danko, H., & Moss, A.H. (2003). ESRD patient quality of life: Symptoms, spiritual beliefs, psychosocial factors and ethnicity. *American Journal of Kidney Diseases, 42,* 713-721. doi:10.1053/S0272-6386(03)00907-7

Kleinpell, R. (2013). Measuring outcomes in advanced practice nursing. In R. Kleinpell (Ed.), *Outcome assessment in advanced practice nursing* (3rd ed., pp. 1-43). New York: Springer.

Mid-Atlantic Renal Coalition and the Kidney End-of-Life Coalition. (2009). *Clinical algorithm and preferred medications to treat pain in dialysis patients.* http://www.kidneysupportivecare.org/Files/PainBrochure9-09.aspx.

Melzack, R. (2005). The McGill Pain Questionnaire: From description to measurement. *Anesthesiology, 103,* 199-202.

Moss, A.H., & Armistead, N. C. (2013). Improving end-of-life care for ESRD patients: An initiative for professionals. *Nephrology News & Issues.* Retrieved on August 5, 2014, from http://www.nephrologynews.com/articles/109673-improving-end-of-life-care-for-esrd-patients-an-initiative-for-professionals

Moss, A.H., Ganjoo, J., Sharma, S., Gansor, J., Senft, S., Weaner, B., … Schmidt, R. (2008). Utility of the "surprise" question to identify dialysis patients with high mortality. *Clinical Journal of the American Society of Nephrology, 3,* 1379-1384. doi:10.2215/CJN.00940208

National Hospice and Palliative Care Organization. (n.d.). *Caring connections.* Retrieved from http://www.caringinfo.org and http://www.nhpco.org

National Association of Clinical Nurse Specialists. (2014). *What is a clinical nurse specialist?* Retrieved from http://www.nacns.org/html/cns-faqs.php

National Quality Forum. (n.d.). *Quality positioning system.* Retrieved from http://www.qualityforum.org/QPS

Newhouse, R., Stanik-Hutt, J., White, K., Johantgen, M., Bass, E., Zangaro, G., …Weiner, J. (2011). Advanced practice nurse outcomes 1990–2008: A systematic review. *Nursing Economics, 29*(5), 1-22.

Nurse Licensure Compact Administrators (2012). *APRN (advanced practice nurse) licensure compact.* National Council of State Boards of Nursing. Retrieved from https://www.ncsbn.org/APRN_Compact_hx_timeline_April_2012_(2).pdf

O'Connor, N.R., & Corcoran, A.M. (2012). End-stage renal disease: Symptom management and advance care planning. *American Family Physicians, 85*(7), 705-710.

Parry, R., Seymour, J., Whittaker, B. Bird, L., & Cox, K. (2013). *Rapid evidence review: Pathways focused on the dying phase in end of life care and their key components.* Final version 1.0. National End of Life Care Programme, University of Nottingham: United Kingdom. https://www.gov.uk/government/uploads/system/uploads/attachment_data/file/212451/review_academic_literature_on_end_of_life.pdf

Renal Physicians Association (RPA). (2010). *Shared decision-making in the appropriate initiation of and withdrawal from dialysis* (2nd ed.). Rockville, MD: Author.

Saylor, R. (2012). *Ethics of ESRD patient care. Weighing the outcomes: Ethical issues in kidney disease.* American Kidney Fund, slides 76-132. Retrieved from http://www.kidneyfund.org/professionals/online-course/

Schell, J.O., Green, J.A., Tulsky, J.A., & Arnold, R.M. (2013). Communication skills training for dialysis decision-making and end-of-life care in nephrology. *Clinical Journal of the American Society of Nephrology, 8*, 675-680. doi:10.2215/CJN.05220512

Swidler, M. (2013). Considerations in starting a patient with advanced frailty on dialysis: Complex biology meets challenging ethics. *Clinical Journal of the American Society of Nephrology, 8*, 1421-1428. doi:10.2215/CJN.12121112

Swidler, M.A. (2012). Geriatric renal palliative care (Translational article: Special issue on the aging kidney). *The Journals of Gerontology Series A: Biological Sciences and Medical Sciences, 67*(12), 1400-1409. doi:10.1093/Gerona/gls202

Tamura, M.K., & Cohen, L.M. (2010). Should there be an expanded role for palliative care in end-stage renal disease? *Current Opinion in Nephrology and Hypertension, 19*(6), 556-560. doi:10.1097/MNH.0b013e32833d67bc

Tamura, M.K., & Meier, K.E. (2013). Five policies to promote palliative care for patients with ESRD. *Clinical Journal of the American Society of Nephrology, 8*, 1783-1790.

United States Renal Data System, 2014 Annual Data Report: Epidemiology of Kidney Disease in the United States. National Institutes of Health, National Institute of Diabetes and Digestive and Kidney Diseases, Bethesda, MD, 2014. Retrieved from http://www.usrds.org/adr.aspx

World Health Organization (WHO). (n.d.) *Home page.* http://www.who.int/cancer/palliative/definition/en

World Health Organization (WHO). (2008). *Scoping document for WHO treatment guideline on non-malignant pain in adults.* Adapted in WHO Steering Group on Pain Guidelines. Retrieved from http://www.who.int/medicines/areas/quality_safety/Scoping_WHOGuide_non-malignant_pain_adults.pdf

Overview of CKD for the APRN

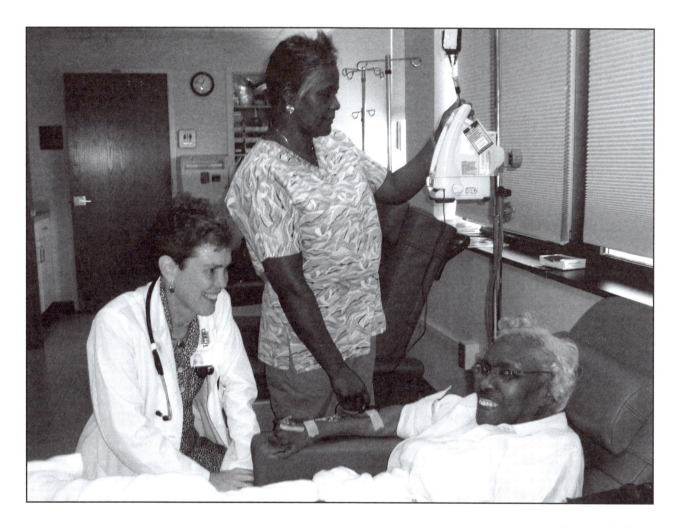

Chapter Editors
Kim Alleman, MS, APRN, FNP-BC, CNN-NP
Katherine Houle, MSN, APRN, CFNP, CNN-NP

Authors
Sally F. Campoy, DNP, ANP-BC, CNN-NP
Andrea Easom, MA, MNSc, APRN, FNP-BC, CNN-NP

CHAPTER **2**

Overview of CKD for the APRN

This offering for **1.4 contact hours with 1.0 contact hour of pharmacology content** is provided by the American Nephrology Nurses' Association (ANNA).

American Nephrology Nurses' Association is accredited as a provider of continuing nursing education by the American Nurses Credentialing Center Commission on Accreditation.

ANNA is a provider approved by the California Board of Registered Nursing, provider number CEP 00910.

This CNE offering meets the continuing nursing education requirements for certification and recertification by the Nephrology Nursing Certification Commission (NNCC).

To be awarded contact hours for this activity, read this chapter in its entirety. Then complete the CNE evaluation found at **www.annanurse.org/corecne** and submit it; or print it, complete it, and mail it in. Contact hours are not awarded until the evaluation for the activity is complete.

Example of reference for Chapter 2 in APA format. Use author of the section being cited. This example is based on Section B – APRN Role in CKD, Stages 4 to 5, Not on Dialysis.

Easom, A. (2015). Overview of CKD for the APRN: APRN role in CKD, stages 4 to 5, not on dialysis. In C.S. Counts (Ed.), *Core curriculum for nephrology nursing: Module 6. The APRN's approaches to care in nephrology* (6th ed., pp. 19-52). Pitman, NJ: American Nephrology Nurses' Association.

Interpreted: Section author. (Date). Title of chapter: Title of section written by that author. In ...

Cover photo by Sandra Cook.

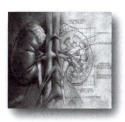

CHAPTER 2

Overview of CKD for the APRN

Purpose

Section A provides the advanced practice registered nurse (APRN) a framework for strategies to assess and treat persons with chronic kidney disease (CKD) stages 1 through 3. Section B enables the APRN to use evidence-based practice to provide care and education to prevent or slow the progression of kidney disease, as well as prepare the patient for kidney replacement therapy when needed.

Objectives

Upon completion of this chapter, the learner will be able to:
1. Define classification of chronic kidney disease (CKD) according to the current nephrology guidelines.
2. Identify persons at risk for CKD.
3. Formulate diagnostic strategies for all stages of CKD.
4. Describe clinical actions that may delay progression of CKD and estimate progression.
5. Diagnose and treat comorbid conditions and complications that commonly occur.
6. Educate and prepare patients for kidney replacement therapy, as appropriate.

> ### SECTION A
> ### APRN Role in Chronic Kidney Disease Stages 1 through 3
> #### Sally F. Campoy

I. Definition and classification of chronic kidney disease (CKD).

A. CKD is defined as the presence of kidney damage or decreased kidney function which has been present for > 3 months with implications for health (KDIGO, 2013a).
   1. Markers of kidney damage: albuminuria, abnormalities detected in urine sediment, tubular disorders, histologic changes or structural findings, or history of kidney transplantation.
   2. Decreased glomerular filtration rate (GFR) < 60 mL/min/1.73 m².
   3. Addition of phrase "with implications for health" was added to provide emphasis on the negative impact of CKD on maintaining optimal health status.

B. Classification of CKD.
   1. Kidney Disease Improving Global Outcomes (KDIGO) (2013a) guidelines recommend classification to offer a guide to management, which includes risk stratification for progression and complications of CKD. Several factors were outlined in classification.
   a. Cause of kidney disease includes presence or absence of systemic disease, location of kidney pathology or anatomic pathology.
      (1) Identification of cause may enable specific therapy directed at preventing further injury.
      (2) Cause may have implications on rate of progression and development of complications.
   b. GFR category. One major change in KDIGO guidelines from the original National Kidney Foundation's (NKF) classification involves splitting CKD stage 3 into 2 separate categories as the presence of complications and greater mortality rise with lower GFR (see Table 2.1) (NKF, 2002).
      (1) G1 is normal-to-high kidney function with GFR > 90 mL/min/1.73 m².

Table 2.1			Persistent albuminuria categories Description and range		
Prognosis of CKD by GFR and Albuminuria Categories: KDIGO 2012			A1	A2	A3
			Normal to mildly increased	Moderately increased	Severely increased
			< 30 mg/g < 3 mg/mmol	30–300 mg/g 3–30 mg/mmol	> 300 mg/g > 30 mg/mmol
GFR categories (mL/min/1.73 m²) Description and range	G1	Normal or high	≥ 90		
	G2	Mildly decreased	60–89		
	G3a	Mildly to moderately decreased	45–59		
	G3b	Moderately to severely decreased	30–44		
	G4	Severely decreased	15–29		
	G5	Kidney failure	< 15		

Dark gray, low risk (if no other markers of kidney disease, no CKD); Light blue, moderately increased risk; Light gray, high risk; Dark blue, very high risk.

Abbreviations: CKD – chronic kidney disease; GFR – glomerular filtration rate; KDIGO – Kidney Disease: Improving Global Outcomes.

Source: Kidney Disease: Improving Global Outcomes (KDIGO) CKD Work Group. KDIGO 2012 Clinical Practice Guideline for the Evaluation and Management of Chronic Kidney Disease. *Kidney International Supplements 2013*; 3: 1–150 (originally figure 9 on page 34). Used with permission.

(2) G2 is mildly decreased GFR with GFR 60 to 89 mL/min/1.73 m².

(3) G3a is mildly to moderately decreased GFR 45 to 59 mL/min/1.73 m².

(4) G3b is moderately to severely decreased GFR 30 to 44 mL/min/1.73 m².

(5) G4 is severely decreased GFR 15 to 29 mL/min/1.73 m².

(6) G5 is kidney failure with GFR < 15 mL/min/1.73 m².

c. Albuminuria level was added because of the increased risk for disease progression, cardiovascular disease, mortality, and kidney failure, independent of GFR. It is described as persistent albuminuria > 3 months.

(1) A1 is normal to mildly increased albuminuria with levels < 30 mg/g or < 3 mg/mmol.

(2) A2 represents moderately increased albuminuria with levels 30 to 300 mg/g or 3 to 30 mg/mmol.

(3) A3 is severely increased albuminuria with levels > 300 mg/g or > 30 mg/mmol.

2. Staging of CKD combines the GFR categories with the albuminuria categories to assess risk of progression.

II. Epidemiology of CKD.

A. Prevalence of CKD.
   1. There are no exact statistics regarding the prevalence of the early stages of CKD.
   2. Estimations of prevalence are made from large representative samples measuring various markers of kidney damage, such as decreased estimated GFR, increased serum creatinine or presence of albuminuria, and extrapolating data to the general population.
   3. Prevalence of CKD from 2007 to 2012 was estimated to be 13.6% (USRDS, 2014).
   4. Barriers to quantifying true prevalence of CKD Stages 1 through 3 (USRDS, 2014).
      a. CKD is largely asymptomatic until the later stages.
      b. There is provider unawareness of CKD.
      c. There is patient unawareness of CKD stages 1 to 3, estimated as less than 10%.

B. Risk factors for CKD (see Table 2.2, Risk Factors for Chronic Kidney Disease, Stages 1 through 3).
   1. Identification of potential risk factors may lead to early detection of kidney disease, allowing for early interventions which may reduce the rate of decline.
   2. U.S Renal Data System (USRDS, 2014) assessed single-sample, cross-sectional estimates of kidney function with data collected by the National Health and Nutrition Examination Survey (NHANES) to determine CKD prevalence estimates, trends, disease burden, and interactions with other conditions, such as diabetes, cardiovascular disease, and albuminuria.
   3. Based on USRDS 2014 annual data report, the leading cause of kidney failure (end-stage renal disease) is diabetes mellitus, followed by hypertension, which accounts for approximately 75% of kidney failure (USRDS, 2014). Given the large prevalence of both of these diseases, which are commonly seen in adult and geriatric primary care APRN practices, special attention to disease management and surveillance of markers of kidney damage should be paramount.
   4. Other risk factors.
      a. Age over 70 years old.
         (1) Prevalence of kidney failure in this age population is increasing.
         (2) Increased risk of kidney disease progression with albuminuria is similar in the older adult compared to younger age.
      b. Race/ethnicity (USRDS, 2014).
         (1) Highest incidence of kidney failure is seen in African Americans, followed by Native Americans, Hispanics, Asian Americans, and Caucasians.
         (2) Hispanics have a higher incidence of kidney failure compared to non-Hispanics.
      c. Acute kidney injury (AKI).
         (1) AKI increases the risk of CKD and kidney failure (Coca et al., 2012).
         (2) Even with recovery from AKI, there is increased future risk (Bucaloiu et al., 2012).
         (3) Those persons who required dialysis to treat AKI have the greatest risk of developing CKD (Chawla et al., 2011).
         (4) Many patients are not referred to nephrologists after AKI.
      d. Cardiovascular disease (Choi & Fried, 2013).
         (1) CKD progression may increase with cardiac dysfunction by a variety of mechanisms including decreased perfusion, endothelial dysfunction, arrhythmias, and left ventricular hypertrophy.
         (2) Vascular disease, both of large and small vessels, may also contribute.

Table 2.2

Risk Factors for Chronic Kidney Disease, Stages 1-3

Definition	Examples
Patient factors that increase susceptibility	Older age, family history of chronic kidney disease, reduction in kidney mass, low birth weight, racial or ethnic minority status, low income
Conditions that can cause direct kidney damage	Diabetes, hypertension, autoimmune diseases, systemic infections, urinary tract infections, urinary stones, lower urinary tract obstruction, drug toxicity, neoplasm
Conditions that can cause worsening of kidney damage and /or faster progression	Uncontrolled high blood pressure, poor glycemic control, higher levels of proteinuria, smoking

Adapted from Stevens, L., A., Stoyucheff, N., & Levey, A.S. (2009). Staging and management of chronic kidney disease. In A. Greenburg (Ed.), *Primer on kidney disease* (5th ed.). Philadelphia: Saunders Elsevier. Used with permission.

   e. History of kidney disease.
      (1) Glomerular, tubular, or interstitial disease.
      (2) Renal calculi, kidney tumors, bladder outlet obstruction.
   f. Autoimmune disorders.
      (1) Systemic lupus erythematosus.
      (2) Sarcoidosis.
   g. Infectious disease.
      (1) HIV.
      (2) Hepatitis C.
      (3) Streptococcus.
   h. Kidney transplant.
   i. Kidney donor.
   j. Family history of CKD/kidney failure.
   k. Exposure to nephrotoxic drugs or procedures with potential for kidney damage.

III. Pathophysiology of CKD.

A. Pathophysiology of CKD involves kidney injury and loss of functioning nephrons, as the result of the underlying cause. Whatever the etiology, once established, the basic mechanism for further progression is the same. The rate of progression varies depending upon the underlying disease, presence or absence of co-morbid conditions, treatments, socioeconomic status, genetics, and ethnicity, to name a few factors (Hallan et al., 2006).
   1. Adaptive hyperfiltration occurs within the remaining glomeruli to increase GFR. While initially beneficial, over time it can result in glomerular damage.

2. Ongoing glomerular stress promotes further injury and more glomerular and tubular destruction which leads to reduced GFR.

B. Predicting prognosis of CKD (Inker et al., 2014).
   1. KDIGO (KDIGO, 2013, pg. 9) recommends incorporating the following factors: cause of CKD, GFR category, albuminuria category, and other risk factors and comorbid conditions.
   2. KDIGO (2013a, pg. 6) recommends the 2009 CKD-EPI creatinine equation or another creatinine-based GFR estimating equation.
   3. In cases when GFR is 45 to 59 mL/min/1.73 m^2 without evidence of kidney damage and confirmation of CKD is needed, KDIGO (2013a) recommends cystatin-C measurement and the use of a GFR estimating equation using cystatin-C.
   4. Predictive models (Choi & Fried, 2013, pg. 241).
      a. Modification of diet in renal disease (MDRD).
         (1) Underestimates GFR when GFR > 60 mL/min.
         (2) Less accurate with extremes in age and weight, amputation, pregnancy, and cirrhosis.
      b. CKD-EPI.
         (1) Overestimates GFR in the older adult and in persons with CKD.
         (2) More accurate than MDRD when GFR > 60 mL/min/1.73 m^2. Generally better for defining persons at risk in the general population and who are younger.
      c. CKD-EPI cystatin C equation.
         (1) Recommended by KDIGO when confirmation of CKD status is needed, such as in the older adult.
         (2) Lack of standardization among different laboratories and general availability of the test have been identified as barriers to routine use of cystitis C.
         (3) May be more useful in older adults, and in persons with malnutrition and/or decreased muscle mass (Ix et al., 2011).
      d. CKD-EPI creatinine-cystatin C equation.
         (1) More accurate than MDRD, CKD-EPI, and CKD-EPI cystatin C in estimating GFR.
         (2) May be more useful in older adults, persons with malnutrition or decreased muscle mass, and persons with GFR 45–74 mL/min/1.73 m^2.
   5 Refer to Table 2.1, KDIGO's Definition and Classification of Chronic Kidney Disease, which correlates risk of progression and prognosis.
   6. Estimation of GFR in pediatric patients requires a different formula. CKiD bedside formula was more accurate than the adult-based formulas.

IV. Diagnosis of CKD.

A. Determination of chronicity (KDIGO, 2013a, pg. 6).
   1. Differentiate from AKI versus CKD.
      a. Review past history and laboratory data to estimate duration.
      b. AKI is potentially reversible.
   2. Duration of impaired kidney function or other markers of kidney damage > 3 months confirms CKD.

B. History.
   1. Personal history.
      a. Exposure to prior kidney insults, such as AKI, nephrotoxic drugs, or procedures that can potentially alter kidney function.
      b. Medical history of kidney disease, diabetes, hypertension, lupus, or other systemic diseases known to affect kidney function.
      c. Obesity.
   2. Family history.
      a. African Americans with a family history of kidney failure are at increased risk of developing CKD (Tareen et al., 2005).
      b. Family history of other known hereditary diseases, such as polycystic kidney disease, Alport's disease, and/or acquired cystic disease.
   3. Social factors.
      a. Socioeconomic factors have implications in CKD risk and healthcare disparities.
      b. Tobacco use may contribute to CKD progression.
   4. Environmental factors.
      a. Exposure to toxic agents, such as lead or heavy metals.
      b. Access to care.
   5. Medications.
      a. Prescribed medications that have potential nephrotoxic side effects.
      b. Medications that are inappropriately dosed for the CKD stage.
      c. Herbals and over-the-counter medications that may have direct negative effects on kidney function as well as potential drug-herb interactions (see Table 2.3).
         (1) Nonsteroidal antiinflammatory (NSAID) drugs.
         (2) Chinese herb aristolochic acid (Combest et al., 2005).

C. Physical examination.
   1. Focused examination to identify pathologic processes caused by existing or suspected primary disease.
      a. In persons with diabetes and/or hypertension, examination for retinal changes, volume status, assessment of lung and heart sounds, presence of edema or ascites, carotid, abdominal and

femoral bruits, and peripheral sensation and circulation.
   b. Skin changes for ecchymosis or rashes commonly seen in collagen vascular disorders.
   c. Examination of bladder and prostate to rule out bladder distention, possible obstruction, or atony.
2. General examination to assess effects, if any, of progression of kidney disease.
   a. Vital signs including orthostatic blood pressures as indicated.
   b. Assessment of mental status to screen for depression, cognitive deficits, or delirium.
   c. Assessment of other body systems as indicated.

D. Laboratory.
   1. Estimation of glomerular filtration rate (eGFR).
      a. Provider should be aware of the estimation formula used by the laboratories encountered in practice.
      b. Provider should be aware of clinical situations in which certain estimation formulas may be less accurate (Shlipak et al., 2013).
         (1) Extremes in body size.
         (2) Heavy muscular build.
         (3) Extremes in age: very young or very old.
         (4) Estimation formulas should be used during steady state, not during AKI.
      c. KDIGO (2013a, pg. 6) recommends the 2009 CKD-EPI creatinine equation or another creatinine-based GFR estimating equation.
      d. In cases when GFR is 45 to 59 mL/min/1.73 m² without evidence of kidney damage and confirmation of CKD is needed, KDIGO (2013a, pg. 7) recommends cystatin-C measurement and the uses of a GFR estimating equation utilizing cystatin-C.
   2. Serologic testing.
      a. Serum creatinine.
      b. Comprehensive metabolic panel including blood urea nitrogen, fasting glucose, liver function, lipid panel, calcium, phosphorus, magnesium, and complete blood count.
      c. Other blood tests as indicated by presence of known or suspected disease (Ferri, 2014).
         (1) Viral infections.
            (a) Hepatitis B and C.
            (b) HIV.
         (2) Intact parathyroid hormone (PTH).
         (3) Other testing as indicated.
            (a) Wegener's (Antineutophil cystoplasmic antibodies P-ANCA, C-ANCA).
            (b) Cryoglobulinemia or membrano-proliferative glomerulonephritis (Complement C-3, C-4).
            (c) Systemic lupus erythematosus (Antinuclear antibodies ANA).

Table 2.3

Herbals That May Contribute To Kidney Injury or Potential Drug-Herb Interactions

Herbal	Potential Effect
Gingko	Bleeding
Asparagus root Juniper berry Lovage root	Diuretic action
Buckthorn bark Cascara Rhubarb root	Hematuria/Albuminuria
Licorice root Cascara Senna Rhubarb	Hypokalemia
Noni Juice Dandelion Stinging nettle Horsetail Alfalfa	Hyperkalemia
Ephedra Bitter orange	Hypertension Cardiovascular events
Rhubarb Star fruit	Kidney stones
Echinacea St. John's wart	Interaction with transplant medications
Aristolochic acid (Chinese Herb) Djenkol Impila Cat's claw	Nephrotoxicity

Source: Campoy & Elwell, 2005; Combest et al., 2005.

            (d) Goodpastures (P-ANCA, antiglomerular basement membrane antibody).
            (e) Erythrocyte sedimentation rate (ESR).
   3. Urine testing.
      a. Early morning specimen is preferred.
      b. Urinalysis (Fogazzi, 2010).
         (1) Presence of RBC > 5/HPF.
            (a) Infection, trauma, cancer, stones.
            (b) Dysmorphic RBC, seen in glomerular disorders.
         (2) Presence of WBC > 5/HPF.
         (3) Casts.
            (a) Red cell casts indicate more acute process which should be investigated immediately.

(b) White cell casts indicate infectious process in the kidney, such as pyelonephritis.

(c) Hyaline casts may be a normal variant but will be increased in CKD.

(d) Granular casts nonspecific finding indicative of CKD.

(e) Broad, waxy casts sign of advanced CKD.

(f) Crystals, such as uric acid or calcium oxalate.

(g) Oval fat bodies and fat casts may be seen in nephrotic syndrome.

(h) Bacteria seen in infectious processes.

c. Urine dipstick.

(1) Standard dipstick records albuminuria > 300 mg/g. Other dipsticks for detection of albuminuria < 300 mg/g are available.

(2) Confirmation of positive dipstick should be made with quantitative laboratory measurement of spot urine albumin or protein and spot urine creatinine.

d. Untimed spot albumin or protein.

(1) Prefer morning specimen.

(2) Urine albumin-to-creatinine ratio (ACR) or urine protein-creatinine ratio (PCR).

(a) KDIGO recommends ACR for spot urine samples (Inker et al., 2014).

(b) ACR more sensitive and specific measure of kidney damage.

(3) Urine protein-to-creatinine ratio most closely corresponds to the 24-hour protein excretion.

(a) The sample is easily obtained.

(b) Confirmation should be done with 24-hour protein collection, if clinically indicated.

e. Timed albumin.

(1) 24-hour protein excretion urine is the gold standard for measurement.

(2) Obtaining an accurate collection can be challenging.

(3) Obtaining urine creatinine can provide a double check on the accuracy of the sample (over-collection versus under-collection). The creatinine excretion should be approximately 20-25 mg/kg/day for a healthy male and 15 to 20 mg/kg/day for a healthy female (Stevens, Shastri, & Levey, 2010).

(4) 24-hour urine measures total proteins, thereby potentially identifying other nonalbumin causes of proteinuria.

(5) KDIGO recommends the elimination of the terminology micro/macro albuminuria (Inker et al., 2014).

f. Measurement of other proteins.

(1) Consider other testing when dipstick is negative but the spot PCR or 24-hour total protein is elevated.

(2) Serum electrophoresis, urine electrophoresis, serum-free light chains, and immunofixaton of free immunoglobulin light chains can help detect other disorders, such as multiple myeloma.

E. Imaging studies (Wymer, 2010).

1. Kidney ultrasound is useful to determine kidney size, symmetry, echogenicity, and the presence of cysts or obstruction.

a. Bilateral small kidney size < 9 cm, which can be an indication of chronic medical kidney disease, congenital abnormalities, or papillary necrosis.

b. Unilateral decreased kidney size may be a result of infection, renal artery stenosis, congenital abnormalities, or radiation nephritis.

2. Computed tomography (CT) can assess for stones, tumors, and complex cysts.

a. Noncontrast CT urography is preferred for stones rather than the kidney, ureter, and bladder x-ray (KUB).

b. With GFR< 30 mL/min/1.73 m², evaluation of risks vs. benefits of IV contrast dye must be done to avoid unnecessary contrast dye exposure, which can negatively affect GFR.

c. With GFR < 60 mL/min/1.73 m², caution with dye exposure should be used.

3. Magnetic resonance imaging can differentiate tumors, detect noncalculus causes of obstruction, and provide better images of vasculature when assessing for renal artery stenosis.

a. Magnetic resonance urography may be the preferred test for pediatric clients as it can be performed rapidly and with less radiation exposure than with a CT.

b. Use of gadolinium is contraindicated when GFR < 15 mL/min due to the risk of nephrogenic systemic fibrosis.

4. Nuclear kidney scan, usually captopril or enalapril-enhanced, is used for determining renal artery stenosis.

a. Angiography is the gold standard and usually is used after a less invasive test indicates a lesion may be present.

b. Other indications for a kidney scan are obstructive uropathy, evaluation of separate function between the two kidneys, and in kidney transplant donor evaluations.

F. Kidney biopsy (Topham & Chen, 2010).

1. Referral to nephrologists for kidney biopsy.

2. Indications for kidney biopsy are nephrotic

syndrome, AKI of unknown cause, systemic disease with kidney dysfunction, unexplained CKD, familial kidney disease, isolated hematuria in the absence of structural lesion, and kidney transplant dysfunction.

3. Contraindications for kidney biopsy.
   a. Kidney related issues such as solitary kidney, small size kidneys < 9 cm, cystic kidneys, kidney neoplasm, acute pyelonephritis, or kidney abscess.
   b. Patient-related issues include uncontrolled bleeding disorder, uncontrolled hypertension, advanced uremia, obesity or an uncooperative patient.

V. General management of CKD stages 1 through 3.

A. It is likely that the person with CKD stage 1 through 3 may not be seen by a nephrology health provider.

B. The role of the nephrology APRN is to increase patients' and other providers' awareness of CKD, provide consultation for kidney issues, and be the advocate for early recognition and diagnosis of CKD.

C. CKD is largely asymptomatic until the late stages.

D. The provider should be aware of the potential for AKI and treat the reversible causes of kidney failure.

E. The goal of care in the early stages is to prevent or delay progression of kidney disease (Schieppati et al., 2005).

F. The complications of CKD usually start when GFR stays < 60 mL/min/1.73 m², with the exception of cardiovascular complications which may be present in CKD stage 1 and 2.

G. Adjustment of drug dosages should be considered when GFR < 50 mL/min/1.73 m².

VI. Preventing CKD progression.

A. Hypertension management.
   1. Hypertension is a cause of CKD as well as a complication of CKD (Svetkey & Tyson, 2013).
   2. Blood pressure (BP) goal (James et al., 2014).
      a. The Eighth Joint National Committee (JNC8) recommended the same thresholds for hypertensive adults with diabetes or nondiabetic CKD as for the general population younger than 60 years.
      b. For adults < 60 years, recommended goal < 140/90.
      c. For adults > 60 years, recommended goal < 150/90.

   3. Individualization of BP goals need to be considered depending upon a person's age, presence of cardiovascular or other co-morbidities, and response to treatment.
   4. Use of angiotensin-converting enzyme inhibitor (ACE-I) or angiotensin receptor blocker (ARB) recommended as first-line or add-on treatment to improve kidney outcomes (JNC8).
      a. Use of ACE-I with ARB is not recommended to be used in treatment of hypertension or nephrotic proteinuria.
      b. Noted increased incidence of complications, such as hyperkalemia, with this combination therapy (Inker et al., 2014).
   5. Special considerations.
      a. Older adults.
         (1) Assessment of drug response, side effects of medications, and adverse reactions to medications, such as electrolyte imbalance and postural hypotension.
         (2) Start low and go slow with careful titration of medications.
      b. Children (KDIGO, 2013a, pg. 9).
         (1) Start BP lowering treatment when BP is consistently above the 90th percentile for age, sex, and height.
         (2) BP goal is to get systolic and diastolic readings consistently ≤ the 50% percentile for age, sex, and height.
         (3) Use of ACEI or ARB should be first-line treatment regardless of level of proteinuria.

B. Reduce risk of AKI.
   1. Prompt recognition of sudden decline from baseline GFR may indicate an underlying process that, if identified and treated early, may be reversible, making recovery back to baseline range possible.
   2. Prerenal insults represent more common causes of AKI, which can lead to decreased renal perfusion that reduces GFR.
      a. Hypovolemia.
      b. Acute GI losses, such as vomiting or diarrhea.
      c. Over-diuresis.
      d. Medications that can alter afferent or efferent glomerular arteriolar tone, such as NSAIDS, ACE-I, ARB, tacrolimus, or cyclosporine (Naughton, 2008; Pham & Scarlino, 2013).
      e. Prerenal exacerbations caused by other disease processes such as heart failure, cirrhosis, or infection.
   3. Intrinsic or kidney injury results in direct damage to the kidney.
      a. Renal ischemia or acute tubular necrosis.
      b. Medications with potential for direct interstitial damage can promote inflammatory response in the renal tubular interstitium that can lead to

interstitial fibrosis and tubular atrophy, such as aminoglycosides or radiocontrast dyes. Drugs that can cause hypersensitivity reactions, such as sulfa or beta lactams, may lead to inflammation and damage to the interstitium (Naughton, 2008; Pham & Scarlino, 2013).

4. Suspect postrenal problems such as urinary tract obstruction in a person with worsening kidney function of unknown cause (Klahr, 1983).
   a. Urinary tract obstruction can be insidious, especially with a slow-developing obstruction as there are usually no symptoms and no changes in urinary output or urinalysis. Prostate hypertrophy and to a lesser extent metastatic cancers are most common causes. A kidney ultrasound should be ordered to rule out.
   b. Certain drugs may cause postrenal obstruction either by their anticholinergic effects, such as diphenhydramine, or by production of crystals which block the tubules or urinary tract, such as acyclovir (Naugton, 2008; Pham & Scarlino, 2013).

5. KDIGO clinical guidelines for AKI (2012a) assist the provider with developing strategies for prompt assessment and management of AKI.
   a. Start action during illness or procedures that can increase risk of AKI.
      (1) Risk Assessment.
      (2) Identification of exposures that may lead to kidney damage.
   b. Kidney sparing activities to reduce risk.
      (1) Temporarily withhold potentially nephrotoxic agents, such as ACEI or ARB, diuretics, lithium, digoxin, and metformin (Vrtis, 2013).
      (2) Maintain hydration and perfusion pressures.
      (3) Avoid hyperglycemia.
      (4) Monitor serum creatinine and urine output.
      (5) Consult with AKI specialist.
   c. Ensure follow-up with nephrology provider after the AKI event.

C. Diabetes control (KDIGO, 2013, pg. 10).
   1. Target hemoglobin A1C of 7.0% is recommended.
   2. Higher hemoglobin A1C targets are acceptable in those individuals who are at risk for hypoglycemia, have multiple comorbidities, and/or have limited life expectancy.
   3. Multiple interventions in management of diabetic complications should be a part of treatment plan, such as hypertension control, reducing cardiovascular risk factors, lipid control, use of ACEI or ARB, and ongoing foot care.

D. Dietary recommendations (KDIGO, 2013, pg. 10).
   1. Protein intake 0.8 g/kg/day.
      a. Adults with diabetes.
      b. Adults without diabetes but GFR < 30 mL/min/173 m².
      c. Avoid high protein intake > 1.3 g/kg/day.
   2. Salt intake.
      a. Adults < 2 g/day.
      b. Children with hypertension or prehypertension should restrict sodium intake based upon the age-based recommended daily intake.
   3. Dietitian referral for education on kidney diet as indicated.
   4. Lifestyle management (KDIGO, 2013).
      a. Achieve and maintain healthy body weight, ideally BMI 20 to 25.
      b. Physical activity, goal at least 30 minutes 3 times per week.
      c. Stop smoking.

E. Medication management.
   1. Determination of drug dosing should be considered when GFR falls < 50 mL/min/1.73 m².
   2. Nephrotoxic drugs (Campoy & Elwell, 2005) (see Table 2.4).
      a. Administration of nephrotoxic drugs may precipitate a sudden decline in kidney function; should be avoided or used with caution if no other option is possible.
         (1) Aminoglycosides, nonsteroidal anti-inflammatory drugs (NSAIDs), and IV radiocontrast dye are most commonly seen offenders.
         (2) If the drug must be used, careful monitoring of kidney function should be done during and after the therapy as well as during dose titration.
   3. Over the counter (OTC) and herbal drugs.
      a. Seek advice of kidney provider or pharmacist before using any OTC product.
      b. Herbals should be avoided in CKD (refer to Table 2.3).
         (1) Lack of safety and efficacy data on many herbals and natural medicines.
         (2) Potential drug-drug interactions or direct kidney toxicity if used.
   4. Radiocontrast dyes (KDIGO, 2013, pg. 12).
      a. Avoid high osmolar agents.
      b. Lowest possible dose.
      c. Hold potentially nephrotoxic drugs, usually before and after the procedure. Typically, these medications are ACE-I, ARB, or diuretics.
      d. IV hydration with normal saline before, during, and after the procedure.
      e. Measure GFR at least 2 to 4 days after the procedure.
   5. Avoid use of oral phosphate bowel preparations when eGFR < 60 mL/min to prevent potential phosphate nephropathy.

VII. Other complications of CKD stages 1 through 3.

A. Cardiovascular (CV) disease.
   1. Disease burden in CKD.
      a. Persons with CKD are at greater risk for CV.
      b. CKD patients are more likely to die than to progress to ESRD (Go et al., 2004).
      c. Most common cause of death in CKD is due to CV events.
      d. Presence of albuminuria denotes greater CV risk.
   2. Aggressive management of traditional CV risk factors should be incorporated in the early CKD stages.
   3. Level of care and usual approaches to care for heart disease or peripheral vascular disease for the person with CKD should be the same as for those in the general population (KDIGO, 2013b).
   4. Monitor for potential side effects of drugs as CKD progresses.
      a. May need to adjust medication doses or change to less nephrotoxic medication as GFR declines.
      b. Assessment of electrolyte disorders.
   5. Lipid management (KDIGO, 2013b).
      a. Development of hyperlipidemia seen in CKD can be result of GFR, severity of proteinuria, diabetes, use of immunosuppressive drugs for transplant, nutritional status, and other co-morbidities.
      b. KDIGO lipid guidelines (2013) recommend baseline evaluation of lipid panel at initiation of CKD assessment.
         (1) Ongoing measurements are not required unless knowledge of result would change management.
         (2) LDL-c does not reliably identify those at low vs. high risk of cardiovascular events and is no longer recommended as a tool to start treatment or follow treatment progress.
            (a) Lack of direct data to support use of LDL-c in persons with CKD.
            (b) Wide variability in LDL-c measurement.
            (c) Potential for medication-related toxicity.
      c. Management of hyperlipidemia when done early in CKD may provide benefit for those at increased risks for coronary events.
         (1) High cardiovascular risk and not elevated LDL-c should be primary indicator to start or adjust lipid-lowering therapy in persons with CKD.
         (2) Use of the 10-year incidence risk of coronary death or nonfatal MI (event rate per 1000 patient-years) is recommended as the marker for determining treatment.
            (a) Risk tools are available on a variety of websites.
            (b) One resource for calculator is the National Institutes of Health National Heart, Lung and Blood Institute at http://cvdrisk.nhlbi.nih.gov/calculator.asp
      d. KDIGO recommends continued treatment of hyperlipidemia for those persons with GFR < 60 mL/min who have high coronary risk factors such as known coronary artery disease, diabetes, prior myocardial infarction (MI), or ischemic cerebral vascular attack.
         (1) Limited data suggests that lipid control may slow rate of progression in CKD.
         (2) There is no data to support same benefits of lipid control on reducing mortality once a person reaches kidney failure.
      e. Treatment recommendation.
         (1) Statin.
         (2) Statin/ezetimibe combination.
         (3) Lifestyle modifications for triglyceride lowering therapy.

B. Anemia.
   1. Cause of anemia in CKD is due to decreased erythropoietin production by diseased kidneys and shortened red blood cell life span seen in uremia.
   2. Anemia becomes more prevalent when eGFR falls < 60 mL/min/1.73 m².
   3. It is typically normocytic and normochromic.
   4. Starting in CKD stage 3a, KDIGO (2013a, pg. 10) recommends checking hemoglobin (Hgb) when it is clinically indicated (< 13 g/dL in males and < 12 g/dL in females) or at least yearly.
      a. CBC with differential and platelets.
      b. Iron panel consisting of ferritin, iron and total iron binding capacity, and transferrin saturation percentage.
      c. Absolute reticulocyte count, as indicated.
      d. If MCV elevated, vitamin B12 and folate levels.
      e. If iron deficiency, stool for occult blood to rule out GI bleeding.
   5. Goals for anemia in CKD are recommended in KDIGO anemia guidelines (KDIGO, 2012b).
      a. Hemoglobin 10 to 11.5 g/dL in adults; 11 to 12 g/dL in children.
      b. Transferrin saturation > 20%.
      c. Ferritin > 100 ng/mL to ≤ 500 ng/mL.
   6. Treatment for anemia.
      a. Iron replacement if iron deficient.
      b. Folate or vitamin B12 replacement if deficient.
      c. Erythropoiesis stimulating agent (ESA).
         (1) Consider use when Hgb < 9 g/dL.
            (a) All other causes of anemia have been ruled out.

(b) Individualize dose based on rate of Hgb decline and other patient-specific factors.

(c) Use lowest dose to reduce the need for blood transfusion.

(d) Increased risks noted with normalization of Hgb, which should be avoided.

(e) Requires frequent lab monitoring and dose adjustments, as indicated.

(2) Avoid use with uncontrolled hypertension, active malignancy, history of malignancy, or history of CVA.

C. Metabolic bone disease (MBD).
1. Abnormalities of calcium (Ca), phosphorus (PO_4) and parathyroid hormone (PTH) levels may be detected as early as CKD stage 3b when GFR falls < 45 mL/min/1.73 m² (KDIGO, 2013a) and will progress in prevalence and severity as GFR declines.
   a. Hyperphosphatemia starts early due to inability of kidney to efficiently excrete phosphate load (Evenepoel et al., 2010; Juppner, 2011).
   (1) This leads to increased fibroblast growth factor-23 (FGF-23) secretion from the bone.
   (2) FGF-23 levels act on the kidney to inhibit phosphate resorption and suppress 1,25 $(OH)_2$ vitamin D levels which lead to increased PTH levels.
   (3) FGF-23 is effective in the early CKD stages to maintain normal phosphorus levels. However, responsiveness to FGF-23 declines in the later CKD stages as functional kidney mass declines. Then higher FGF-23 levels may lead to other complications, such as left ventricular hypertrophy, faster CKD progression, and premature mortality.
   b. Hypersecretion of PTH initially can correct both hypocalcemia and hyperphosphatemia, in the early CKD stages, so serum levels

Table 2.4

Drugs Associated with Nephrotoxicity

Drug class/drug(s)	Pathophysiologic mechanism of renal injury
Analgesics	
Acetaminophen	Chronic interstitial nephritis
Nonsteroidal antiinflammatory drugs	Acute interstitial nephritis, altered intraglomerular hemodynamics, chronic interstitial nephritis, glomerulonephritis
Antidepressants/mood stabilizers	
Amitriptyline (Elavil*), doxepin (Zonalon®), fluoxetine (Prozac®)	Rhabdomyolysis
Lithium	Chronic interstitial nephritis, Glomerulonephritis, rhabdomyolysis
Antihistamines	
Diphenhydramines (Benadryl®), doxylamine (Unisom®)	Rhabdomyloysis
Antimicrobials	
Acyclovir (Zovirax®)	Acute interstitial nephritis, crystal nephropathy
Aminoglycosides	Tubular cell toxicity
Amphotericin B (Fungizone* deoxycholic acid formulation more so than the lipid formulation)	Tubular cell toxicity
Beta lactams (penicillins, cephalosporins)	Acute interstitial nephritis, glomerulo-nephritis (ampicillin, penicillin)
Foscarnet (Foscavir®)	Crystal nephropathy, tubular cell toxicity
Ganciclovir (Cytovene®)	Crystal nephropathy
Pentamidine (Pentam®)	Tubular cell toxicity
Quinolones	Acute interstitial nephritis, crystal nephropathy (Ciprofloxacin [Cipro®])
Rifampin	Acute interstitial nephritis
Sulfonamides	Acute interstitial nephropathy, crystal nephropathy
Vancomycin (Vancocin®)	Acute interstitial nephritis
Antiretrovirals	
Adefovir (Hepsera®), cidofovir (Vistide®), tenofovir (Viread®)	Tubular cell toxicity
Indinavir (Crixivan®)	Acute interstitial nephritis, crystal nephropathy
Benzodiazepines	Rhabdomyolysis
Calcineurin inhibitors	
Cyclosporine (Neoral®)	Altered intraglomerular hemodynamics, chronic interstitial nephritis, thrombotic microangiopathy
Tacrolimus (Prograf®)	Altered intraglomerular hemodynamics

Continues on next page

of Ca and PO$_4$ may remain within normal limits often through CKD stage 3b.
  c. This over-secretion of PTH is an early sign of osteitis fibrosis, a type of bone disease caused by secondary hyperparathyroidism (Rivera & Smith, 2013).
2. Early prevention strategies in CKD stage 3.
  a. Obtain baseline status by monitoring serum Ca, PO4, alkaline phosphatase, and PTH levels at least once when GFR < 45 mL/min/1.73 m² (KDIGO, 2013a).
  b. Dietary phosphate restriction to maintain PO$_4$ levels within normal limits (Kalantar-Zadeh et al., 2010).
    (1) Organic phosphorus from dietary protein is less absorbable in the GI tract. Dairy products are a major source of dietary phosphorus.
    (2) Inorganic phosphorus seen in food additives. However, is almost 100% absorbable.
  c. If diet ineffective, add phosphate binders taken with meals to block dietary phosphorus absorption.
  d. Use of vitamin D analog usually is not given in CKD stage 3 but may be considered if PTH is progressively rising despite implementation of above interventions.
  e. Only use vitamin D supplements only if there is evidence of 25 hydroxy vitamin D deficiency.

D. Metabolic acidosis (KDIGO, 2013).
  1. Recommended serum bicarbonate concentration > 22 mmol/l.
  2. The use of oral bicarbonate supplements to maintain serum bicarbonate levels is also recommended unless there are contraindications for its use.
  3. Generally, metabolic acidosis is more prevalent in CKD stages 4 and 5.

E. Infection risk.
  1. Persons with CKD have altered immune system, making them more susceptible to infection.

| **Table 2.4** | *Continued from previous page* |

Drugs Associated with Nephrotoxicity

Cardiovascular agents	
Angiotensin-converting enzyme inhibitors, angiotensin receptor blockers	Altered intraglomerular hemodynamics
Clopidogrel (Plavix®), ticlopidine (Ticlid®)	Thrombotic microangiopathy
Statins	Rhabdomyolysis
Chemotherapeutics	
Carmustine (Gliadel®), semustine (investigational)	Chronic interstitial nephritis
Cisplatin (Platinol®)	Chronic interstitial nephritis, tubular cell toxicity
Interferon-alfa (Intron® A)	Glomerulonephritis
Methotrexate	Crystal nephropathy
Mitomycin-C (Mutamycin®)	Thrombotic microangiopathy
Contrast dye	Tubular cell toxicity
Diuretics	
Loops, thiazides	Acute interstitial nephritis
Triamterene (Dyrenium®)	Crystal nephropathy
Drugs of abuse	
Cocaine, heroin, ketamine (Ketalar®), methadone, methamphetamine	Rhabdomyolysis
Herbals	
Chinese herbals with aristocholic acid	Chronic interstitial nephritis
Proton pump inhibitors	
Lansoprazole (Prevacid®), omeprazole (Prilosec®), pantoprazole (Protonix®)	Acute interstitial nephritis
Others	
Allopurinol (Zyloprim®)	Acute interstitial nephritis
Gold therapy	Glomerulonephritis
Haloperidol (Haldol®)	Rhabdomyolysis
Pamidronate (Aredia®)	Glomerulonephritis
Phenytoin (Dilantin®)	Acute interstitial nephritis
Quinine (Qualaquin®)	Thrombotic microangiopathy
Ranitidine (Zantac®)	Acute interstitial nephritis
Zoledronic acid (Zometa®)	Tubular cell toxicity

*Brand not available in the United States

Used with permission from American Academy of Family Physicians. From article by Naughton, C.A. (2008). Drug induced nephropathy. *American Family Physician, 78*(6), 743-775.

2. There is an increased risk of infection-related hospitalizations and mortality associated with CKD (Fried et al., 2005).
3. Persons with CKD in the early stages may have a greater risk of pulmonary and genitourinary infections (Dalrymple, 2012).
4. KDIGO (2013a) recommends immunizations in persons with CKD.
  a. Annual influenza.
  b. Pneumococcal vaccine.

c. Hepatitis B when eGFR < 30 mL/min/1.73 m².
d. Pediatrics as recommended by CDC guidelines for children.

SECTION B
APRN Role in Chronic Kidney Disease Stages 4 and 5, Not on Dialysis
Andrea Easom

I. Evidence-based practice.

Both American Kidney Disease Outcomes Quality Initiative (KDOQI) and International Kidney Disease Improving Global Outcomes (KDIGO) guidelines outlining evidence-based practice for many aspects of CKD are available to guide clinical decisions.

The initial National Kidney Foundation (NKF) KDOQI guidelines, published in 1997, focused on dialysis and later progressed to provide evidence-based clinical practice guidelines for all stages of CKD. In 2003, KDIGO was established as an independent nonprofit foundation governed by an international board and managed by the NKF. All of the guidelines, with their dates of publication, are listed to provide both an up-to-date and historical review of each topic.

A. KDOQI (Kidney Disease Outcomes Quality Initiative). Initially published in the *American Journal of Kidney Disease* (AJKD) and available at http://www.kidney.org/professionals/KDOQI/ guidelines at no cost. Guidelines are graded as evidence-based or opinion and followed by discussion.
1. Update of Diabetes and CKD (2012).
2. Diabetes and CKD (2007).
3. Anemia in CKD (2006).
4. Anemia in CKD: Update of Hemoglobin Target (2007).
5. CKD: Evaluation, Classification & Stratification (2000).
6. Bone Metabolism and Disease in CKD (2003).
7. Bone Metabolism and Disease in Children with CKD (2005).
8. Hypertension and Antihypertensive Agents in CKD (2004).
9. Managing Dyslipidemia in CKD (2002).
10. Nutrition in Children with CKD (2008).
11. Nutrition in CKD (2000).
12. Clinical Practice Guidelines: Hemodialysis, Peritoneal Dialysis, Vascular Access, Anemia, and Nutrition (1997).
13. Updates: Hemodialysis, Peritoneal Dialysis, and Vascular Access (2006).
14. Cardiovascular Disease in Dialysis (2005).

B. KDIGO (Kidney Disease Improving Global Outcomes). All but one of the KDIGO guidelines were published in Kidney International. The Care of the Kidney Transplant Recipient was published in the American Journal of Transplantation. All are available at http://www.kdigo.org/home/guidelines at no cost. If the level of evidence is strong, the guideline is worded, "we recommend…." If the evidence is weak or discretionary, it is worded, "we suggest." Some are "not graded." All are followed by discussion. See Tables 2.5 and 2.6 for how the group grades and reports the strength of the evidence for their guidelines.
1. Hepatitis C in CKD (2008).
2. Care of the Transplant Recipient (2009).
3. Mineral and Bone Disorder (2009).
4. Anemia in CKD (2012).
5. Acute Kidney Injury (2012).
6. Glomerulonephritis (2012).
7. Blood Pressure in CKD (2012).
8. CKD Evaluation & Management (2013).
9. Lipid Management in CKD (2013).

II. Staging, definition, and prevalence.

A. CKD Staging (KDIGO: CKD, 2013).
1. Based on cause, GFR category, and albuminuria level (1B).
2. Evaluate duration of disease. CKD is confirmed if duration is > 3 months (not graded).
3. Use serum creatinine and a GFR estimating equation for initial assessment (1A).

B. Stage 4.
1. Severely decreased glomerular filtration rate (GFR), range 29 to 15 mL/min.
2. First stage of very high risk over all ranges of albuminuria range (refer to Table 2.1 in Section A).
3. Estimate 10% of the US adult population has CKD, more than 20 million people (CDC, 2013).
   a. Figure 2.1 shows the prevalence of CKD by stage (USRDS, 2014).
   b. Major cause of death thought to be due to cardiovascular deaths.
4. Monitor progression of CKD 3 times a year unless albuminuria over 300 mg/g and then monitor 4 times a year (not graded) (KDIGO: CKD, 2013).

C. Stage 5 ND (Not on dialysis).
1. Kidney failure, estimated glomerular filtration rate (eGFR) less than 15 mL/min.
2. Monitor progression 4 times a year (not graded) (KDIGO: CKD, 2013).
3. Estimated 2.4% of the U.S. population has CKD stage 5. At the end of 2011, there were 602,000 Americans on dialysis, who would be included in stage 5. The U.S. population at the same time was 311.6 million.

Table 2.5

Final Grade for Overall Quality of Evidence

Grade	Quality of Evidence	Meaning
A	High	We are confident that the true effect lies close to that of the estimate of the effect.
B	Moderate	The true effect is likely to be close to the estimate of the effect, but there is a possibility that it is substantially different.
C	Low	The true effect may be substantially different from the estimate of the effect.
D	Very Low	The estimate of effect is very uncertain, and often will be far from the truth.

A level 1 grade implies that a recommendation should be followed on the basis of the assumption that a well informed consumer would almost always want to pursue the recommended course of action. By contrast, many patients may want to pursue a level 2 recommendation but a substantial number of patients may not. This means that the risks and benefits must be weighed in each specific situation, taking into account the patient's preferences and values. Level 1 recommendations can be examined to determine their suitability for use in developing a clinical performance measure. On the other hand, a level 2 grade inherently indicates uncertainty, and future research may provide higher quality evidence or more precise estimates or yield opposing findings.

Table 2.6

KDIGO Nomenclature and Description for Grading Recommendations

Grade*	Implications		
	Patients	**Clinicians**	**Policy**
Level 1 "We recommend"	Most people in your situation would want the recommended course of action and only a small proportion would not.	Most patients should receive the recommended course of action.	The recommendation can be evaluated as a candidate for developing a policy or a performance measure.
Level 2 "We suggest"	The majority of people in your situation would want the recommended course of action, but many would not.	Different choices will be appropriate for different patients. Each patient needs help to arrive at a management decision consistent with her or his values and preferences.	The recommendation is likely to require substantial debate and involvement of stakeholders before policy can be determined.

Tables 2.5 and 2.6 are used with permission from Kidney Disease: Improving Global Outcomes (KDIGO) Blood Pressure Work Group. (2012). KDIGO clinical practice guideline for the management of blood pressure in chronic kidney disease. *Kidney International, Supplements, 2*(5), 337–414.

III. Prevention and treatment.

A. Continue plan from previous stages CKD. The healthcare provider may need to make further reductions or changes of medications per recommended renal dosing. Metabolic and pathologic comorbidities by stage of CKD can be seen in Figure 2.2.

B. Estimate progression.
   1. Teach "Know your number."
      a. Provide eGFR as the key measure of kidney function.
         (1) Based on a percentage (0 to 100%).
         (2) Dialysis generally, but not always, needed when function decreases to 10% and patient has symptoms of uremia.
         (3) Provide a handout or flowchart for tracking labs.
      b. Estimate time to dialysis using Kidney Failure Risk Calculator.
         (1) Available on QxMD (free medical app).
         (2) Developed & validated in Canada (Tangri, et. al., 2011).
         (3) Variables: age, sex, GFR, urine albumin: creatinine ratio, calcium, phosphorus, albumin, and bicarbonate.
         (4) Risk of progression to kidney failure requiring dialysis or transplantation given in a percentage at 2 years and 5 years with

an explanation. Example: For patients in stage 4, a 2-year risk factor of 0% to10% is low risk, 10 to 20% is intermediate risk, and > 20% is high risk.

2. Use rate and risk of progression as a guide for response to therapy and preparation for kidney replacement therapy education.

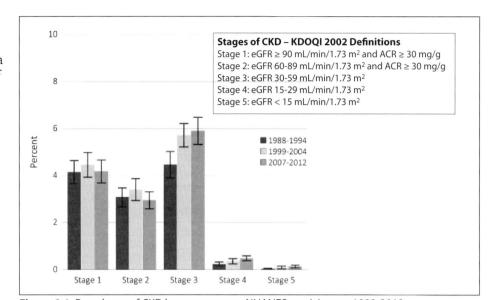

Figure 2.1. Prevalence of CKD by stage among NHANES participants, 1988-2012.

Data source: National Health and Nutrition Examination Survey (NHANES), 1988–1994, 1999–2004, and 2005–2012 participants age 20 and older. Whisker lines indicate 95% confidence intervals. *Abbreviations*: CKD = chronic kidney disease. *Figure source*: CKD in the United States: An Overview of USRDS Annual Data Report, Volume 1, 2014, Slide, Figure i.1.

C. Predictors of progression (KDIGO: CKD, 2013).
  1. Cause of CKD.
  2. Level of GFR.
    a. Small fluctuations in eGFR are common and may not indicate progression (not graded).
    b. Progression is based on the following.
      (1) A drop in eGFR category accompanied by a 25% drop in GFR from baseline (not graded).
      (2) Sustained decline of eGFR of more than 5 mL/min/1.73 m²/year (not graded).
  3. Level of albuminuria/proteinuria (see section IV).
  4. Other variables that predict risk (not graded).
    a. Nonmodifiable.
      (1) Age.
      (2) Sex.
      (3) Race/ethnicity.
      (4) History of cardiovascular disease.
    b. Modifiable.
      (1) Level of blood pressure (see section V).
      (2) Hyperglycemia (see Section VI).
      (3) Dyslipidemia (see Section VII).
      (4) Smoking (see Section XIII).
      (5) Obesity (see Section XI).
      (6) Ongoing exposure to nephrotoxic agents (see Section XIII).

D. Proteinuria/albuminuria (KDIGO: CKD, 2013).
  1. May develop as kidney function declines; if preexisting, needs continued monitoring by the following.
    a. Urine albumin: creatinine (Cr) ratio (ACR).
    b. Urine protein: Cr ratio.
    c. 24-hour urine collection.
    d. Serum albumin.
      (1) Increased risk for hypoalbuminemia and malnutrition as declines.

      (2) Increased risk of thrombotic events if serum albumin falls to less than or equal to 2.5g/dL.
  2. The greater the amount of proteinuria, the more rapid progression of kidney loss.
  3. Continue or start treatment with an angiotensin-converting enzyme inhibitor (ACE-I) and/or an angiotensin receptor blocker (ARB).
    a. Recommended for both diabetic and nondiabetic adults with CKD and urine albumin excretion > 300 mg/24 hours (1B).
    b. Can reduce proteinuria by 40–50%.
    c. Monitor for hyperkalemia; if uncontrollable, discontinue ACE-I and/or ARB.
    d. Monitor for elevated serum creatinine (Scr); if greater than 30% increase from baseline, discontinue ACE-I and/or ARB.
    e. Monitor for cough; if present, discontinue ACE-I and start an ARB (accumulation of bradykinin).
    f. There is insufficient evidence to recommend combining an ACE-I with ARB to prevent progression of CKD (not graded).
  4. Diet.
    a. Maintain patient on salt restriction (2 grams/day) (1C).
    b. Cautious use of low protein diet as it increases risk of malnutrition. In CKD stages 4 and 5: 0.8 grams/kg/day (2B).
    c. Avoid high protein intake (> 1.3 grams/kg/day) in adults with CKD risk of progression (2C).

E. Medical nephrectomy (KDIGO: CKD, 2013).
   1. Only in cases of severe proteinuria (generally in children).
   2. Patient at risk of dying from the protein malnutrition.

F. Hypertension (KDIGO: Blood Pressure, 2012).
   1. Individualize BP targets & agents according to (not graded).
      a. Age.
      b. Coexisting cardiovascular disease & other comorbidities.
      c. Risk of CKD progression.
      d. Presence or absence or retinopathy (in CKD patients with diabetes).
      e. Tolerance of treatment.
         (1) Risk and benefit of increasing medications versus episodes of postural hypotension.
         (2) Side effect profile of agent.
   2. Encourage lifestyle modification to lower BP and improve long-term cardiovascular and other outcomes.
      a. Maintain healthy weight (BMI 20-25) (1D).
         (1) Use caution when recommending weight loss in late stages of CKD.
         (2) Malnutrition may be linked to poorer outcomes.
         (3) Higher weights have been shown to be protective in some patients with stage 5 CKD.
      b. Lower salt intake to < 2 grams daily of sodium, unless contraindicated.
      c. Exercise 30 minutes 5 times per week (1D).
      d. Limit alcohol to no more than two standard drinks per day for men and one for women (standard drink size varies by country) (2D).
         (1) Alcohol has shown to produce both acute and chronic increases in BP.
         (2) Restricting alcohol resulted in a 3.8 mmHg reduction in systolic and 3.2 mmHg diastolic BP in a review of 4 trials.
   3. Inquire about symptoms of and assess for postural hypotension regularly (not graded).
      a. Gradual escalation of treatment and close attention to adverse events due to BP treatment, especially in older adults.
      b. Balance risk and benefit. May need to tolerate a slightly higher BP to decrease risk.
   4. Recommend treating with BP-lowering drugs those whose office BP is consistently > 140 mmHg or diastolic > 90 mmHg, have CKD, and urine albumin excretion is < 30 mg/24 hours (1B).
   5. When urine albumin excretion exceeds 30 mg/24 hours and BP is consistently over 130/80 (respectively), BP lowering drugs should be started (2D).
   6. ARB or ACE-I should be used in patients with CKD and albuminuria (diabetics 30 to 300 mg/24

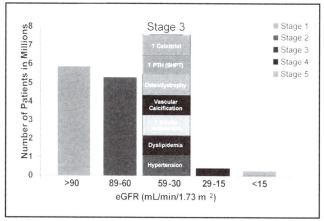

Figure 2.2. Metabolic and pathologic comorbidities as they begin to apear in CKD stage 3.

(Andress, 2005; Becker et al., 2005; Elder, 2002; Kramer et al., 2005). Used with permission from AbbVie, North Chicago, IL.

hours(2D) and nondiabetic adults > 300 mg/24 hours(1B).
   7. Adult kidney transplant recipients should be treated to have a BP consistently > 130/80 regardless of level of albuminuria (2D).
   8. Average number of antihypertensives required to meet goal is three or more of different classes.
   9. Except for using ACE-I or ARBS for patients with high levels of urinary albumin or protein excretion, there is not strong evidence to guide preferential use of a particular class of antihypertensive.
   10. Tailor therapy to the individual patient.
      a. Absence or presence of high urine albumin excretion.
      b. Comorbidities. (See Table 2.7, which lists the preferred antihypertensive agents for CVD).
      c. Concomitant medications/drug interactions.
      d. Adverse side effects and allergies.
      e. Availability of the medication (including cost).
      f. Drug half-life especially in CKD stages 4 and 5.
      g. Dose or interval adjustments may be needed in CKD stages 4 and 5.
   11. Actual reduction in BP achieved is more important than the agent used.
   12. Consider evening dosing.
      a. CKD patients who do not have the usual decrease in BP during sleep have worse cardiovascular and kidney outcomes compared to those that do.
      b. Research is being done, but has not yet proven, if evening dosing to produce blood pressure dipping will improve CKD outcomes.
   13. Consider home BP monitoring.
      a. Though automated ambulatory BP (ABMP) monitoring is the "gold standard," self-BP measurements using automated devices provide readings more in line with ABMP than office measurements.

Table 2.7

Preferred Antihypertensive Agents for CVD

Types of CVD	Thiazide or Loop Diuretics	ACE Inhibitors or ARBs	Beta-Blockers	Calcium-Channel Blockers	Aldosterone Antagonists
Heart Failure with Systolic Dysfunction	X	X	Xª		X
Post MI with Systolic Dysfunction		X	X		X
Post MI			X		
Chronic Stable Angina			X	X	
High-Risk for Coronary Artery Disease	X	X	X	X	
Recurrent Stroke Prevention	X	X			
Supraventricular Tachycardias			X	Xᵇ	

ªOnly some beta-blockers (carvedilol, bisoprolol, metaprolol succinate).
ᵇNondihydropyridine calcium-channel blockers.

Used with permission from National Kidney Foundation (2002). K/DOQI Clinical Practice Guidelines on Hypertension and Antihypertensive Agents in Chronic Kidney Disease, Guideline 7: Pharmacological therapy: use of antihypertensive agents in CKD, Originally Table 86.

  b. Office BP measurements.
    (1) Overestimate BP in white-coat hypertension.
    (2) Underestimate BP in masked hypertension.
  c. Self-BP measurements can have inaccuracies in patients with the following.
    (1) Atrial fibrillation.
    (2) Very high pulse pressures.
  d. Recalibrate home equipment against traditional equipment.
14. Antihypertensive agents.
  a. Agents that inhibit the renin-angiotensin-aldosterone system (RAAS) include the following.
    (1) ACE-I and ARBs.
      (a) Protect the kidney by relaxing (vasodilating) of the efferent arteriole of the nephron, hence decreasing intraglomerular pressure and decreasing proteinuria.
      (b) Inhibit fibrosis and enhance vascular and cardiac remodeling.
      (c) Drug of choice for congestive heart failure, for use soon after myocardial infarction (MI) and stroke, and for patients with high cardiovascular risk.
      (d) Considerations for use.
        i. Monitor for hyperkalemia.
        ii. Monitor for increasing serum creatinine (decreasing eGFR). Expect a small (< 30%) change when starting an ACE-I or ARB (from the drop in intraglomerular pressure). This is a hemodynamic effect and is reversible with drug discontinuation (shows the drug is working). If the change is larger than 30%, suspect underlying renal artery stenosis and discontinue the drug.
      (e) These agents should not be used during pregnancy. (Most are category D.)
    (2) Aldosterone agonists.
      (a) Includes ACE-I and ARBs (50% patients showed reduction).
      (b) Spironolactone and eplerenone not used in CKD stages 4 or 5.
    (3) Direct renin inhibitors (aliskiren).
      (a) FDA counseled against the combination with ACE-I and ARBS due to increased risks of adverse events.
      (b) See considerations for ACE-I and ARB use above.
  b. Calcium channel blockers.
    (1) Used to treat hypertension, angina, and supraventricular tachycardia.
    (2) Major subclasses.
      (a) Nondihydropyridine (diltiazem and verapamil).

i. Decrease proteinuria.

ii. Use with beta blockers can cause severe bradycardia.

iii. Use increases calcineurin inhibitor and sirolimus levels.

(b) Dihydropyridine (e.g., amlodipine, nifedipine).

i. Cause more vasodilation and less action on myocardium than nondihydropyridines.

ii. Fluid retention, dizziness, headaches, and redness of the face can be problematic.

iii. Nicardipine and nimodipine accumulate with impaired kidney function and should be used with caution in both CKD and the older adult.

c. Beta blockers.

(1) Used widely for hypertension, angina, and heart failure.

(2) Atenolol and bisoprolol can accumulate in advanced CKD causing bradycardia and arrhythmias.

d. Diuretics.

(1) Thiazides and potassium-sparing diuretics are not generally used in CKD stages 4 and 5 ND. The following are exceptions.

(a) Chlorthalidone – avoid with creatinine clearance (CrCl) < 10.

(b) Indapamide – use with caution.

(c) Metolazone – give 30 minutes before loop diuretic if given IV.

(d) Note all have many drug interactions.

(2) Loop diuretics (furosemide, bumetanide, torsemide, and ethacrynic acid).

(3) All used to treat edema and high blood pressure.

e. Direct vasodilators (e.g., hydralazine and minoxidil).

(1) Used for resistant hypertension.

(2) Cause compensatory reactions including tachycardia, edema, flushing, and headaches.

(3) Concomitant use of a beta-blocker and a loop diuretic may reduce these side effects.

(4) Monitor for pericardial effusions with minoxidil use.

(5) Hirsutism may preclude use of minoxidil in women who are unwilling to deal with increased facial hair.

15. Experimental therapies.

a. Catheter-based radiofrequency ablation of renal sympathetic nerves (renal sympathetic denervation) (Papademtriou, 2014).

(1) Lowers BP in patients with resistant hypertension on three or more antihypertensives.

(2) Six devices in use.

(3) Symplicity was one proof-of-concept study in 50 patients.

(4) Initial BP reduction was modest and improved over time (6 months).

(5) Multiple other studies have been done with various devices.

(6) Disparity between office and ambulatory BP monitoring reductions persist in most. Some studies had negative results.

(7) Procedure done in cardiac catheterization laboratory or interventional radiology.

b. Electrical stimulation of carotid sinus baroceptors (Baroreflex activation therapy or BAT) (Bisognano, 2011).

(1) Rheos Pivotal Trial.

(2) 265 patients with resistant hypertension (5 reading 160/80 or above, mean ABPM 135 mmHg despite on three antihypertensives, including a diuretic).

(3) Device implanted in operating suite.

(4) Patients receiving BAT were significantly more likely to achieve a goal systolic pressure of 140 mmHg or lower (42% vs. 24%).

(5) Within 1 month, 35% of the patients had a serious procedure-related adverse event, including nerve damage. Most events resolved spontaneously.

G. Diabetes and insulin resistance (KDIGO: CKD, 2013a).

1. Goal Hhemoglobin A1C 7%, and no lower due to risk of increased episodes of hypoglycemia (1A).

2. May extend target AIC in patients with comorbidities, limited life expectancy, and risk of hypoglycemia (1B).

3. Insulin is excreted by the kidney. As GFR decreases, patients are at increased risk of hypoglycemia.

4. Beta-blockers may mask symptoms of hypoglycemia, also putting patients at increased risk.

5. Note glyburide can cause increased hypoglycemia when GFR is < 50 mL/min due to a buildup of active metabolites and is therefore not recommended for these patients.

6. Note metformin is contraindicated when the creatinine is > 1.5 in males or > 1.4 in females or the CrCl is < 60–70 mL/min, due to the increased risk of lactic acidosis.

7. Increased renal insulin resistance and hyperinsulinemia have been reported in CKD patients who are neither diabetic nor hypertensive.

H. Dyslipidemias (KDIGO: Lipid, 2013b).
   1. Monitor and manage dyslipidemias.
      a. Evaluate lipid profile on newly identified CKD patients (1C).
      b. Follow-up measurements of lipid levels are not required for the majority of patients (not graded).
         (1) Rule out remediable causes of secondary dyslipidemia.
         (2) Determine if treatment is necessary. If yes, select agent and dose.
         (3) Treat by "fire and forget" strategy. Do not repeat LDL-C unless the results would alter management.
      c. Secondary causes include the following.
         (1) Comorbidities such as hypothyroidism, diabetes mellitus, nephrotic syndrome, alcohol excess, and chronic liver disease.
         (2) Medications such as beta-blockers, diuretics, corticosteroids, calcineurin inhibitors, sirolimus, oral contraceptives, anticonvulsants, and antiretroviral therapy.
      d. Treating dyslipidemia.
         (1) Adults age > 50 years treat with a statin or statin/ezetimibe combination (1A).
         (2) Adults ages 18 to 49 suggest treatment with a statin in people with one or more of the following (2A).
            (a) Known coronary disease.
            (b) Diabetes mellitus.
            (c) Prior ischemic stroke.
            (d) Estimated 10-year incidence of coronary death or nonfatal myocardial infarction > 10%.
         (3) Adult kidney transplant recipients should be treated with a statin (2B).
         (4) Adults with hypertriglyceridemia should be advised on therapeutic lifestyle changes (2D).
         (5) 2013 ACC-AHA cardiovascular prevention guidelines drop cholesterol treatment goals and focus on four groups whom moderate (30 to 49% LDL reduction) to high intensity (> 50% LDL reduction) statin therapy is recommended along with an increased focus on CV risk lifestyle modifications. These groups include patients who have the following.
            (a) Clinical atherosclerotic cardiovascular disease (ASCVD).
            (b) A primary elevation of LDL-C of 190 mg/dL or higher.
            (c) Diabetes, ages 40 to 75 years, with no ASCVD and LDL levels of 70 to 189 mg/dL.
            (d) No clinical ASCVD or diabetes, ages 40 to 75, with an LDL of 70 to 189 and an estimated 10-year risk of ASCVD of at least 7.5% (global cardiovascular risk assessment score/see guideline).
            (6) Note some agents such as fluvastatin, simvastatin, and lovastatin recommend dose adjustments when eGFR is < 30 mL/min.

I. Cardiovascular disease (CVD).
   1. Use evidence-based knowledge to educate and motivate patients to adhere to their plan of care.
      a. Decreased GFR is a risk factor for CVD.
      b. CVD is thought to be the leading cause of death in patients with advanced CKD.
      c. Albuminuria is associated with increased risk for CVD.
      d. 2013 ACC/AHA Cardiovascular prevention guidelines (Goff, et.al., 2013).
      e. 2013 ACC/AHA/TOS Guideline for the management of overweight and obesity in adults (Jenson, et.al., 2013).
   2. Lifestyle Modification.
      a. Assessment of cardiovascular risk.
      b. Weight management.
         (1) BMI goal (18.5-25) (1D).
         (2) Waist circumference (< 40 inches).
      c. Regular exercise.
      d. Healthy diet.
   3. Treatment with an agent that inhibits the renin-angiotensin aldosterone system (RAAS) should be considered.
      a. Drugs of choice for treatment of congestive heart failure.
      b. Drugs of choice for treatment of proteinuria.
      c. Preferred agents for slowing GFR decline.
   4. If patient is on digoxin, note that the dose adjustment for CKD begins at a GFR of less than 50.
      a. Reduce dose by 25% to 75% depending on the GFR.
      b. Monitor for digoxin toxicity.

J. Anemia of chronic disease (KDIGO: Anemia, 2012).
   1. CKD anemia management programs.
      a. Excellent initial program for CKD management clinics.
      b. APRN managed.
      c. Model after Dialysis Anemia Management programs.
      d. Protocol driven for both erythropoiesis stimulating agents (ESA) and IV iron titrations done by office staff nurse, when possible.
      e. Outliers reviewed by APRN for further orders.
      f. Medicare and other payor reimbursement generally available.
         (1) Varies by state and payor.
         (2) General Medicare guidelines: Creatinine 2 or above or creatinine clearance (CrCl) less

than 45 mL/min and a hemoglobin less than 10 g/dL with symptoms of anemia. Treat iron deficiency prior to initiating ESA.
2. Anemia of CKD should be normocytic and normochromic. If not, then do the following.
   a. Check for iron deficiency, if found, correct.
      (1) Balance benefit versus risk (not graded).
      (2) Suggest trial of iron (oral or IV) if transferrin saturation (Tsat) is < 30% and ferritin is < 500 ng/mL (2C).
   b. Check for obvious blood losses. If diagnosed, treat or refer as appropriate.
   c. If other, refer to hematology for workup. Obtain vitamin B12, folate levels.
3. Testing for patients with CKD 4 and 5 ND.
   a. Measure hemoglobin (Hb) when clinically indicated and at least twice per year for patients without anemia (not graded).
   b. Measure hemoglobin (Hb) when clinically indicated and at least every 3 months for patients with anemia (not graded).
   c. Diagnose anemia at the following Hb concentrations.
      (1) < 13.5 g/dL in adult males.
      (2) < 12.0 g/dL in adult females.
   d. Anemia frequently diagnosed in stage 3 CKD.
4. Initial assessment includes the following tests (not graded).
   a. Complete blood count.
   b. Absolute reticulocyte count.
   c. Serum ferritin level.
   d. Transferrin saturation (Tsat).
   e. Serum B12 and folate levels.
5. Use of ESAs to treat anemia.
   a. Balance benefit vs. risk of therapy.
   b. Address all correctable causes prior to initiation of ESA (not graded).
   c. Use with great caution in patients with the following.
      (1) Active malignancy, especially when cure is anticipated (1B).
      (2) A history of stroke (1B) or malignancy (2C).
   d. Decide on therapy when Hb is < 10 g/dL based on (2C).
      (1) Rate of fall of Hb concentration.
      (2) Prior response to iron therapy.
      (3) Risk of needing a transfusion.
      (4) Risks related to ESA therapy.
      (5) Presence of anemia-related symptoms.
   e. Individualization of therapy to start ESA when Hb levels at or above 10 g/dL are reasonable for some patients who have improvement of quality of life (QOL) at higher Hb levels (not graded).
   f. Suggest ESAs not be used to maintain Hb levels above 11.5 g/dL (2C).

   g. Individualization will be necessary for some patients that have improvements of QOL at Hb levels above 11.5 g/dL and are willing to accept the risks (not graded).
   h. Recommend that ESAs not be used to intentionally increase Hb levels above 13 g/dL (1A).
   i. Serious adverse events have been seen with Hb > 13 g/dL.
      (1) Cerebrovascular accidents.
      (2) Thrombosis.
      (3) Myocardial infarctions.
      (4) See black box warning in package insert.
6. ESA dosing.
   a. Recommend dosing based on (1D):
      (1) Patient's Hb level.
      (2) Body weight.
      (3) Clinical circumstances.
   b. Recommend ESA dose adjustments be made based on (1B):
      (1) Patient's Hb level.
      (2) Rate of change in Hb level.
      (3) Current ESA dose.
      (4) Clinical circumstances.
   c. Suggest decreasing ESA dose in preference to holding ESA when a decrease in Hb is needed (2C).
   d. Reevaluate ESA dose if (not graded):
      (1) Patient suffers an ESA-related event.
      (2) Patient has an illness that may cause ESA hyporesponsiveness.
   e. Suggest subcutaneous ESA dosing for patients with CKD ND (2C).
   f. Available ESAs.
      (1) Erythropoetin (initial dose: 50 to 100 units/kg up to 3 times a week).
      (2) Darbopoetin (initial dose: 0.45 mcg/kg every 4 weeks).
         (a) Half-life is ~ 3 times as long as epoetin alpha.
         (b) Do not increase dose more frequently than every 4 weeks.
7. ESA hyporesponsiveness.
   a. Initial.
      (1) Defined as no increase in Hb concentration from baseline after first month of appropriate weight-based dosing (not graded).
      (2) Avoid repeated escalation in dose beyond double the weight-based dose (2D).
   b. Subsequent.
      (1) Defined as requirement of two increases in ESA dose up to 50% beyond the dose at which they had been stable to maintain a stable Hb concentration (not graded).
      (2) Avoid repeated escalation in dose beyond double the weight-based dose at which they had been stable (2D).

c. Poor ESA responsiveness.
   (1) Evaluate patients with either initial or acquired hyporesponse for specific cause (not graded).
   (2) In patients who remain hyporesponsive, suggest individualization accounting relative risk and benefits of (2D).
      (a) Decline in Hb level.
      (b) Continuing ESA, if needed to maintain Hb, with due consideration of dose required.
      (c) Blood transfusion.
d. Evaluate for pure red cell aplasia (PRCA) when a patient on ESA therapy for more than 8 weeks develops the following (not graded).
   (1) Sudden rapid decrease in Hb level at a rate of 0.5 to 1.0 g/dL per week or requires a blood transfusion at the rate of 1 to 2 per week AND has normal platelet count and white cell counts, AND absolute reticulocyte count less than 10,000/ul.
   (2) Contact the manufacturer of the ESA that the patient is receiving for details on PRCA collection and processing.
8. Considerations when treating with iron (KDOQI, 2006).
   a. Target transferrin saturation 20% or above. When the total iron binding capacity (TIBC) is less than 200, the Tsat may be falsely elevated, which will not reflect true iron status.
   b. Content of hemoglobin in reticulocytes (CHr) if above 29 denotes sufficient available iron. There is no value that denotes iron overload.
   c. Target ferritin 100 ng/dL or above.
      (1) No upper limit of ferritin is recommended.
      (2) When ferritin is above 500, the patient's clinical status, ESA responsivness, Hb and Tsat levels should be considered.
      (3) When ferritin is above 500 or below 100, the clinical status of the patient should be evaluated.
         (a) History and physical.
         (b) Laboratory workup including: C reactive protein, WBC and CHr (if not routinely done).
         (c) Differentiate between the following (Easom, 2006).
            i. Absolute iron deficiency: Insufficient iron for effective erythropoiesis (low Tsat and ferritin).
            ii. Inflammatory iron blockade: Iron is blocked from leaving the reticular endothelial system (RES) usually from infection or inflammation. (TIBC may be reduced.) Intravenous iron should not be

given during an active infection.
            iii. Functional iron deficiency: Iron is mobilized too slowly from the RES to keep up with the demands of EPO-driven erythropoiesis (TIBC is generally normal to elevated). Intravenous iron will correct.
            iv. Patients with a high ferritin should be evaluated for secondary causes such as infection and inflammatory states, including malignancies, which need to be diagnosed and treated.
            v. A trial of intravenous iron may be helpful in patients without active infection. If hemoglobin does not increase or ESA dose does not decrease after 1 month, then discontinue.
   d. Treat with iron supplementation, as needed.
      (1) Oral iron once or twice a day.
      (2) Intravenous iron may still be necessary to attain and maintain targets.
   e. Monitor iron indices at least every 3 months during ESA therapy, depending on iron status, ESA responsiveness, and the stability of the patient.
9. Adjunctive therapies for ESA treatment (KDIGO: Anemia, 2012).
   a. Recommend not using androgens (1B).
   b. Suggest not using vitamin C, vitamin D, vitamin E, folic acid, L-carnitine, or pentoxifylline (2D).
10. Use of red blood cell (RBC) transfusions to treat anemia in CKD.
   a. Recommend avoiding RBC transfusions whenever possible to avoid risks related to their use (1B).
   b. In patients eligible for organ transplantation, recommend avoiding, when possible, to minimize the risk of allosensitization (1C).
   c. Benefits may outweigh the risks in patients in whom ESA therapy is ineffective and when the risks of ESA therapy outweigh its benefit (2C).
11. Suggest the decision to transfuse nonacute anemia not be based on any arbitrary Hgb threshold, but be determined by anemia-related symptoms (2C).

K. CKD-mineral and bone disease (MBD). Management of MBD has been an area of both great interest and controversy. The grading system was modified to allow guidance even if the evidence was weak. Many areas are not graded, and the lack of evidence that is 1A suggests limited opportunity to develop clinical performance measures from this guideline. Please read the discussion in the guidelines for areas of interest.

1. Definition of CKD-MBD: a systemic disorder of mineral and bone metabolism due to CKD manifested by one or more of the following (KDIGO: Bone, 2009) (see Figure 2.3 showing the consequences of SHPT).
   a. Abnormalities of calcium, phosphorus, PTH, or vitamin D metabolism.
   b. Abnormalities in bone turnover, mineralization, volume, linear growth, or strength.
   c. Vascular or other soft tissue calcification.
2. Definition of renal osteodystrophy.
   a. An alteration of bone morphology in patients with CKD.
   b. A measure of a skeletal component of the systemic disorder of CKD-MBD that is quantifiable by histomorphometry of bone biopsy.
3. Common disturbances in mineral and bone metabolism in CKD.
   a. Secondary hyperparathyroidism (SHPT).
   b. Hypocalcemia.
   c. Hyperphosphatemia.
   d. Altered vitamin D metabolism.
   e. Defective intestinal absorption of calcium.
   f. Renal osteodystrophy.
   g. Soft tissue calcifications including vascular calcifications.
   h. Altered handling of phosphate, calcium, and magnesium by the kidney.
   i. Proximal myopathy.
   j. Skin ulcerations and soft-tissue necrosis.
4. CKD-MBD management programs.
   a. Excellent addition for CKD management clinics.
   b. APRN managed.
   c. Model after Dialysis MBD Management programs.
   d. Protocol driven for both vitamin D and binder, titrations done by office staff nurse or kidney dietitian, when possible, with APRN support and guidance.
   e. All protocol outliers reviewed by APRN for further orders.
5. Secondary hyperparathyroidism (SHPT)/CKD-MBD.
   a. As GFR decreases, 1,25-dihydroxycholecalciferol production decreases, serum calcium decreases, and phosphate retention develops, resulting in secondary hyperplasia of the parathyroid glands and increased production of parathyroid hormone. The prevalence of an elevated iPTH by eGFR intervals is shown in Figure 2.4.
   b. A decrease in the number of vitamin D receptors (VDR) develops, and they become

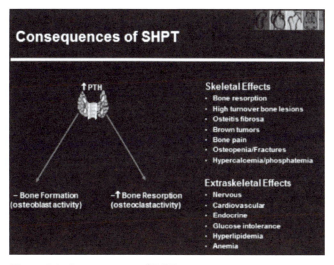

Figure 2.3. Consequences of SHPT

Used with permission from AbbVie, North Chicago, IL.

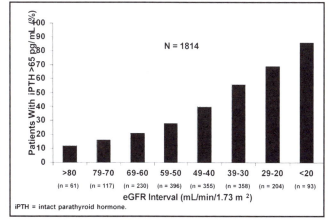

Figure 2.4. Prevalence of elevated iPTH by eGFR intervals.

Used with permission from AbbVie, North Chicago, IL.

   more resistant to the action of vitamin D and calcium.
   c. Progressive parathyroid gland hyperplasia and nodularity are associated with declining levels of vitamin D.
   d. Start screening for SPTH/CKD-MBD in CKD Stage 3 (1C) and continue in later stages. Do not wait for the change in Ca and P. These changes occur later. (See Figure 2.5, which addresses the prevalence of abnormal corrected Ca and P levels.)
   e. Base frequency of monitoring (calcium, phosphorus, and PTH) on presence and abnormalities and the rate of progression of CKD (not graded). Reasonable monitoring intervals are as follows.
      (1) CKD stage 4: calcium and phosphorus every 3–6 months and PTH every 6 to 12 months.

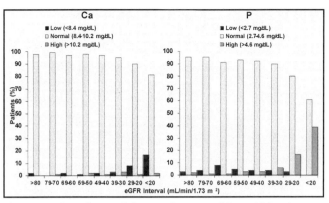

Figure 2.5. Prevalence of abnormal corrected Ca and P levels.

Used with permission from AbbVie, North Chicago, IL.

(2) CKD stage 5: calcium and phosphorus every 1–3 months and PTH every 3 to 6 months.

(3) CKD stages 4–5: alkaline phosphatase every 12 months, or more frequently if PTH is elevated.

f. Measure 25(OH)D levels (2C) and correct vitamin D deficiency and insufficiency using treatment strategies recommended for the general population (2C).

g. Base therapeutic decisions on trends rather than a single laboratory value, taking into account all available CKD-MBD assessments (1C).

6. Diagnosis of CKD-MBD: bone.

a. Reasonable to perform bone biopsy for the following: unexplained fracture, persistent bone pain, unexplained hypercalcemia, unexplained hypophosphatemia, possible aluminum toxicity, and prior to therapy with bisphosphonates in patients with CKD-MBD (not graded).

b. Bone mineral density testing is not routinely recommended since it does not predict fracture risk or type of renal osteodystrophy (2B).

c. Measurement of PTH or bone-specific alkaline phosphatase can be used to evaluate bone disease; markedly high or low levels predict underlying bone turnover (2B).

7. Diagnosis of CKD-MBD: vascular calcification.

a. Lateral abdominal radiograph can be used to predict presence or absence of vascular calcification (see x-ray) (2C).

b. An echocardiogram can be used to detect presence or absence of valvular calcification (reasonable alternative to CT-based imaging) (2C).

c. Suggest CKD patients 3-5D with known vascular or valvular calcifications be considered at highest cardiovascular risk (2A).

d. It is reasonable to use this information to guide management of CKD-MBD (not graded).

e. Vascular calcifications. See Figure 2.6 that focuses on vascular calcification and CKD.

(1) Medial calcification.

(a) Common CKD-related calcification caused from calcium and phosphorus buildup in the medial layer of the vessel due to SHPT.

(b) The vessel appears as bone on imaging studies.

(2) Intimal calcification.

(a) Caused from atherosclerosis related to classic CV risk factors such as hypertension, dyslipidemia, diabetes, smoking, obesity, and age.

(b) Leads to vessel occlusion.

(3) Both cause increased CV morbidity and mortality.

(4) Most CKD patients are at risk for both due to their comorbid conditions and cause of CKD.

8. Treatment of CKD-MBD.

a. Suggest maintaining phosphorus in the normal range (2C).

b. Suggest maintaining calcium in the normal range (2D).

c. Suggest using phosphorus binders to treat hyperphosphatemia (2D).

d. Reasonable to base choice if binder on CKD stage, presence of other components of CKD-MBD, concomitant therapies, and side-effect profile (not graded).

e. Recommend restricting the dose of calcium based binders and/or the dose of calcitriol or vitamin D analog in the presence of persistent or recurrent hypercalcemia (1B).

f. Recommend avoiding the use of aluminum-containing phosphate binders (1C).

g. Suggest limiting dietary phosphate intake in the treatment of hyperphosphatemia alone or in combination with other treatments (2D).

9. Treatment of abnormal PTH levels.

a. Optimal level of PTH is unknown in CKD stages 3–4 ND. In patients with PTH levels above the upper-limit of normal, suggest evaluation for hyperphosphatemia, hypocalcemia, and vitamin D deficiency (2C).

b. Correct any abnormalities found (not graded).

(1) Limit phosphorus intake.

(2) Consider phosphorus binder if phosphorus is elevated despite dietary restrictions.

(3) Risk of death increased 18% for every 1 mg/dL increase in phosphorus concentration.

(4) No association was seen with either calcium or PTH and all-cause mortality.

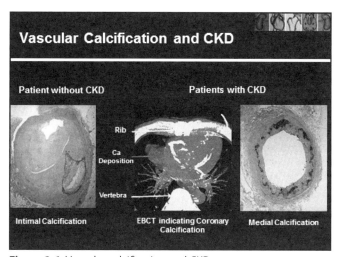

Figure 2.6. Vascular calcification and CKD.
Used with permission from AbbVie, North Chicago, IL.

(5) In the MESA study, each 1 mg/dL increase in serum phosphate was associated with a 21% to 62% greater prevalence of various CV calcifications.

c. Suggest treatment with calcitriol or vitamin D analogs for persistently elevated PTH levels despite correction of modifiable factors (2C).

d. Suggest parathyroidectomy for patients with severe SHPT who fail to respond to medical and pharmacologic therapy (2B).

10. Vitamin D therapies.
   a. Calcitriol.
      (1) Active form of D3 (animal source).
      (2) Increases gut absorption of calcium and phosphorus, especially at higher doses.
      (3) Approved in the 1970s with the purpose to correct hypocalcemia.
      (4) Increases urinary calcium excretion over 100%, still in normal range.
      (5) Elimination half-life 3–8 hours.
   b. Doxercalciferol (Coburn, et.al., 2004).
      (1) Inactive D2 (plant source).
      (2) Must be hydroxalated in the liver to become active (Prodrug).
      (3) Pivotal study showed an increased need for phosphate binders to maintain targets. Patients requiring binders increased from 22% to 44% over the 24-week study.
      (4) Elimination half-life 32–37 hours with a range up to 96 hours.
      (5) Increases urinary calcium excretion over 100%, still in normal range.
      (6) Pivotal study showed 74% of patients achieved less than 30% in their PTH from baseline at weeks 20 to 24.
   c. Paricalcitol (Coyne et al., 2004).
      (1) Active D2 (plant source).

(2) Minimal calcemic and phosphatemic effects on the intestines as shown in preclinical studies.
(3) Urinary calcium excretion nonsignificant.
(4) Elimination half-life 17 hours.

d. In the pivotal study, 91% of the patients obtained two consecutive > 30% reductions in iPTH (24-week study).

e. Goals of therapy.
   (1) Efficacy: reduce or maintain iPTH in target range.
   (2) Minimal or no effect on calcium, phosphorus, and urinary calcium levels.
   (3) Prevent hyperplasia/hypertrophy and nodularity of the parathyroid gland.
   (4) Minimize bone resorption, promote bone formation, and prevent bone loss.

11. Early, optimal management of SHPT can prevent and/or minimize the risks associated with MBD associated with CKD.

L. Metabolic acidosis (Kdigo: CKD, 2013a).
   1. Suggest bicarbonate concentrations < 22 mmol/l be treated with oral bicarbonate supplementation to within the normal range unless contraindicated (2B).
   2. High bicarbonate levels are associated with an increased risk of death no matter what the level of kidney function.
   3. Chronic acidosis is associated with:
      a. Increased protein metabolism.
      b. Uremic bone disease.
      c. Muscle wasting.
      d. Chronic inflammation.
      e. Impaired glucose hemostasis.
      f. Impaired cardiac function.
      g. CKD progression.
      h. Increased mortality.
   4. Caution should be used when treating acidosis with sodium bicarbonate or sodium citrate to avoid sodium loading. Patients with dietary sodium intake near maximum levels may need to reduce their sodium chloride intake to maintain sodium balance.

M. Nutritional concerns (KDOQI: Nutrition, 2000).
   1. Screening for undernutrition in CKD (1C). Defined as:
      a. Less than 85% of ideal body weight (IBW).
      b. Reduction in edema-free body weight of 5% or more in 3 months or 10% or more in 6 months.
      c. BMI < 20 kg/m².
      d. Subjective global assessment (SGA) (B or C on 3-point scale or 1 to 5 on 7-point scale).
      e. The above measures have been linked to increased mortality and other adverse events.
   2. Frequency of screening recommended every 2 to 3

months for outpatients with eGFR < 20, not on dialysis (1D).

3. Additional assessment methods for undernutrition.
   a. Include bioimpedance analysis, anthropometry, handgrip strength, and assessment of nutritional intake.
   b. Low serum albumin is a strong predictor of adverse outcomes but is largely unrelated to nutritional status. It is an acute phase reactant.

4. Protein calorie malnutrition (PCM).
   a. Factors associated with PCM include the following.
      (1) Proteinuria.
      (2) Anorexia.
      (3) Uremia (nausea & vomiting).
      (4) Depression.
      (5) Socioeconomic issues.
      (6) Comorbid conditions.
   b. Dietary protein intake.
      (1) Though the Modification of Diet and Renal Disease (MDRD) study did not conclusively show that protein restriction slows progression of kidney disease, ad hoc analyses indicated it may retard the progression or delay the onset of renal replacement therapy in individuals with severe (stage 4) CKD.
      (2) Frequently, patients have spontaneous decrease in protein and energy intake when GFR falls below 50 mL/min and even more so when GFR falls below 25 mL/min.
      (3) A positive correlation between energy intake and GFR has been found regardless of prescribed diet.
      (4) Malnutrition is linked to poor clinical outcomes.
         (a) Caution should be used when instructing patients to decrease protein. NKF K/DOQI recommends 0.75 grams/protein/kg body weight/day in stage 4–5 ND CKD.
         (b) The majority of the protein should come from high-biologic-value sources such as meat and egg whites.
         (c) Calorie intake should be 30 to 35 kcal/kg/d depending on age and physical activity (2B).
   c. Support from a kidney dietitian is invaluable.

5. Obesity (overnutrition) in CKD.
   a. Obesity related disorders that cause CKD.
      (1) Focal segmental glomerulosclerosis (FSGS).
      (2) Stone disease.
      (3) Obesity-related glomerulopathy (ORG).
      (4) Metabolic syndrome.
      (5) Diabetic (type 2) nephropathy.
   b. Persons most at risk.
      (1) Those with central adiposity.
      (2) Those with high waist-to-hip ratios.
      (3) Suggest measurements not be routinely collected at this time (2C).
   c. Assessment and monitoring by BMI recommended (1C).
   d. Dietary modifications for weight loss.
      (1) Must be individualized and appropriate for the stage of CKD.
      (2) Goal is to lighten the kidney's load of the products of metabolism while helping the kidney maintain normal equilibrium.
      (3) Weight loss of 5% to 10% of body weight lowers blood pressure and cholesterol levels.
      (4) Healthy eating habits and exercise are essential.
      (5) If no kidney dietitian is available, the Dietary Approaches to Stop Hypertension (DASH) diet is appropriate for earlier stages of CKD but needs modification for protein and phosphorus as GFR decreases.

6. Vitamin D.
   a. Vitamin D levels start to fall early in CKD (review Figure 2.2).
   b. Serum levels of 25-hydroxyvitamin D (25[OH]D) should be measured at the first visit. If normal (> 30), repeat annually.
   c. If 25(OH)D is less than 30, supplement with vitamin D2 or D3 (ergocalciferol or cholecalciferol).
   d. Discontinue use of Vitamin D supplements if calcium is above 10.2.

7. Electrolytes and minerals.
   a. Potassium.
      (1) May be elevated or decreased depending on underlying medical condition and medications.
      (2) Recommended intake 40 to 70 mEq/day if serum levels are elevated.
      (3) If elevated, avoid salt substitutes since these contain potassium.
      (4) Should be monitored closely for hyperkalemia if patient is on an ACEI or ARB or a potassium sparing diuretic such as spironolactone.
      (5) Should be monitored closely for hypokalemia when patient is taking other diuretics.
   b. Sodium.
      (1) Recommended intake 2000 mg or less a day.
      (2) Some patients are salt sensitive; limiting sodium may decrease both their blood pressure and edema.
   c. Phosphorus.

(1) Generally not elevated until CKD stage 4 and 5, yet bones are being demineralized.

(2) Phosphate has a direct effect on the parathyroid gland.

(3) In bone, phosphate retention increases FGF-23. High FGF-23 levels correlate with mortality in CKD patients (Silver, 2013).

(4) Limiting phosphorus intake early (eGFR 40) can in itself reduce PTH levels.

(5) If phosphorus is trending up or is elevated, limit dietary phosphorus to 800 to 1000 mg/day adjusted for dietary protein needs.

d. Calcium.

(1) Generally not low until stage 3 or 4 CKD, yet bones are being demineralized.

(2) Goal-corrected calcium should be in the normal range for the laboratory used, preferably toward the lower end.

(3) Total elemental calcium intake including both diet and medications should not exceed 2,000 mg a day (1500 mg from binders and 500 mg from diet).

(4) If serum albumin is low, calcium will need to be corrected (4 – serum albumin) x 0.8 + serum calcium = corrected calcium).

N. Acute kidney injury (AKI) (KDIGO: CKD, 2013).

1. All people with CKD are considered to be at increased risk for AKI (1A).

2. Follow AKI guidelines for risk management (not graded).

a. During concurrent illness.

b. When undergoing investigation or procedure likely to increase AKI.

O. Miscellaneous drug issues.

1. Polypharmacy is a common problem in CKD. Medication review for any drug that could be discontinued should be done at each clinic visit.

2. Nonsteroidal antiinflammatory drugs (NSAIDs) should be avoided. They affect prostaglandins, causing vasoconstriction of the afferent arteriole of the nephron.

a. May cause a drop in GFR, especially with concomitant use of ACEi or ARBs.

b. May cause or worsen hypertension.

3. Many drugs are excreted by the kidneys and require dose and/or interval adjustments as GFR declines.

4. Bisphosphonates such as alendronate should be avoided when the eGFR is less than 35. Bone biopsy is suggested prior to any bisphosphonate use in stage 4 or 5.

5. Antihistamines such as cetirizine and hydroxyzine should be decreased by 50% when the GFR is less than 50.

6. Antibiotics such as gentamicin and vancomycin should be decreased according to GFR and blood levels monitored, as appropriate.

7. Avoid magnesium-containing drugs such as milk of magnesia, Mylanta, and Maalox. As GFR decreases, so does the ability of the kidney to excrete magnesium.

8. Avoid enemas and laxatives that contain phosphorus.

9. Herbals, especially those gotten from foreign sources, have been associated with kidney failure and most should be avoided.

10. Insulin is metabolically cleared by the kidney and may require dose adjustment as CKD worsens.

11. Avoid using sulfonylureas that are mainly excreted by the kidneys; for example, glyburide.

12. Check reliable sources to see if dose adjustments are needed or agent is contraindicated before prescribing drugs or herbals.

13. All patients with CKD should be offered annual influenza vaccinations (KDIGO: CKD, 2013).

14. All patients with CKD stage 4 or 5 and at risk of continued progression should be immunized against hepatitis B (1B) (KDIGO: CKD, 2013).

15. All patients with CKD stage 4 or 5 should be vaccinated with pneumococcal vaccine or revaccinated if it has not been given within the last 5 years (KDIGO: CKD, 2013).

P. Education and preparation for kidney replacement modalities.

1. Consult published guidelines.

a. American Nephrology Nurses' Association (ANNA).

b. Renal Physicians Association (RPA).

c. National Kidney Foundation (NKF) KDOQI.

d. American Society of Nephrology (ASN).

e. Fistula First Initiative.

2. There is no absolute level of CKD (eGFR) that requires dialysis to be started.

a. Dialysis usually is started when eGFR is around 10 and the patient has subjective symptoms of uremia.

b. There is conflicting evidence on survival benefit with early initiation of dialysis.

c. Kidney replacement therapy choice will also help determine timing for interventions such as access so the patient can be ready for dialysis or transplant when needed.

3. Patient and family psychosocial preparation.

a. Introduce kidney replacement therapy options early.

b. Will require multiple repeated conversations.

c. Encourage participation in multidisciplinary educational offerings.

d. Patients and families need time to adjust to change in lifestyle. Spousal abandonment has occurred.

e. Focus on positives and provide constant encouragement and hope.

f. Acknowledge fear, anxiety, and sense of loss.

g. Refer to social worker for assessment, coping strategies, and financial assistance.

h. Identify and treat depression.

4. Peritoneal dialysis (PD).

a. Preferred therapy at initiation of dialysis when there is residual kidney function.

b. Requires peritoneal catheter placement.

c. Normal serum albumin desirable.

d. May require transfer to another modality if adequacy is not achieved.

e. Challenge to achieve adequacy of dialysis in a person with excessive body mass index and no residual kidney function.

f. Possibility of peritonitis if aseptic technique is broken.

g. Patient desires home therapy and unable to do home hemodialysis.

h. Allows freedom in schedule.

   (1) Continuous ambulatory peritoneal dialysis (CAPD).

      (a) Usually four manual exchanges of dialysis fluid daily requiring ~ 30 minutes each to complete.

      (b) Generally 4 to 6 hours between exchanges.

   (2) Automated peritoneal dialysis (APD).

      (a) Uses a machine to cycle fluid through the night and then leave fluid in for a daytime exchange.

      (b) Generally connected to the cycler 9 to 10 hours nightly.

   (3) Times for both can be adjusted to meet scheduling needs.

   (4) Table 2.8 shows comparisons of the two main types of PD.

i. PD contraindicated/not recommended in the following.

   (1) Severe malnutrition or morbid obesity.

   (2) Fresh intraabdominal foreign body.

   (3) Bowel disease or other sources of chronic infection.

j. Cost effective.

k. Fosters independence, no partner needed.

l. Easier to arrange backup travel support.

5. In-center hemodialysis.

a. Requires an available spot in a dialysis center and placement on a schedule of days and time.

b. Usually requires 3.5 to 4 hours, three times per week to achieve desired Kt/V.

c. May require additional treatments for fluid management.

d. Childcare issues.

e. Requires transportation to and from dialysis center.

f. Access to the blood circulation is required and involves surgery to create an A-V Fistula (preferred) or A-V Graft. Central venous catheters can be used until permanent vascular access is available but is not a preferred permanent access.

6. Home hemodialysis (HHD).

a. Requires space for equipment and supplies.

b. A trained support person available during treatments is preferred.

c. Requires specialized training.

d. Medical compliance.

e. Cost less than in center but more than PD.

f. Allows greater freedom in schedule.

g. May do daily (5 to 6 days a week) for 2 to 3

Table 2.8

Comparison of the Two Main Types of Peritoneal Dialysis

Continuous Ambulatory Peritoneal Dialysis (CAPD)	Automated Peritoneal Dialysis (APD)
4 exchanges a day	Generally done overnight for 9 to 10 hours. Takes 10 to 15 minutes at the beginning and end to get things ready and start and then disconnect and clean up at the end.
Preferably 4 to 6 hours apart	
7 days a week	
No machines needed	Uses simple machine
Flexible schedule	Flexible schedule
Takes about 30 min. per exchange (2 hours a day)	May start out at 5 to 6 nights a week but when residual kidney function goes down will increase to 7 days a week
Takes ~2 weeks to train	Takes ~2 weeks to train
No helper needed	No helper needed

Table 2.9

Differences Between Hemodialysis Performed In-Center or at Home

In-center Hemodialysis (HD)	Home Hemodialysis (HHD)
3 times a week	5 to 6 times a week
3 to 4.5 hours per treatment	2 to 3 hours per treatment for short daily HHD
Fixed schedule	Note may also do conventional HD, # days weekly, for 3 to 4.5 hours.
No helper needed	Flexible schedule
Staff present	Helper needed
Kidney MD or APRN/PA sees you on dialysis	Monthly visits to Kidney MD office
	Takes about 3 to 6 weeks to train

hours or conventional 3 days a week HD for 3 to 4.5 hours per treatment.

h. Hemodialysis can be done in a center or at home. The differences are outlined in Table 2.9.

7. Transplantation.
   a. Performed preemptively or after initiation of dialysis. The sources of kidneys used for transplant can be seen in Table 2.10.
   b. Surgically acceptable candidate.
      (1) Cardiac stability.
      (2) Infection free.
      (3) Cancer free (usually for 2 years, but varies dependent on the type of cancer and by transplant program).
      (4) Medically compliant.
      (5) Financial resources available for surgery and medications.
   c. Consider age, family support, lifestyle, cognitive ability, and substance abuse.
   d. Start conversation about living donors.
   e. Refer to Medicare approved transplant center for formal evaluation usually when eGFR is approximately 20 mL/min.
      (1) Medical evaluation by transplant nephrologists and/or APRN.
      (2) Surgical evaluation by transplant surgeon.
      (3) Psychosocial evaluation by social worker.
      (4) Nutritional evaluation by dietitian.
8. Nondialysis management and palliative care.
   a. Patients may choose no kidney replacement therapy. Need to support this decision.
   b. Advance directive obtained. Patients have the option to change their minds at any time.
   c. Involve family, clergy, as appropriate.
   d. Involve primary care health provider and nurses caring for patient.
   e. Provide education and assistance to make process as comfortable as possible.
   f. Provide palliative care and/or refer for hospice care.

Table 2.10

Sources of Kidneys for Transplant

- Living-related donor
- Emotionally-related donor
- Paired donor
- Deceased donor

9. Access for dialysis.
   a. For hemodialysis, save an arm when CrCl < 30 mL/min. This means no phlebotomy, IV's, PICC lines in chosen extremity. Be aware of magnitude of possible complications (e.g., significant subclavian vein stenosis caused by subclavian vein catheterization).
   b. Arrange hemodialysis access 6 months in advance when AV fistula placement is planned or 3 to 6 weeks in advance for AV grafts.
      (1) AV Fistula preferred (see Table 2.11). PTFE grafts are the next preferred type of vascular access (see Table 2.12).
      (2) Timely placement obviates need for temporary catheters.
      (3) Order vein mapping.
      (4) Refer to vascular access surgeon.
      (5) Educate patient and family to understand the need for timely placement.
   c. Monitor access for development, stenosis, patency, steal syndrome, and infection at every clinic visit. Refer back to surgeon immediately for any problems.
   d. Refer for peritoneal catheter placement if doing PD 3 to 4 weeks in advance. *Note*: The PD catheter may be placed earlier if it is left buried in the subcutaneous tissue until needed.
   e. Prepare patient psychologically for body image changes.

Table 2.11

The AV Fistula

- Uses your own blood vessels
- Is the preferred hemodialysis access
- Need 6 weeks to 3 months to mature (be ready for use)
- Buttonhole creation can be done (allows use of dull needles)
- Ideally placed 3-6 months before dialysis needed
- Least number of complications
- Do not allow blood pressures or blood draws to be done in the access arm

Table 2.12

The AV Graft

- Uses a synthetic material
- Needs ~ 2 weeks to mature (Be ready to use)
- Ideally placed about a month before needed
- Compared to a fistula, higher clotting and stenosis rates
- Do not allow blood pressures or blood draws to be done in the access arm

f. Lack of advance planning or late presentation emergency situations will require vascular catheter. Temporary or tunneled dialysis catheters are considered short-term and prone to infection. Also cause increased cost, discomfort, venous stenosis, and thrombosis. See Figure 2.7, The Hemodialysis Vascular Access from Fistula First, to compare and contrast vascular accesses. Educate on risks of catheter placement whenever possible.

10. Urgent start PD may be an option for eligible patients.

11. Patient and family education.
   a. Identify resources and encourage patients and family members to be proactive in seeking out resources.
      (1) Community resources in nephrology offices, kidney centers, and universities.
      (2) CKD education clinics.
         (a) Medicare funding for up to 6 sessions for patients in CKD stage 4.
         (b) APRN, PA, or physician is required to do education for Medicare billing.
         (c) Both group and individual rates available.
      (3) Internet websites.
         (a) Home Dialysis Central, http://www .homedialysis.org

         (b) American Kidney Fund, http://www .akfinc.org
         (c) American Association of Kidney Patients, http://www.aakpnat@aol.com
         (d) Kidney Care partners, http://www .kidneycarepartners.org.
         (e) Renal Support Network, http://www .RSUhope.org.
         (f) National Kidney Foundation, http:// www.kidney.org.
         (g) Life Options, http://www.Life Options.org.
         (h) Kidney School, http://www.Kidney School.org.
         (i) eKidney Clinic, http://www.ckd .vacloud.us.
         (See Table 2.13 for more resources.)
      (4) Audiovisual materials.
   b. Providers give education with every visit. Keep teaching sessions short and reinforce previous teachings.
   c. Family members need to expect changes such as:
      (1) Decreased energy and an increased difficulty maintaining the same level of ADLs as uremic symptoms develop.
      (2) Initiation of disability or increased absence from work and possible reduction in financial income.
      (3) Encourage continued contact with kidney social worker as lifestyle changes occur.
   d. Follow-up nephrology clinic visits are essential and increase in frequency for monitoring of kidney function and management of complications.
   e. As GFR decreases, problems with infertility can occur, but birth control and prevention of pregnancy is frequently advised.
   f. Continue to reinforce taking prescribed medications and review rationale. If income drops or insurance becomes a problem, be cognizant of costs of medications.
   g. Encourage patient to maintain ongoing healthcare visits with primary care, diabetologist, cardiologist, dentist, etc., to maintain optimal health.
   h. Encourage and teach importance of continued exercise.
   i. Keep up appearances and hygiene.

12. Education for hospitals and primary care providers.
   a. Refer to nephrology specialty clinic recommended by KDOQI for the following reasons (1B) (KDIGO, CKD, 2013).
      (1) AKI or an abrupt fall in GFR.
      (2) When eGFR < 30 mL/min/1.73 m^2.
      (3) Consistent finding of significant albuminuria.
      (4) Progression of CKD.

Hemodialysis Vascular Access

Hemodialysis cleans your blood through a fistula, graft or catheter. If you have kidney failure, one of these will be your **LIFELINE!**

Talk with your doctor to decide which type of vascular access is best for you.

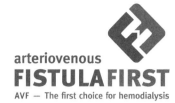

arteriovenous
FISTULAFIRST
AVF — The first choice for hemodialysis

Fistula

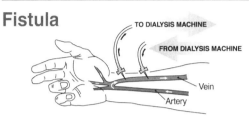

A fistula directly connects an artery to a vein. The vein stretches over time, allowing needles to be put in it.
Fistulas are the gold standard for hemodialysis.

Advantages

✔ Permanent
✔ Beneath the skin
✔ Lasts longest, up to 20 years
✔ Provides greater blood flow for better treatment
✔ Fewer infections & other complications
✔ Fewer hospitalizations
✔ Better survival (lower risk of dying than patients with catheters)

Disadvantages

✘ May not mature/develop
✘ Not possible for all patients
✘ Usually cannot be used for at least 6–8 weeks

Graft

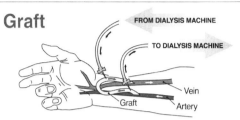

A graft is a tube, usually made of plastic, that connects an artery to a vein, allowing needles to be put in it. Grafts are the second best way to get access to the bloodstream for hemodialysis.

Advantages

✔ Permanent
✔ Beneath the skin
✔ May be used after 2 weeks, in some cases
✔ May work in patients with poor veins

Disadvantages

✘ Increased hospitalizations
✘ Increased risk for clotting
✘ Increased risk for serious infections
✘ Increased risk for other complications and repair procedures
✘ Does not last as long as a fistula

Catheter

A catheter is a tube inserted into a vein in the neck or chest to provide vascular access for hemodialysis. The tip rests in your heart. It is usually a **temporary** access. It is the third choice for getting access to the bloodstream for hemodialysis. For some patients it is the only choice and it will need to be used as a permanent access.

Advantages

✔ Can be used immediately after placement

Disadvantages

✘ Higher infection rates, which can be very serious or fatal
✘ Increased hospitalizations
✘ Does not last long, usually less than one year
✘ May require longer treatment times
✘ Prolonged use may lead to inadequate dialysis
✘ Cannot shower without special appliance
✘ High rate of clotting requiring frequent procedures
✘ Risk of destroying important vein

Adapted with modifications from a flyer produced by the Roanoke Vascular Access Center, 4/10. This material was prepared by the Mid-Atlantic Renal Coalition as part of the Fistula First Breakthrough Initiative Special Project; further updates prepared by the End Stage Renal Disease Network Coordinating Center, 4/11; under contract with the Centers for Medicare & Medicaid Services (CMS), an agency of the U.S. Department of Health and Human Services. The contents presented do not necessarily reflect CMS policy. CMS Contract Number: HHSM-500-2010-NW002C.

Figure 2.7. The hemodialysis vascular access by Fistula First.

Adapted with modifications from a flier produced by the Roanoke Vascular Access Center, 4/10. This material was prepared by the Mid-Atlantic Renal Coalition as part of the Fistula First Breakthrough Initiative Special Project; further updates prepared by the End Stage Renal Disease Network Coordinating Center, 4/11; under contract with the Centers for Medicare & Medicaid Services (CMS), an agency of the U.S. Department of Health and Human Services. The contents presented do not necessarily reflect CMS policy. CMS Contract Number: HHSM-500-2010-NW002C.

Table 2.13

Resources on Kidney Replacement

No	Topic	Websites	Comments
1	Understanding CKD	http://www.rsnhope.org/ https://www.aakp.org/ http://nkdep.nih.gov/ http://www.kidney.org/kidneydisease/ http://www.davita.com/kidney-disease http://www.renalinfo.com/ http://www.kidneyfund.org/ http://www2.niddk.nih.gov/ http://www.kidneycarepartners.org http://www.LifeOptions.org	Patients, healthcare professionals and members of the public concerned with kidney disease have helped put these sites together for general information, education, and self-help forums. Additional resources are available on these sites.
2	Forums	http://www.kidney.org/patients/peers/index.cfm http://ihatedialysis.com/forum/	Additional online forums where you can find people with similar problems, and share experiences.
3	Emergency prep	http://www.davita.com/kidney-disease/overview/living-with-ckd/emergency-preparedness-for-people-with-kidney-disease/e/4930 http://www.uptodate.com/contents/chronic-kidney-disease-beyond-the-basics	Plan for severe happenings. What to do in case of emergencies.
4	Diet	http://kidney.niddk.nih.gov/kudiseases/pubs/eatright/	Food choices and how to manage your diet.
5	Travel	http://www.kidney.org/atoz/content/traveltip.cfm	How to plan a trip and make happy and safe travel plans. Information about your needs when you plan to go out of your city.
6	Family support	http://www.kidney.org/patients/pfc/caregiver.cfm http://www.davita.com/kidney-disease/overview/living-with-ckd/caregiver-stress-and-chronic-kidney-disease/e/4915	If you are the person taking care of a CKD patient, you need to have some information and help regarding the challenge you face.
7	National Kidney Foundation Patient Information Help Line	1-855-NKF-CARES (855-653-2273)	Speak with a trained person about kidney disease, organ donation, or transplantation.
8	Financial support	http://www.kidneyfund.org/	Charitable assistance to dialysis/CKD patients who need help with the costs associated with treating kidney failure.
9	Home dialysis	http://www.homedialysis.org	Learn more about home dialysis here. The site has education and covers every aspect of home dialysis. Must see for home dialysis patients and families.
10	More education	http://www.KidneySchool.org	Online education program with audio books; more education for you!

(5) Urinary RBC casts, RBC > 20 per high power field sustained and not readily explained.

(6) CKD and hypertension refractory to treatment with four or more antihypertensive medications.

(7) Recurrent or extensive nephrolithiasis.

(8) Hereditary kidney disease.

b. What to expect with referral.

　(1) Establish diagnosis and/or perform kidney biopsy, if needed, and if not done earlier.

　(2) Provision of specific therapy based on diagnosis.

　(3) Evaluation and treatment of comorbid conditions.

　(4) Identification, prevention, and

Table 2.14

Early versus Late Referral: Consequences and Benefits

Consequences of late referral	Benefits of early referral
Anemia and bone disease	Delay need to initiate KRT
Severe hypertension and fluid overload	Increased proportion with permanent access
Low prevalence of permanent access	Greater choice of treatment options
Delayed referral for transplant	Reduced need for urgent dialysis
Higher initial hospitalization rate	Reduced hospital length of stay and costs
Higher 1-year mortality rate	Improved nutritional status
Less patient choice of RRT modality	Better management of CVD and comorbid conditions
Worse psychosocial adjustment	Improved patient survival

Abbreviations: CVD = cardiovascular disease; KRT = kidney replacement therapy.

Source: Kidney Disease: Improving Global Outcomes (KDIGO) CKD Work Group. (2013). KDIGO 2012 clinical practice guideline for the evaluation and management of chronic kidney disease. *Kidney International Supplements, 3*(1), 1–150 (Table 35, page 114).

management of CKD-related complications.

(5) Prepare for and initiate dialysis when needed.

(6) Provide surveillance of polypharmacy and potential drug interactions, especially with multiple providers, i.e., PCP, cardiologists, etc.

(7) Adjust drug dose and/or educate regarding avoidance of certain drugs as GFR declines.

(8) Plot progression of kidney disease and implement care for prevention of progression of kidney disease.

(9) Psychological support and/or provision of conservative or palliative care if needed.

c. Early referral can delay progression of CKD and comorbidities and improve patient survival (see Table 2.14).

References

Bucaloiu, I.D., Kirchner, H.L., Norfolk, E.R., Hartle, J.E., & Perkins, R.M. (2012). Increased risk of death and de novo chronic kidney disease following reversible acute kidney injury. *Kidney International, 81*(5), 477-485.

Campoy, S., & Elwell, R. (2005). Pharmacology and CKD: How chronic kidney disease and its complications alter drug response. *American Journal of Nursing, 105*(9), 60-71.

Chawla, L.S., Amdur, R.L., Amodeo, S., Kimmel, P.L., & Palant, C. E. (2011). The severity of acute kidney injury predicts progression to chronic kidney disease. *Kidney International, 79*(12), 1361-1369.

Choi, M.J., & Fried, L.F. (Eds.). (2013). Chronic kidney disease and progression. *Journal of the American Society of Nephrology: NephSAP, 12*(4)(Suppl.), 236-264.

Coca, S.G., Singanamala, S., & Parikh, C.R. (2012). Chronic kidney disease after acute kidney injury: A systematic review and meta-analysis. *Kidney International, 81*(5), 442-448.

Combest, M., Newton, M., Combest, A., & Kosier, J.H. (2005). Effects of herbal supplements on the kidney. *Urology Nurse, 25*(5), 381-386.

Dalrymple, L.S., Katz, R., Kestenbaum, B., deBoer, I.H., Fried, L., Sarnak, M.J., & Shlipak, M.G. (2012). The risk of infection-related hospitalization with decreased kidney function. *American Journal of Kidney Diseases, 59*(3), 356-363. doi:10.1053/j.ajkd.2011.07.012

Evenpoel, P., Meijers, B., Viaene, L., Bammens, B., Claes, L., Kuypers, D., … Vanrenterghem, Y. (2010). Fibroblast growth factor-23 in early chronic kidney disease: Additional support in favor of a phosphate-centric paradigm for the pathogenesis of secondary hyperparathyroidism. *Clinical Journal American Society of Nephrology, 5*, 1268-1276.

Ferri, F.F. (2004). *Ferri's best test: A practical guide to clinical laboratory medicine and diagnostic imaging.* Philadelphia: Elsevier Mosby.

Fried, L.F., Katz, R., Sarnak, M.J., Shlipak, M.G., Chaves, P.H., Jenny, N.S., … Newman, A.B. (2005). Kidney function as a predictor of noncardiovascular mortality. *Journal of the American Society of Nephrology, 16*(12), 3728-3735.

Fogazzi, G.B. (2010). Urinalysis. In J. Floege, R.J. Johnson, & J. Feehally (Eds.), *Comprehensive clinical nephrology* (pp. 39-55). St. Louis: Elsevier Saunders.

Go, A.S., Chertow, G. M., Fan, D., McCulloch, C.E., & Hsu, C.Y. (2004). Chronic kidney disease and the risks of death, cardiovascular events, and hospitalization. *New England Journal of Medicine, 351*, 1296-1305.

Hallan, S.I., Coresh, J. Astor, B.C., Asberg, A., Powe, N.R., Romundstad, S., … Holmen, J. (2006). International comparison of the relationship of chronic kidney disease prevalence and ESRD risk. *Journal of the American Society of Nephrology, 17*(8), 2275-2284.

Inker, L.A., Astor, B.C., Fox, C.H., Isakova, T., Lash, J.P., Peralta, C. A., … Feldman, H.I. (2014). KDOQI US commentary on the 2012 KDIGO clinical practice guideline for the evaluation and management of CKD. *American Journal of Kidney Disease, 63*(5), 713-735.

Ix, J.H., Wassel, C.Z., Stevens, L.A., Beck, G. J., Froissart, M., Navis. G., ... Levey, A.S. (2011). Equations to estimate creatinine excretion rate: The chronic kidney disease epidemiology collaboration. *Clinical Journal of the American Society of Nephrology, 6*(1), 184-191.

James, P.A., Oparil, S., Carter, B.L., Cushman, W.C., Dennison-Himmelfarb, C., Handler, J., ... Ortiz, E. (2014). Evidence-based guidelines for the management of high blood pressure in adults: Report from the panel members appointed to the Eighth Joint National Committee (JNC8). *JAMA,* 311 (5), 507-520.

Juppner, H. (2011). Phosphate and FGF-23. *Kidney International, 79* (Suppl 121), S24-S27.

Kalantar-Zadeh, K., Shah, A., Duong, U., Hechter, R.C., Dukkipati, R., & Kovesdy, C. P. (2010). Kidney disease and mortality in CKD: Revisiting the role of vitamin D, calcimimetics, alkaline phosphatase, and minerals. *Kidney International, 78,* S10-S21.

Kidney Disease: Improving Global Outcomes (KDIGO) CKD–MBD Work Group. (2009). KDIGO clinical practice guideline for the diagnosis, evaluation, prevention, and treatment of chronic kidney disease–mineral and bone disorder (CKD–MBD). *Kidney International, 76* (Suppl.), 113, S1-S130.

Kidney Disease: Improving Global Outcomes (KDIGO) Acute Kidney Injury Work Group. (2012a). KDIGO clinical practice guideline for acute kidney injury. *Kidney International, 2*(Suppl. 1), 1-138.

Kidney Disease: Improving Global Outcomes (KDIGO) Anemia Work Group. (2012b). KDIGO clinical practice guideline for anemia in chronic kidney disease. *Kidney International, 2*(Suppl.), 279-335.

Kidney Disease: Improving Global Outcomes (KDIGO) CKD Work Group. (2013a). KDIGO 2012 clinical practice guideline for the evaluation and management of chronic kidney disease. *Kidney International, 3*(1, Suppl. 3), 1-150.

Kidney Disease: Improving Global Outomes (KDIGO) Lipid Work Group. (2013b). KDIGO clinical practice guideline for lipid management in chronic kidney disease. *Kidney International, 3*(Suppl. 3), 259-305.

Klahr, S. (1983). Pathophysiology of obstructive nephropathy. *Kidney International, 23,* 414-420.

Levey, A.S., Stevens, L.A., Schmid, C.H., Zhang, Y.L., Castro, A.F. 3rd, Feldman, H.I., ... CKD-EPI (Chronic Kidney Disease Epidemiology Collaboration). (2009). A new equation to estimate glomerular filtration rate. *Annals of Internal Medicine, 150*(9), 604-612.

National Institutes of Health National Heart, Lung and Blood Institute. (2013). *Risk assessment tool for estimating your 10 year risk of having a heart attack.* Retrieved from http://cvdrisk .nhlbi.nih.gov/calculator.asp

National Kidney Foundation (NFK). (2002). NKF/KDOQI clinical practice guidelines for chronic kidney disease: Evaluation, classification and stratification. *American Journal of Kidney Diseases, 39*(Suppl. 1), S1-S246.

Naughton, C.A. (2008). Drug-induced nephrotoxicity. *American Family Physician, 78*(6), 743-750.

Pham, A.Q., & Scarlino, C. (2013). Diphenhydramine and acute kidney injury. *Pharmacy and Therapeutics, 38*(8), 453-461.

Rivera, S.L., & Smith, L.F. (2013). CKD mineral and bone disorders: An evidence-based approach. *The Journal for Nurse Practitioners, 9*(5), 301-305.

Schieppati, A., Pisoni, R., & Remuzzi, G. (2005). Pathophysiology and management of chronic kidney disease. In A. Greenburg (Ed.). *Primer of kidney diseases* (4th ed., pp. 444-454). Philadelphia: Elsevier Saunders.

Shlipak, M.P., Matsushita, K., Ärnlöv, L., Inker, L.A., Katz, R., Polkinghorne, K.R., ... Gansevoort, R.T. (2013). Cystatin C versus creatinine in determining risk based on kidney function. *The New England Journal of Medicine, 369,* 932-943. doi:10.1056/NEJMoa1214234

Stevens, L.A., Shastri, S., & Levey, A.S. (2010). Assessment of renal function. In J. Floege, R.J. Johnson, & J. Feehally (Eds.), *Comprehensive clinical nephrology* (pp. 31-38). St. Louis: Elsevier Saunders.

Stevens, L., A., Stoyucheff, N., & Levey, A.S. (2009). Staging and management of chronic kidney disease. In A. Greenburg (Ed.), *Primer on kidney disease* (5th ed.). Philadelphia: Saunders Elsevier.

Svetkey, L.P., & Tyson, C.C. (2013). Treatment of hypertension in patients with chronic kidney disease. *Kidney News, 5*(9), 6.

Tareen, N., Zadshir, A., Martins, S., Pan. S., Nicholas, S., & Norris, K. (2005). Chronic kidney disease in African American and Mexican American populations. *Kidney International, 97,* S137-S140.

Topham, P.S., & Chen, Y. (2010). Renal biopsy. In J. Floege, R.J. Johnson, & J. Feehally (Eds.), *Comprehensive clinical nephrology* (pp. 75-84). St. Louis: Elsevier Saunders.

U.S. Renal Data System. (2014). USRDS 2014 annual data report: Atlas of chronic kidney disease and end-stage renal disease in the United States. National Institutes of Health, National Institute of Diabetes and Digestive and Kidney Diseases, Bethesda, MD.

Vrtis, M.C. (2013). Preventing and responding to acute kidney injury: How to recognize the incremental changes in kidney function that adversely affect patient outcomes. *American Journal of Nursing, 113*(4), 38-47.

Walser, M. (1987). Creatinine excretion as a measure of protein nutrition in adults of varying age. *Journal of Parenteral and Enteral Nutrition, 11*(Suppl. 5), 73S-78 S.

Wymer, D.C. (2010). Imaging. In J. Floege, R.J. Johnson, & J. Feehally (Eds.), *Comprehensive clinical nephrology* (pp. 56-74). St. Louis: Elsevier Saunders.

Overview of Treatment Options for CKD for the APRN

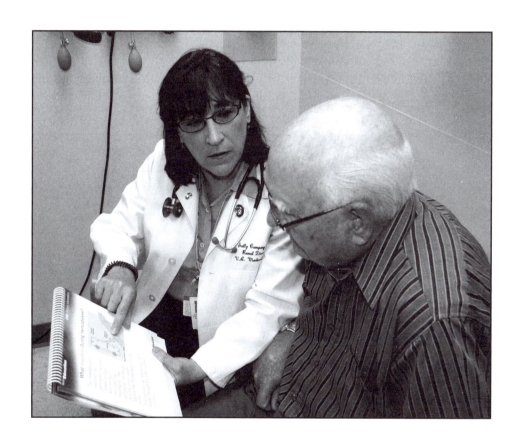

Chapter Editors

Kim Alleman, MS, APRN, FNP-BC, CNN-NP

Katherine Houle, MSN, APRN, CFNP, CNN-NP

Authors

Donna Bednarski, MSN, RN, ANP-BC, CNN, CNP

Colleen M. Brown, MSN, APRN, ANP-BC

Elaine Go, MSN, NP, CNN-NP

Katherine Houle, MSN, APRN, CFNP, CNN-NP

Carol L. Kinzner, MSN, ARNP, GNP-BC, CNN-NP

Mary M. Zorzanello, MSN, APRN

CHAPTER **3**

Overview of Treatment Options for CKD for the APRN

This offering for **2.1 contact hours with 1.0 contact hour of pharmacology content** is provided by the American Nephrology Nurses' Association (ANNA).

American Nephrology Nurses' Association is accredited as a provider of continuing nursing education by the American Nurses Credentialing Center Commission on Accreditation.

ANNA is a provider approved by the California Board of Registered Nursing, provider number CEP 00910.

This CNE offering meets the continuing nursing education requirements for certification and recertification by the Nephrology Nursing Certification Commission (NNCC).

To be awarded contact hours for this activity, read this chapter in its entirety. Then complete the CNE evaluation found at **www.annanurse.org/corecne** and submit it; or print it, complete it, and mail it in. Contact hours are not awarded until the evaluation for the activity is complete.

Example of reference for Chapter 3 in APA format. Use author of the section being cited. This example is based on Section D – Approaches to Care by the APRN in Peritoneal Dialysis.

Zorzanello, M.M. (2015). Overview of treatment options for CKD for the APRN: Approaches to care by the APRN in peritoneal dialysis. In C.S. Counts (Ed.), *Core curriculum for nephrology nursing: Module 6. The APRN's approaches to care in nephrology* (6th ed., pp. 53-110). Pitman, NJ: American Nephrology Nurses' Association.

Interpreted: Section author. (Date). Title of chapter: Title of section written by that author. In ...

Cover photo supplied by Sally Campoy.

The author would like to express her gratitude to Spencer Martin PharmD, BCPS, for his expertise and assistance in development of the pharmacologic component of the chapter.

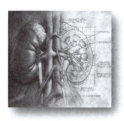

CHAPTER 3

Overview of Treatment Options for CKD for the APRN

Purpose

The purpose of this chapter is to provide a foundation for the Advanced Practice Registered Nurse (APRN) in the area of kidney replacement therapy (KRT). All treatment modalities are addressed, as well as the option of no treatment. Information is offered on transplant, the treatment of choice for the majority of individuals with advanced chronic kidney disease (CKD) (Gupta et al., 2010). The chapter discusses hemodialysis, the dialysis prescription, and ways to maintain optimal health for the patient on hemodialysis from the perspective of the APRN. An overview of the APRN's role in the preparation for the creation, management, and maintenance of hemodialysis access is presented. Additionally, the options of peritoneal dialysis and home hemodialysis as well as role of the APRN are reviewed.

Objectives

Upon completion of this chapter, the learner will be able to:
1. Discuss methods to manage the patient receiving a kidney transplant that will enable a successful transplant.
2. Outline the hemodialysis prescription and its components and rationale for choices.
3. Identify the components of patient evaluation and management to determine an individualized dialysis vascular access plan.
4. Manage patients on peritoneal dialysis (PD) and troubleshoot complications of PD in both inpatient and outpatient settings.
5. Discuss the care of patients on home dialysis and recognize components of a successful program.

SECTION A
Role of the APRN in the Care of the Kidney Transplant Recipient
Colleen Brown

I. The APRN in transplant care.

A. According to the American Academy of Nurse Practitioners (AANP, 2014), "Nurse Practitioners assess patients, order and interpret diagnostic tests, make diagnoses, and initiate and manage treatment plans – including prescribing medications," which is needed throughout the continuum of transplant care.

B. Nurse practitioners have the greatest impact in self-management, decision support, and delivery system design, and therefore possess the skills that are essential in caring for patients with chronic illness (Watts et al., 2008).

C. The nurse practitioner is in the ideal position to enhance patient compliance (Sherry et al., 2007), which is an important part of transplant care.

D. Nurse practitioners practice from a holistic approach and are an integral part of the collaborative approach needed in transplant care (Bolton, 1998).

E. Nurse practitioners function in each phase of transplant care.

II. History of kidney transplantation.

A. Technical developments.
1. The first attempted kidney transplant occured in 1906 when Jaboulay transplanted goat and pig kidneys into humans.
2. Yu Yu Voronoy performed the first human-to-human kidney transplants in 1936.
3. In 1951, the technique of placing the kidney extraperitoneally in the iliac fossa while using the external iliac vessels was described.

4. The first successful kidney transplant was performed by Dr. Joseph Murray between identical twins in 1954 (Watson & Dark, 2012).

B. Advances in immunology.
1. Research conducted by Medawar during World War II was instrumental in understanding the immune system.
2. In the 1950s, total body irradiation was used without success.
3. Azathioprine was the first successful chemical immunosuppressant.
4. In 1970s, the introduction of cyclosporine revolutionized transplantation by dramatically improving outcomes (Watson & Dark, 2012).

C. Improvements in organ preservation.
1. Cold storage refers to the flushing of kidneys with a cold intracellular solution and packing the kidney in sterile containers on ice.
2. Preservation solutions have been developed to counter the effect of lack of circulation on the procured kidney. The aim of the solutions is to "minimize" cellular swelling; minimize the metabolic process; provide adequate oxygenation and hydration; minimize ischemia and reperfusion injury by stabilizing cell permeability; and if possible, remove any accumulation of metabolic waste incurred during the recovery preservation period" (LaPointe et al., 2006, p. 893).
3. Various storage techniques are being used and there is not an established consensus on optimal practice (Watson & Dark, 2012).
4. Pulsatile perfusion is the use of a machine that pumps cool solutions through the kidney vasculature to allow for longer storage times.

D. Kidney transplant statistics.
1. The incidence of kidney failure has started to level off after years of continually increasing. Currently, the adjusted incidence of kidney failure is near 350 per million (NKUDIC, 2014).
2. The advancements in immunosuppressive agents have led to the current 1-year to 2-year patient survival of up to 95% (Marcen, 2009).
3. The 5-year survival rate for transplant recipients is 85.5%, which is more than double the 35.8% for patients on dialysis (NKUDIC, 2014).
4. The annual cost of dialysis treatments is nearly three times the cost of transplant care (NKUDIC, 2014).
5. There are over 120,000 registrants on the kidney transplant waitlist (UNOS, 2014).
6. Unfortunately, the number of patients on the wait list continues to increase annually while the number of donors has remained relatively constant, resulting in a shortage of kidneys for transplant (OPTN/SRTS 2011 Annual Data Report).

E. Phases of transplant care. Care of the kidney transplant recipient can be divided into three stages: pretransplant, wait list, and posttransplant. The APRN plays a critical role throughout this continuum.

III. Transplant immunology.

A. Overview.
1. Immune system recognizes self from nonself.
2. Two types of immune responses.
   a. Cellular response occurs through communication between cells.
   b. Humoral response occurs through antibody production.
3. Kidney transplant is defined as an allotransplant because the donor and recipient are genetically different but of the same species.
4. The transplanted kidney is defined as an allograft.
5. Human leukocyte antigen (HLA).
   a. Protein markers located on surface of most cells.
   b. Immunological identity of the individual.
6. Immune cascade.
   a. Antigen-presenting cell (APC) activates T cells through stimulation and costimulation leads to proliferation of T cells and B cells.
   b. Activated APC releases interleukins which activate further APC cells and lymphocytes.
   c. Interleukin-2 (IL-2) triggers cytotoxic T cells.
   d. Rejection occurs through lysis of the graft cells, antibody production and reactions to the allograft (Van Geler & Ohler, 2013). Figure 3.1 graphically demonstrates the mechanisms of rejection.
7. Immunologic testing.
   a. Screen for risk factors for the development of antibodies which includes history of prior transplant, blood transfusions, and pregnancy.
   b. Blood type – ABO (see Table 3.1).
      (1) Identification and verification is imperative.
      (2) ABO matching follows the same system for blood transfusions.
      (3) Since Rh antigens are not on tissue cells, they are not taken into account.
   c. HLA tissue typing.
      (1) Uses DNA technology.
      (2) Identifies antigens on six major loci.
      (3) Antigens are compared with those of potential donor to determine the number of mismatched antigens.
   d. Cross-match.

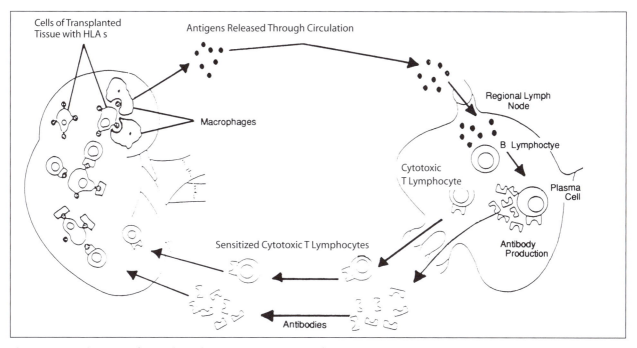

Figure 3.1. Mechanisms of transplanted tissue rejection. Macrophages recognize and process foreign HLAs, and antigenic material is released into the circulation. Lymphocytes in lymph nodes produce activated cytotoxic T lymphocytes and antibodies, which then destroy the transplanted tissue.

Source: Counts, C.S. (2008). *Core curriculum for nephrology nursing* (5th ed.). Pitman, NJ: American Nephrology Nurses' Association.

(1) Donor lymphocytes are mixed with serum from the potential recipient.

(2) Determines if the recipient has antibodies against the door antigens.

(3) Positive crossmatch is a contraindication to transplant under routine circumstances.

e. Panel of reactive antibodies (PRA).

(1) Identifies preformed antibodies against a sample of donors.

(2) Antibodies develop from prior transplant, pregnancy, and blood transfusions.

(3) Monthly samples are followed while a potential recipient is listed.

(4) Reported as percentage and represents probability of rejection.

(5) The higher the PRA, the greater probability of a positive cross-match (Van Geler & Ohler, 2013).

IV. Pretransplant evaluation.

A. Transplant referral.

1. The nephrology clinician typically makes the transplant referral; however, patients, primary care physicians, and specialists may initiate the referral process. There is not an established consensus on the timing of transplant referral. It is recognized that when an individual's glomerular filtration rate (GFR) is less than or equal to 30 mL/min, referral to a transplant center should be considered. In general, early referrals are recommended to allow for the potential of the individual to undergo preemptive live donor kidney transplantation since this affords the individual the most optimal outcome.

2. The evaluation of the potential kidney transplant recipient requires a multidisciplinary approach. The patient is evaluated by a team typically comprised of nurse practitioners, transplant nephrologists, transplant surgeons, social workers, dietitians, financial coordinators, pharmacists, and transplant coordinators. A psychologist or psychiatrist may also be part of the team.

B. Transplant team members.

1. The nurse practitioner and transplant nephrologist

Table 3.1

ABO Matching

Donor Blood Type	Compatible Recipient Blood Type
O	O, A, B, AB
A	A, AB
B	B, AB
AB	AB

typically are responsible for the medical evaluation of the potential recipient. A comprehensive history and physical (H&P) is conducted. In addition to a standard H&P, attention is given in the social history to identify risk for nonadherence posttransplant. Screening for risk factors for sensitization, including history of prior transplant, pregnancies, and blood transfusions, are sought. Immunization history is reviewed and helps guide plans for pretransplant immunizations. Travel history and environmental risk factors are reviewed to determine postinfection risks. The nurse practitioner and transplant nephrologist interpret laboratory and diagnostic studies.

2. The transplant surgeon renders a clinical opinion about the potential recipient's overall transplant candidacy and determines the technical feasibility of the transplant operation. The transplant surgeon will determine if advanced screening techniques such as computerized tomography scan (CT scan) are required to identify the patient's anatomy. The transplant surgeon assists in interpreting diagnostic studies.

3. Social workers have an important role in the pretransplant evaluation. Since nonadherence is a significant cause of graft loss, social workers perform an extensive psychosocial screen. The screening focuses on identification of risk factors for nonadherence, determination of the patient's support system, and review of mood and mental health history. A thorough substance use history is taken. The social worker will determine if further mental health evaluation and intervention is indicated and assist with such referrals within the team or community.

4. The transplant dietitian meets with the patient for a dietary assessment to ensure the potential recipient is ready for surgery from a nutritional perspective. The transplant dietitian determines if the patient's body mass index (BMI) meets the criteria set by the center's policy.

5. The financial coordinator verifies that the potential recipient has adequate transplant benefits to provide for transplant care. Focus is given to determine that the individual has adequate coverage for posttransplant immunosuppression. This is an imperative step since immunosuppression is essential to successful transplantation.

6. The transplant pharmacist conducts a thorough review of the patient's medications to screen for potential drug-drug interactions and risks for nonadherence. The transplant pharmacist assists with patient education on medication management.

7. The transplant coordinator is typically a nurse who focuses on patient education and case management of the workup. The transplant coordinator is the central team member who often acts as the point of contact for the potential recipient.

C. The objectives of the pretransplant evaluation include the following.
   1. Ensure that technically the operation can be performed.
   2. Rule out contraindications to transplantation.
   3. Ensure the potential recipient's survival is not limited by premature death.
   4. Identify opportunities to maximize the health of the potential recipient.
   5. Educate the patient about risks and benefits (The Renal Association, 2011).

D. Determining kidney transplant eligibility is transplant center-specific. However, there are general guidelines that are common among centers. Potential recipients should be encouraged to seek an evaluation at as many centers as is feasible. Potential recipients may be listed in more than one center.

E. Ensure there are no contraindications to kidney transplantation per the policy of the transplant center. Absolute contraindications include the following.
   1. Untreated malignancy.
   2. Untreated infection.
   3. Untreated severe cardiac or pulmonary disease.
   4. Nonadherence to medications or treatment plans.
   5. Severe psychiatric illness that limits the recipient's ability to manage his or her care.
   6. Active substance abuse.
   7. Lack of insurance or inability to pay for medications (Bartucci, 2006).

F. Determine if kidney function meets criteria to proceed with kidney transplantation (UNOS, 2013).
   1. GFR < 20%.
   2. CKD stage 5 requiring kidney replacement therapy.

G. Identify the cause of kidney failure through review of the potential recipient's history and review of any pretransplant native kidney biopsies. It is important to determine that the cause of the kidney failure is irreversible. It is necessary to establish the potential for the disease to reoccur posttransplant. Focal segmental glomerulosclerosis, membrano-proliferative types 1 & 2, diabetic nephropathy, oxalosis, immunoglobulin A nephropathy, membranous nephropathy, antiglomerular basement membrane disease, hemolytic uremic syndrome, and lupus nephritis have varying rates of reoccurrence posttransplant. Autoimmune diseases should be quiescent before proceeding with transplant (Alleman & Longton, 2008).

H. Review the potential for live donors since it will avoid the need for a wait time and is associated with improved outcomes. Patients are offered education and tools to assist them with speaking to others about potentially donating. Donor coordinators are typically nurses who oversee the workup of potential donors and assist in providing community education about live donor kidney transplantation.

I. Laboratory evaluation.
   1. Identification of ABO on two separate occasions.
   2. Identification of Human Leukocyte Antigen (HLA) and panel reactive antibody (PRA).
   3. If there is a live donor, a cross-match is performed.
   4. Infectious disease screening for HIV, hepatitis, CMV, EBV, herpes, toxoplasma, and tuberculosis. Further testing is center-specific.

J. Cardiac testing.
   1. Review cardiac risk factors.
   2. Obtain EKG and echocardiogram.
   3. Evaluate need for nuclear stress test or cardiac catheterization.

K. Pulmonary evaluation.
   1. Obtain screening chest x-ray.
   2. Evaluate need for pulmonary function tests and pulmonary consult.

L. Vascular evaluation. Review need for carotid ultrasound and bilateral lower extremity noninvasive studies based on risk factors.

M. Urologic evaluation. Determine need for urologic studies and urology consult.

N. Health maintenance.
   1. All patients are required to have health screening per age guidelines, including colonoscopy.
   2. Male patients will have screening PSA per standard.
   3. Female patients will have screening Pap smear and mammogram per standard.

O. Abdominal imaging is performed to assess the kidneys. The surgical evaluation will determine if further imaging is indicated to identify the patient's anatomy.

P. Screen for obesity through height and weight to determine body mass index (BMI) (KDIGO, 2009).

V. Prekidney transplant education.

A. Education of the potential recipient is conducted by the entire team and is an ongoing process. It typically starts with a pretransplant class during the patient's first encounter with the transplant program. Education is tailored to meet the needs of the individual, and significant others are involved whenever feasible.

B. Education content.
   1. Evaluation process.
   2. Risks and benefits of transplantation.
   3. Explanation of surgical procedure.
   4. Potential posttransplant complications.
   5. Posttransplant medications.
   6. Care while waiting for an organ.
   7. Organ allocation system.
   8. Posttransplant follow-up care (Ford & John, 2008).

VI. Allocation of deceased donor kidneys.

A. Terminology related to deceased donors.
   1. *Standard criteria donors* are heart-beating donors that meet the criteria for brain death.
   2. *Expanded-criteria donors* are donors of an advanced age or donors who have a medical condition that could impact the function of the graft.
   3. *Donor after cardiac death* (DCD) are the donors who do not meet brain death criteria where ventilatory support is discontinued in a controlled environment and then cardiopulmonary arrest ensues (Alleman & Longton, 2008).
   4. As defined by the Centers for Disease Control (CDC), *high risk donors* are those who carry a higher risk of transmission of infection.

B. Medical criteria for deceased donors.
   1. Absence of malignancy (except some primary brain tumors and skin cancers).
   2. Absence of significant systemic infection or transmissible disease.
   3. Good kidney function.

C. Goals of deceased donor care.
   1. The principal goal of deceased donor care is to maintain adequate blood pressure and urine output with intravenous solutions, such as crystalloids, colloid, and inotropic medications.
   2. Support of the donor family or significant others is critical (Alleman & Longton, 2008).

D. Allocation of kidneys is managed through the United Network for Organ Sharing (UNOS). Average wait times vary depending on the region where the transplant center is located. In general, wait times have extended because of the increase in number of registrants on the wait list with a relatively constant number of donors.

E. The Organ Procurement and Transplantation Network (OPTN)/UNOS board has approved revisions to the deceased donor kidney allocation policy that were implemented in 2014. The new policy provides for national allocation rules and therefore eliminates the present local variances. The changes are intended to improve outcomes, increase years a recipient may have a graft, and increase use of available kidneys. Two clinical formulas are used.
   1. Kidney Donor Profile Index (KDPI) will estimate how long a kidney is likely to function once it is transplanted.
   2. Estimated posttransplant survival formula (EPTS) will estimate the number of years a candidate on the wait list would likely benefit from transplant.

F. Additional changes to the policy include:
   1. Kidney offers estimated to have the shortest potential length of function are shared over a greater geographic area.
   2. Waiting time is calculated from the first date the patient had a GFR of < 20 mL/min.
   3. Facilitation of offers from donors with certain blood subtypes.
   4. A sliding scale of additional priority to patients who are sensitized.

VII. Live donor kidney transplant.

A. Advantages to the recipient.
   1. Ability to plan surgery optimally.
   2. The donor kidney does not undergo the physiological impact of brain death.
   3. Reduced organ storage time.
   4. Improved outcomes (Holechek & Armstrong, 2008).

B. Donor evaluation is conducted to ensure the donor is healthy and donating a kidney of his/her own volition.

C. Donor workup includes the following.
   1. ABO typing and histocompatibility testing to determine matching.
   2. History and physical.
   3. Laboratory evaluation includes health screening and serologies.
   4. Evaluation of kidney function through urine analysis and 24-hour urine collection.

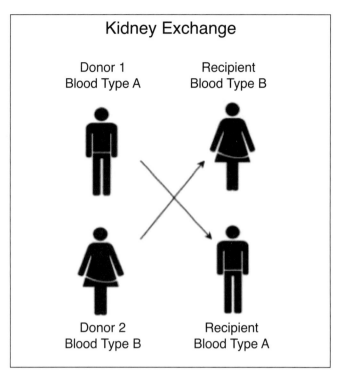

Figure 3.2. Kidney exchange.
Courtesy of Colleen Brown.

   5. Insure routine health maintenance is up to date and within acceptable parameters.
   6. Cardiac evaluation is guided by history and age of the potential donor.
   7. Abdominal imaging is done to evaluate kidneys and define anatomy.
   8. Psychosocial evaluation.
   9. Independent Living Donor Advocate (ILDA) is a member of the transplant team who is not responsible for direct care of the donor or recipient.
      a. Protects the rights of the donor.
      b. Responsible for ensuring the donor is educated about the risk, benefits, and alternatives of donation, donating without coercion, prepared for donation from a psychosocial (OPTN.Transplant.HRSA.gov).

VIII. Paired kidney exchange programs.

A. Paired Kidney Exchange Programs provide an option for individuals who have potential donors that are immunologically incompatible (Ferrari & Klerk, 2009).

B. Computer databases are used to match a donor and recipient with another donor and recipient pair. The event has been referred to as a "kidney swap." An example of the kidney exchange is demonstrated in Figure 3.2.

IX. Operative procedure.

The kidney transplant operation takes approximately 3 hours. The renal graft is placed in the pelvis through an incision extending from the iliac crest to the symphysis pubis. The graft is placed in the iliac fossa. The donor renal artery is anastomosed to the recipient iliac artery and the donor renal vein is anastomosed to the recipient iliac vein. The donor ureter is tunneled through the recipient bladder and a ureteral stent may be placed (Holechek & Armstrong, 2008). The position of the transplanted kidney can be seen in Figure 3.3.

X. Postoperative care.

A. Routine postsurgical care with an emphasis on early ambulation and excellent pulmonary toileting is imperative to prevent postoperative complications.

B. Strict monitoring of intake and output and administration of intravenous fluids is required to maintain adequate fluid balance. Daily weights, central venous pressure monitoring, and physical exam aid in the assessment of fluid balance.

C. Monitoring of kidney function is conducted through urine output measurements and laboratory parameters. It is important to determine the recipient's presurgery urine output and factor this into the evaluation of postoperative urine output.

D. Evaluation of electrolytes includes sodium, potassium, magnesium, phosphorous, and calcium. Any abnormalities should be corrected promptly.

E. Postoperative transplant education is needed to develop a well-informed recipient who is able to manage self-care.

F. Vigilant monitoring is necessary to screen for postkidney surgical transplant complications.
   1. Urine leak, which can be identified by decrease in kidney function, pain over the incision, leakage of urine through the wound, or a dramatic loss of kidney function. The diagnosis may be established through imaging such as a kidney scan. The drainage may be collected and analyzed for creatinine, and if it is higher than the recipient's serum creatinine, the diagnosis can be confirmed.
   2. Lymphocele may be suspected with a decline in kidney function, leg swelling on the side of the transplant, and incisional discomfort. Imaging is needed to establish the diagnosis. Treatment is determined by the size and location of the lymphocele. A small lymphocele may be monitored where a large one may require a percutaneous drain or surgical drainage with

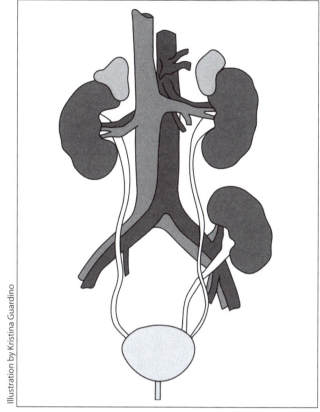

Figure 3.3 Kidney transplant placement.

Illustration by Kristina Guardino

marsupialization into the peritoneum to prevent it from recurring.
   3. Arterial or venous thrombosis are rare events but critical to identify. Symptoms may include sudden loss of kidney function, hematuria, incisional pain, and swelling. Emergent surgery is required to determine if the graft can be salvaged. Thrombosis is a cause of early graft loss and allograft nephrectomy.
   4. Ureteral obstruction is a more common complication and can occur from blood clots or anastomotic complications. It can be identified when there is a decline in kidney function. If the recipient has a foley catheter in place, irrigation may be required. Imaging will aide in the diagnosis, and treatment is dependent on the cause.
   5. Renal artery stenosis is identified through uncontrolled blood pressure, decline in kidney function, and possibly a bruit over the anastomosis. Imaging establishes the diagnosis. Treatment options include angioplasty, stenting, and surgical repair.

G. Early removal and avoidance of catheters and central venous lines are keys in preventing infection.

H. Pain management is necessary to allow early ambulation. It is important to avoid agents that are nephrotoxic or are metabolized through the kidneys (Holechek & Armstrong, 2008).

XI. Immunosuppression.

A. The goal of immunosuppression is to adequately "suppress the immune response to prevent rejection while maintaining sufficient immunity to prevent overwhelming infection" (Bartucci, 2006, p. 402). See Table 3.2 for an overview of current immunosuppressants.

B. Induction therapy.
   1. Induction refers to the use of a biologic agent at the time of transplant or immediately posttransplant. The goal of induction therapy is to deplete or modulate T-cell responses at the time of antigen presentation. This approach is taken to reduce the risk of acute rejection in high risk individuals or in an effort to reduce maintenance immunosuppression. High risk individuals include but are not limited to individuals with a high PRA, younger recipient age, degree of HLA mismatch, African-American ethnicity, delayed graft function, and longer cold ischemic times.
   2. Interleukin-2 receptor antagonists (IL2-RA) are recommended as first line over lymphocyte-depleting antibody preparations because lymphocyte-depleting antibody preparations have a higher incidence of serious side effects (KDIGO, 2009).

XII. Maintenance immunosuppression.

A. A combination of immunosuppressive medications are used per the transplant center protocol. Multiple drug regimens allow for dose reduction to minimize toxicities and improve efficacy with differing mechanisms of action.
   1. Calcineurin inhibitors (CNI) include both cyclosporine and tacrolimus. The primary mechanism of action of CNIs is suppression of activation of T lymphocytes through the inhibition of interleukin-2 (IL-2) (Ohler & Cupples, 2008). Tacrolimus is considered first-line therapy (KDIGO, 2009).
   2. Antiproliferative agents include azathioprine and mycophenolate mofetil and exert their mechanism of action primarily through blocking purine synthesis and preventing B-cell and T-cell proliferation (Ohler and Cupples, 2008). Mycophenolate mofetil is considered first line therapy (KDIGO, 2009).
   3. Corticosteroids act through binding to receptors that alter RNA and DNA synthesis and inhibit the secretion of interleukin-1 (IL-1) from macrophages and IL-2 secretion from T cells and inhibition of cytotoxic T cells. According to the KDIGO 2009 guidelines, patients who receive induction therapy and are considered at a low immunologic risk can have corticosteroids discontinued. The decision to withdraw or avoid corticosteroids is center-specific and a determinate of the balance of the risk of higher acute rejection rates vs. higher steroid associated toxicities.
   4. Sirolimus is a mammilian target of rapamycin (mTOR) and works by blocking the inhibition of this kinase. An advantage of sirolimus is that it has antineoplastic effects. If sirolimus is going to be used for maintenance therapy, it should not be started until wounds are healed due to the effect of delaying wound healing (KDIGO, 2009).
   5. There are numerous medications which interact with immunosuppressive agents through the Cytochrome P-450 System 3A (CYPA3A4) Isozyme. It is important to consider these drug-drug interactions when patient's medication regimen is being adjusted (see Table 3.3).

XIII. Rejection.

A. Hyperacute rejection occurs when the recipient has preformed antibodies to the donor. It causes necrosis of the graft, a toxic status, and signs of disseminated intravascular coagulation. Ensuring a negative pretransplant crossmatch can prevent hyperacute rejection.

B. Acute rejection can occur any time posttransplant but is more likely to occur in the first 6 months posttransplant. It is a T-cell mediated immune response that causes an abrupt deterioration in graft function. Clinical and laboratory parameters will identify the possibility of acute rejection, and a kidney graft biopsy is an important step in the diagnostic process. Corticosteroids are recommended for first-line therapy. Lymphocyte depleting antibodies are used in steroid resistant rejection. Maintenance immunosuppression regimens are altered after an episode of acute rejection such as adding or restoring corticosteroid dose or changing the antiproliferative agent (KDIGO, 2009).

C. Chronic allograft injury is caused by a host of factors including hypertension, calcineurin inhibitor toxicity, and chronic antibody-mediated rejection. A kidney biopsy is necessary to rule out any reversible causes of declining kidney function. Consideration should be given to reducing the dose or eliminating the CNI. Replacing the CNI with mTor is another treatment option (KDIGO, 2009).

Table 3.2

Immunosuppressive Medications

Name of Agent	Purpose	Dose	Method of Administration	Side Effects
Alemtuzumab (Campath®) Recombinant DNA-derived humanized monoclonal antibody (unlabeled use in transplant)	Induction therapy	30 mg	Intravenously over 2 hours as a single dose at the time of transplant. Premedicate with diphenhydramine 50 mg and acetaminophen 500–1000 mg 30 minutes before each infusion. Currently only available through Campath® distribution program	*Rare:* Anaphylactoid/hypersensitivity reaction Flu-like symptoms Anemia Leukopenia Thrombocytopenia Dizziness Hyper/hypotension Headache Nausea Dyspepsia Stomatitis Skin irritation Opportunistic infections
Antithymocyte globulin (Thymoglobulin®) (rabbit) Polyclonal antibody preparation	Induction or rescue therapy (unlabeled use)	Based on adequacy of WBC/platelet/lymphocyte count Induction: 1.5–2.5 mg/kg daily for 5–10 days or per center protocol. Treatment of acute rejection: 1.5 mg/kg/day for 7–14 days or per center protocol.	Premedicate with diphenhydramine and acetaminophen and, for first dose, with corticosteroids. Intravenous infusion with in-line 0.22 micron filter over 6 hours (first dose) through central line. Subsequent doses may be given over 4 hours. May be given at a slow rate peripherally when mixed with heparin and hydrocortisone	Anaphylaxis Cytokine release syndrome Fever and hyperpyrexia Hypo/hypertension Opportunistic infections Increased incidence of malignancy Hematologic toxicity: neutropenia; thrombocytopenia
Azathioprine (Imuran®) Generic available	Maintenance immunosuppression	1–3 mg/kg/day orally maintenance 50 mg tablets 100 mg vials for IV use	Orally IV as indicated	Bone marrow suppression: anemia thrombocytopenia bleeding leukopenia Hair thinning and loss Infections Gastrointestinal problems Mouth ulcers Hepatic dysfunction; hepatitis Malignancies
Basiliximab (Simulect®) Anti-Interleukin-2 receptor humanized monoclonal antibody	Induction therapy	20 mg	Intravenously through a peripheral vein. Administered day of transplant and postop day 4.	*Rare:* Anaphylactoid/hypersensitivity reaction Flu-like syndrome Opportunistic infections Increased incidence of diabetes
Belatacept (Nulojix®) Selective T-cell costimulation blocker	Maintenance therapy	Dosing based on actual body weight at time of transplantation. If change in weight is > 10%, dosing will change. Prescribed dose must be evenly divisible by 12.5 mg Initial phase: 10/mg/kg/dose on Day 1 and Day 5, Week 2, 4, 8, and 12 following transplantation Maintenance phase: 5 mg/kg/dose q 4 weeks beginning at Week 16	IV infusion over 30 minutes using a 0.2–1.2 micron low protein-binding filter	Increased incidence of lymphoproliferative disorders, and therefore contraindicated in EBV negative patients. Increased incidence of other malignancy and infections Anemia Leukopenia Constipation Diarrhea Nausea, vomiting Fever Headache Hyper/hypotension Hyper/hypokalemia Peripheral edema Urinary tract infection *Rare:* hypersensitivity reactions

Table continues

Table 3.2

Immunosuppressive Medications (page 2 of 3)

Name of Agent	Purpose	Dose	Method of Administration	Side Effects
Cyclophosphamide (Cytoxan®) (Rarely used)	Maintenance immunosuppression if unable to tolerate azathioprine or mycophenolic acid. Used in nontransplant patients with immune-mediated disease	50–75 mg/day	Orally once a day in the morning Available as intravenous solution	Leukopenia Thrombocytopenia Bladder fibrosis GI disturbances Hemorrhagic cystitis Bladder cancer (periodic cystoscopic screening per center protocol)
Cyclosporine Generics available Modified: Neoral®, Gengraf® Cyclosporine modified-micro-emulsion allowing for more consistent absorption. Nonmodified: Sandimmune® Variable rate of absorption. Use same dose to convert from one formulation to another and adjust dose to attain appropriate therapeutic trough level. (Lexicomp, 2013)	Maintenance immunosuppression	Adjusted to serum drug levels per center protocol; usually 3–4 mg/kg as maintenance dose. 25 mg and 100 mg capsules Also available in oral and intravenous solutions	Usually twice daily dosing based on trough level	Nephrotoxicity Hepatotoxicity Hand tremors Hypertrichosis Gingival hyperplasia Seizures Flushing Hyperesthesia Nausea/vomiting Anorexia Diarrhea Feeling of fullness Headaches Mild anemia Hyperkalemia Hypertension Malignancies Hirsutism Hyperlipidemia
Methylprednisolone Prednisone	Oral maintenance and IV induction and rescue immunosuppression	Oral maintenance: 0.2 mg/kg Methylprednisolone: 4 mg, 8 mg, 16 mg, 32 mg tablets Prednisone: 2.5 mg, 5 mg, 10 mg, 20 mg, 50 mg tablets IV induction and rescue dosing per center protocol	Intravenous for induction or rescue. Oral taper in divided doses, then daily for maintenance	Cushingoid appearance Increased appetite Na^+/H_2O retention Hypertension Peptic ulcers Easy bruising Impaired wound healing Acne Diaphoresis Infections Hyperlipidemia Osteoporosis Avascular joint necrosis Diabetes Cataracts Pancreatitis Anemia Thrombocytopenia Leukopenia Mood lability Increased incidence of malignancies
Mycophenolate mofetil (CellCept®) Generics available Mycophenolic acid delayed release (Myfortic ®) Generic available	Maintenance immunosuppression	Based on GI tolerance and WBC. Mycophenolate mofetil 250 mg, 500 mg capsules 1000–1500 mg twice daily Also available in an oral suspension 200 mg/mL Mycophenolic acid delayed release 180 mg, 360 mg tablets 720–1040 mg twice daily	Orally twice daily	Bone marrow suppression: anemia leukopenia thrombocytopenia GI distress

Table continues

Table 3.2

Immunosuppressive Medications (page 3 of 3)

Name of Agent	Purpose	Dose	Method of Administration	Side Effects
Rituximab (Rituxan®)	Treatment of antibody-mediated acute rejection (unlabeled use)	Per center protocol. Approximately 375 mg/m²	Pretreatment with acetaminophen and diphenhydramine is recommended. Start infusion at 50 mg/hr, if no reaction, increase rate by 50 mg/hr increments every 30 minutes, to maximum rate of 400 mg/hour	Infusion hypersensitivity reactions (occasionally fatal) Serious and potentially fatal infections Bowel obstruction/perforation Hepatitis B virus reactivation Mucocutaneous reactions Progressive multifocal leukoencephalopathy Peripheral edema Hyper/hypotension Fever, chills Fatigue Headache Nausea, diarrhea
Sirolimus (Rapamune ®)	Maintenance immunosuppression	Adjust to serum trough concentrations per center protocol. 0.5 mg, 1 mg and 2 mg tablets Available in oral solution 1 mg/mL	Orally once daily	Hyperlipidemia Hypercholesterolemia Diarrhea Anemia Arthralgia Acne Thrombocytopenia Delayed wound healing Mouth sores Rash
Tacrolimus (Prograf®, Hecoria®) Immediate release Generics available	Maintenance immunosuppression	Adjusted to trough level per center protocol. 0.1-0.2 mg/kg in two divided doses 0.5 mg, 1 mg, 5 mg capsules Available in an intravenous solution	Orally twice daily	Nephrotoxicity Hypertension Diabetes Infections Neurotoxicity: Tremors Tingling in hands or feet Paresthesias Insomnia Headache Tinnitus Visual light sensitivity Sleep disturbances/nightmares Mood changes Increased incidence of malignancies
Tacrolimus extended release (Astagraf XL ®)		Adjusted to trough level per center protocol 0.15–0.2 mg/kg/once daily 0.5 mg, 1 mg, 5 mg capsules	Orally once daily in the morning	

Source: Lexicomp®, 2013.

D. Antibody-mediated rejection is caused by donor specific antibodies. The criteria for antibody-mediated rejection include positive C4D stain, circulating donor-specific antibodies, and graft biopsy revealing polymorphonuclear cells in the peritubular capillaries. Treatment options for antibody-mediated rejection include plasma exchange, intravenous immunoglobulin, anti-CD20 antibody, and lymphocyte-depleting antibodies (KDIGO, 2009).

XIV. Graft monitoring.

Serum creatinine is measured frequently in the early postoperative period and then less frequently as the recipient is further out from the date of surgery. After the acute period, serum creatinine is measured every 2 weeks for 4 to 6 weeks, monthly for months 7 to 12, and thereafter every 2 to 3 months. Urine protein excretion is measured in the first month postoperatively, every 3 months during the first year, and annually thereafter (KDIGO, 2009).

XV. Nonadherence.

Nonadherence is defined as "deviation from the prescribed medication regimen sufficient to adversely influence the regimen's intended effect" (Fine et al., 2009, p. 36). Education throughout the transplant continuum is imperative in addressing nonadherence.

Table 3.3

Possible Drug-Drug Interactions Related to the Cytochrome P-450 System 3A (CYP3A4) Isozyme Substrates *

CYP3A4 Substrates	CYP3A4 Inhibitors	CYP3A4 Inducers
Alprazolam	Amiodarone	Carbamazepine
Amiodarone	Amprenavir	Dexamethasone
Amlodipine	Aprepitant	Efavirenz
Atazanavir	Atazanavir	Naficillin
Atorvastatin	Clarithromycin	Phenobarbital
Buprenorphine	Conivaptan	Phenytoin
Bupropion	Cyclosporine	Rifabutin
Carbamazepine	Darunavir	Rifampin
Clarithromycin	Diltiazem	St. John's wort
Clonazepam	Erythromycin	
Clopidogrel	Fluconazole	
Colchicine	Fluoxetine	
Cyclophosphamide	Fosamprenavir	
Cyclosporine	Grapefruit Juice	
Dapsone	Isoniazid	
Diltiazem	Itraconazole	
Efavirenz	Ketoconazole	
Eplerenone	Posaconazole	
Erythromycin	Ritonavir	
Everolimus	Saquinavir	
Fentanyl	Verapamil	
Finasteride	Voriconazole	
Indinavir		
Itraconazole		
Ketoconazole		
Lopinavir		
Midazolam		
Nicardipine		
Nifedipine		
Oxycodone		
Paricalcitol		
Pioglitazone		
Ritonavir		
Saquinavir		
Sildenafil		
Simvastatin		
Sirolimus		
Tacrolimus		
Tadalafil		
Tamsulosin		
Topiramate		
Verapamil		

* Not an all-inclusive list
   CYP3A4 substrates will compete with each other at the active-binding site of the CYP3A4 isozyme; theoretically, concentrations of both medications may increase.
   CYP3A4 inhibitors prevent metabolism of CYP3A4 substrates resulting in increased concentrations of substrate-medications.
   CYP3A4 inducers may enhance the metabolism of CYP3A4 substrates resulting in decreased concentrations of substrate-medications.
(Adapted from Horn & Hansen, 2008).

Nonadherence is a significant cause of graft loss; therefore, it is important to use a team approach. Identification of those recipients who are at risk for nonadherence and increased monitoring of these individuals is recommended.

XVI. Infection.

Infection is a common problem postkidney transplantation, and recipients' presentations are often atypical due to their dampened immune response. Therefore, clinicians need to maintain a high level of suspicion and conduct early investigation to allow for better patient outcomes.

A. BK polyoma virus (BKV).
   1. BKV can cause kidney dysfunction and graft failure.
   2. All recipients should be screened for BKV with quantitative plasma NAT.
   3. Reduction in immunosuppression is the main therapeutic modality.
   4. Consideration can be given to antiviral therapies.

B. Cytomegalovirus (CMV).
   1. CMV is a common cause of morbidity and mortality postkidney transplant.
   2. Chemoprophylaxis strategy is the use of valganciclovir for at least 3 months posttransplant.
   3. Surveillance strategy is the monitoring of viral loads at predefined intervals.
   4. CMV disease can present as viremia or tissue invasive disease, and the extent of the disease determines treatment.

C. Epstein-Barr virus (EBV).
   1. EBV is associated with posttransplant lymphoproliferative disease.
   2. Reduction in immunosuppression is the mainstay of therapy.

D. Herpes simplex virus (HSV) 1 and 2 and varicella-zoster virus (VZV). Antiviral therapies are used according to clinical presentation.

E. *Pneumocystis jirovechi* pneumonia (PCP). All kidney transplant recipients should receive prophylaxis with trimethoprim-sulfamethoxazole for 3 to 6 months after transplantation.

F. Urinary tract infections (UTI). Kidney recipients should receive trimethoprim-sulfametoxazole for at least 6 months posttransplant for UTI prophylaxis (KDIGO, 2009).

XVII. Malignancy.

Kidney transplant recipients are at an increased risk for both common and uncommon cancers. Skin cancer and lymphoma are related to the immunosuppressive agents used posttransplant.

A. Routine health screening is critical for early detection of malignancy.

B. Patient education regarding symptoms to report will aid in early recognition.

C. When a malignancy has been diagnosed, posttransplant immunosuppression needs to be reduced in conjunction with oncologic care (KDIGO, 2009).

XVIII. Managing cardiac risk factors.

Cardiovascular disease is a major cause of morbidity and mortality after kidney transplant. Recipient pretransplant risk factors are often compounded by side effects of immunosuppressive medications. Therefore, vigilance must be taken in addressing each cardiac risk factor and driving efforts toward meeting treatment targets. A transplant nurse practitioner is in a key position to coordinate care among the many specialists involved in the care of the transplant recipient. Coordination of care allows for better outcomes and improved patient satisfaction.

A. Posttransplant hypertension.
1. Lifestyle modification should be initiated in the prekidney transplant phase and be a part of all transplant related visits.
2. Multiple medication regimens are often needed to achieve target levels posttransplant.
3. Consider adding ACE-I or ARB when urine protein excretion is > 1g/day (KDIGO, 2009).

B. Posttransplant diabetes.
1. Blood sugars are variable in the early postoperative period as dosages of immunosuppressive agents are altered.
2. Patient education is critical toward the goal of glycemic control.
3. Integration of a diabetologist into patient's care team in important.
4. Insulin is often required to achieve target levels (KDIGO, 2009).

C. Dyslipidemia.
1. Medication therapy is routinely needed to achieve target levels.
2. Treatment strategies are based on the KDOQI Dyslipidemia Recommendations (KDIGO, 2009).

D. Obesity.
1. BMI should be measured at every visit.
2. Weight reduction programs should be offered to all obese kidney transplant recipients (KDIGO, 2009).

E. Smoking cessation. Assistance with smoking cessation should be addressed at each visit (KDIGO, 2009).

XIX. Metabolic bone disease (MBD).

A. Monitor serum calcium, phosphorous, and PTH levels.

B. Consider treating with vitamin D, calcitriol/alfacalcidiol, or bisphosphonates if eGFR is greater than 30.

C. Consider bone biopsy.

D. Postkidney transplant recipients with MBD and CKD stages 4 to 5 should be managed as the patient who is on kidney replacement therapy (KDIGO, 2009).

XX. Hematologic complications.

A. Posttransplant erythrocytosis. ACE-I or ARBs are first-line therapy.

B. Anemias.
1. CBC with differential should be monitored.
2. Evaluate for underlying causes.
3. Review medications for potential causes (KDIGO, 2009).

XXI. Psychological functioning.

A. Adjustment disorder is common posttransplant and should be screened for in routine visits.

B. Immunosuppressive medications may alter mood and coping.

C. Kidney transplant recipients may need to adapt to the loss of their network associated with a dialysis unit.

D. Kidney transplant recipients may need to adjust to the loss of the sick role and changes in their social roles posttransplant.

E. An interdisciplinary approach is required to meet the mental health needs of the postkidney transplant recipient.

I. CKD Stage 5 as defined by the National Kidney Foundation – Kidney Dialysis Outcomes Quality Initiative and by the KDIGO 2012 Clinical Practice Guidelines for the Evaluation and Management of Chronic Kidney Disease (NKF/KDOQI) (KDIGO, 2012; NKF/KDOQI, 2002).

A. Severely decreased estimated glomerular filtration rate (eGFR) as determined by a validated measuring method.
   1. Cockcroft-Gault.
   2. Modification of Diet in Renal Disease either 4 or 6 variables.
   3. 2009 CKD-EPI creatinine equation (KDIGO, 2012).

B. eGFR of < 15 mL/min/1.73 m^2.

II. Hemodialysis – removal of waste products and water from the blood while maintaining electrolyte balance by diffusion and osmosis through a semipermeable membrane as the blood is being circulated outside the body (Henrich, 2009) (Schmidt & Holley, 2012).

A. Solute removal.
   1. Diffusion – movement of a molecule from an area of higher solute concentration to lower solute concentration across a semipermeable membrane (dialyzer membrane).
   2. This is affected by the following.
      a. Molecule size.
      b. Dialysate membrane pore size.
      c. Concentration of molecules on blood side vs. dialysate side of membrane.
      d. Countercurrent flow – blood and dialysate flow going in opposite directions, thus keeping the diffusion gradient in the blood higher than in the dialysate.
   3. Convective transport.
      a. Augments diffusion.
      b. Solutes are dragged along with the fluid as it moves across the dialysate membrane.

B. Water removal.
   1. Ultrafiltration.
   2. This is affected by the following.
      a. Osmosis.
         (1) Removal of water across the semipermeable membrane.
         (2) Moves from area of lesser solute to higher solute.
         (3) Osmotic pressure – opposes water movement and is done by the plasma proteins.
      b. Hydraulic pressure – pressure exerted on the membrane to force water from one compartment to another.
         (1) On the blood side, due to the positive pressure as measured by the venous pressure.
         (2) On the dialysate side, due to the negative pressure applied by the dialysis machine to draw water from the blood side.
      c. Two forces combined are called the transmembrane pressure (TMP).

III. Hemodialysis prescription.

A. Dialysis machine (Schmidt & Holley, 2012).
   1. Allows the dialysis to take place and to monitor its safety.
   2. This includes the following.
      a. Blood pump to move blood between the patient and the dialyzer.
      b. Delivery system to transport the dialysis solution to the dialyzer.
      c. Monitoring devices.
         (1) Venous pressure monitor.
         (2) Arterial pressure monitor.
         (3) Conductivity monitor – ensuring that the dialysate solution is appropriately portioned.
         (4) Temperature sensor.
         (5) Blood pressure monitor.
   3. Numerous brands and unit-specific.

B. Dialysis solution (Schmidt & Holley, 2012).
   1. The characteristics of the dialysate are vital for a safe and effective dialysis treatment.
   2. Free of metabolic waste products.
   3. The dialysis machine mixes the different components with water to produce the final product.
   4. Water.
      a. Needs to be purified to remove the potential contaminants such as aluminum, copper, chloramine, bacteria, and endotoxins.
      b. Several different types of purification are used with reverse osmosis being most common.
   5. Sodium.
      a. Generally 136 to 140 meq/L.
      b. Can be adjusted by the machine.
      c. Sodium modeling.
         (1) Being used less often due to potential for increased interdialytic thirst and fluid gain.
         (2) The sodium may be increased in an attempt to achieve hemodynamic control.

6. Potassium content ordered to meet the needs of the patient based on current laboratory values.
   a. K–0 or no potassium is used only in cases of severe hyperkalemia and is used cautiously to prevent hypokalemia. It can only be considered if safety measures are in place such as cardiac monitoring or in an intensive patient monitoring environment, even if used for just part of the HD treatment.
   b. K–1 to K–3 are most common concentrations of potassium used. Solutions come commercially prepared.
   c. K–4 used in cases of hypokalemia and used cautiously because not commercially prepared and requires adding potassium to the solution.
7. Calcium – between 2.0 and 3.0 meq/L commercially prepared.
8. Magnesium – between 0.5 and 1.0 meq/L and rarely manipulated.
9. Glucose – between 150 and 200 mg/dL.
10. Bicarbonate.
    a. Used to buffer the dialysate solution.
    b. Can be varied between 30 and 40meq/L dependent on patient.
11. Considerations for prescription.
    a. Interpret patient's current laboratory values.
    b. Availability of the solutions.

C. Dialyzers (hollow fibers that are like capillaries) (Schmidt & Holley, 2012).
   1. Two compartments – blood side and dialysate side.
   2. Fibers that are bundled together are porous and serve as the dialyzer's semipermeable membrane.
   3. Factors that can affect the dialyzer's performance.
      a. Type of membrane (e.g., synthetic, cellulose, or modified cellulose).
      b. Membrane surface area.
      c. Blood volume capacity.
      d. Ultrafiltration coefficient and predictability for the removal of water.
      e. Pore size and distribution that affects the clearance of the waste products.
      f. Resistance to clotting.
      g. Biocompatibility – the ability to induce a mild inflammatory response.
   4. Numerous brands and are unit-specific.
   5. Considerations for prescription.
      a. NKF/KDOQI target for Kt/V_{urea}: minimum of 1.3 (NKF, 2006b).
      b. Availability of dialyzers.
      c. Patient characteristics.
      d. Dialyzer characteristics.
      e. Type of delivery system to be used.

D. Vascular access (Bander & Schwab, 2012; Henrichs, 2013; Oliver, 2012).

1. Double-lumen temporary hemodialysis catheter that can be inserted in various sites.
   a. Femoral vein.
   b. Subclavian vein.
   c. Internal jugular vein.
2. Permanent vascular accesses.
   a. Arteriovenous fistula (AVF).
      (1) Considered to be the best form of vascular access.
      (2) Created by side-to-side or end-to-side vein to artery anastomosis.
      (3) Cephalic vein to radial artery at the wrist.
      (4) Brachial artery to cephalic vein at elbow.
      (5) Brachial artery to basilic vein at the elbow.
   b. Synthetic arteriovenous grafts (AVG).
      (1) Generally polytetrafluoroethylene (PTFE) material.
      (2) Forearm loop graft – brachial artery to basilic vein.
      (3) Forearm straight graft – distal radial artery to basilic vein.
      (4) Upper arm graft – brachial artery to basilic or cephalic vein.
      (5) Chest wall – axillary artery to axillary vein or axillary artery to jugular vein.
      (6) Thigh – femoral artery to femoral vein.
   c. Tunneled cuffed catheters.
      (1) Double-lumen synthetic catheter with a felt cuff.
      (2) Inserted through a subcutaneous tunnel.
      (3) Done under ultrasound and fluoroscopy guidance.
      (4) Placement.
         (a) Internal jugular vein (most common and on the right).
         (b) External jugular vein.
         (c) Subclavian vein.
         (d) Femoral vein.
      (5) Not intended to be used for long-term use.

E. Duration of treatment – prescription considerations.
   1. Patient characteristics.
   2. NKF/KDOQI target for Kt/V_{urea}: minimum of 1.3 (opinion-based) (NKF, 2006b).
   3. Current laboratory values.
   4. Dialyzer characteristics.
   5. Type of delivery system.
   6. Patient's fluid and cardiovascular status.

F. Flow rates – considerations for prescription.
   1. Blood flow rate (BFR).
      a. To achieve the NKF/KDOQI Kt/V_{urea} target.
      b. Type of vascular access to be used.
      c. Patient characteristics to include, but not limited to, cardiovascular status.
      d. Solutes to be removed.

(1) Small solutes will reach a plateau once a certain rate is achieved.

(2) Large solutes will always maintain a gradient.

2. Dialysate flow rate (DFR).
   a. To achieve the NKF/KDOQI Kt/V_{urea} target.
   b. Type of delivery system.
   c. BFR that can be achieved.
      (1) Lower BFR (300) required lower DFR (500) to maintain gradient.
      (2) Higher BFR (500) required higher DFR (800) to maintain gradient.

G. Anticoagulation (Kovalik, 2013).
   1. When blood comes in contact with the foreign surfaces of the dialysis system, such as the bloodlines and dialyzer, the clotting mechanism is activated.
   2. Heparin, usually porcine, is the most common drug used for anticoagulation.
      a. Bolus given at beginning of treatment and an infusion given throughout the remainder of the treatment.
      b. Bolus at beginning of treatment and extra boluses given during the treatment.
   3. Other anticoagulation options are:
      a. Heparin free.
      b. Regional citrate-anticoagulation used in acute situations.
   4. Considerations for prescription.
      a. Comorbid conditions that might affect bleeding.
      b. Type of access to be used.
      c. Patient medications and possible interactions.
      d. Allergies.
      e. Patient's size – heparin is dosed by patient's body weight.

H. Fluid removal/estimated dry weight – considerations for prescription include assessment of patient's volume status to include but not be limited to the following.
   1. Edema.
   2. Blood pressure.
   3. Cardiovascular status.
   4. Breath sounds, respiratory rate.
   5. Jugular venous distention.
   6. Patient complaints, i.e., dyspnea, orthopnea, orthostatic hypotension.
   7. Recent laboratory data.
   8. Characteristics of dialyzer to be used.
   9. Amount of time for dialysis.

I. Medications to be given during the hemodialysis treatment – considerations for prescription.
   1. Erythropoiesis-stimulating agents such as erythropoietin alfa or darbepoietin alfa.

a. NKF/KDOQI guidelines and goals of therapy: hemoglobin (Hgb) 11 to 12 g/dL (evidence-based) (NKF/KDOQI, 2007).
      b. Current laboratory data for hemoglobin/hematocrit.
      c. Manufacturer's product insert for dosing guidelines.
      d. Medicare guidelines for maximum dosing and reimbursement.
      e. Unit-specific protocols.
   2. Vitamin D analogs.
      a. NKF/KDOQI guidelines and goals for therapy (NKF/KDOQI, 2003).
      b. Intact parathyroid hormone (PTH) results.
      c. Corrected serum calcium level.
      d. Serum phosphorus level.
      e. Manufacturer's product insert for dosing guidelines.
      f. Unit-specific protocols.
   3. Iron replacement therapy.
      a. NKF/KDOQI guidelines and goals of therapy: Transferrin saturation (TSAT) > 20% and Ferritin > 200 ng/dL (evidence based) (NKF, 2006b).
      b. Current laboratory values for iron, TSAT, and ferritin.
      c. Signs and symptoms of inflammatory or infectious process.
      d. Type of iron infusion product to be used.
      e. Manufacturer's product insert for dosing guidelines.
      f. Unit-specific protocols.
   4. Laboratory values to be drawn.
      a. Data to monitor adequacy of therapy for clearances, anemia, mineral bone disease.
      b. Data to monitor patient specific illness, i.e. diabetes.
      c. Electrolytes.
      d. Unit-specific protocols.

IV. Interventions for complications during dialysis to include, but not limited to, the following (Russell, 2008; Henrich, 2013).

A. Pruritus.
   1. Antihistamines.
   2. Lotions.
   3. Evaluate for serum phosphorus control and educate as needed.

B. Nausea and vomiting.
   1. Antiemetics.
   2. Normal saline if related to hypotension.

C. Hypotension.
   1. Normal saline bolus.
   2. Decrease ultrafiltration and blood flow rate.

3. Medication review of hypertensive medications and assess timing of drugs in relation to treatment times. Educate as needed.
4. Salt poor albumin infusion in acute situations, generally not available in outpatient situations but is available in hospital or intensive care units.
5. Assess appropriateness of estimated dry weight listed.
6. Assess for excessive weight gain and need for patient education of its consequences.
7. Avoid eating during dialysis treatments.
8. Midodrine prior to treatment.

D. Cramping.
   1. Normal saline bolus.
   2. Decrease ultrafiltration.
   3. Pressure on extremity with cramp.

V. Ongoing assessment and management of the hemodialysis patient (NKF, 2006b; Russell, 2008).

A. Vascular access.
   1. AVF or AVG to include but not limited to the following.
      a. Pain or tenderness.
      b. Sensations of coldness, numbness, tingling in access extremity.
      c. Bleeding or drainage from cannulation sites.
      d. Swelling
      e. Fever or chills.
      f. Erythema.
      g. Bruising or hematoma.
      h. Rash.
      i. Aneurysm or pseudoaneurysm.
      j. Auscultation for bruit noting changes in pitch and amplitude.
      k. Pressures recorded during dialysis.
   2. Hemodialysis catheter.
      a. Absence of facial or neck edema.
      b. Erythema at exit site or along tunnel.
      c. Induration or swelling at exit site.
      d. Bruising.
      e. Rashes.
      f. Bleeding or drainage at exit site.
      g. Fever or chills.
      h. Respiratory distress.
      i. Catheter occlusion by thrombus or fibrin sheath.
      j. Integrity of catheter.

B. Dialysis adequacy (NKF, 2006b) (Russell, 2008).
   1. Assessment – to include but not limited to the following.
      a. Interpret results of kinetic modeling.
      b. Review NKF/KDOQI Clinical Guidelines for Hemodialysis Adequacy (NKF, 2006b).
      c. Assess for signs and symptoms of dialysis inadequacy.

d. Monitor prescribed and delivered dose of treatment.
e. Monitor patient's response to treatments.
f. Monitor patient's adherence to dialysis prescription.
g. Assess patient's residual kidney function.
h. Monitor vascular access function.
i. Assess patient's cardiovascular status.
j. Monitor patient's nutritional status.
k. Monitor patient's anemia status.
l. Evaluate technical difficulties during treatment.

2. Interventions.
   a. Adjust the dialysis prescription to achieve target Kt/V_{urea}.
   b. Adjust the dialysis prescription based on patient's response to treatment and kinetic modeling date.
   c. Adjustments to the dialysis prescription could include but not limited to: change in dialyzer, increase/decrease in BFR or DFR, increase/decrease in treatment time, change in gauge of dialysis needle to achieve prescribed BFR.
   d. Initiate consults or referrals as necessary, i.e. vascular surgeon, interventional radiology, social work services.
   e. If indicated, educate patient regarding adherence to dialysis prescription.

C. Anemia.
   1. Assessment.
      a. Interpret current laboratory values to include Hgb and iron panel and achievement of the target goals set.
      b. Monitor patient's response to therapy.
      c. Monitor hypo-response and its causes.
         (1) Inflammation or infection.
         (2) Blood loss.
         (3) Secondary hyperparathyroidism.
         (4) Vitamin deficiencies to include B12 or folic acid.
         (5) Cancers.
         (6) Malnutrition.
         (7) Inadequate dialysis dose.
         (8) Medication interactions.
   2. Intervention.
      a. Treat anemia according to the NKF/KDOQI guidelines (NKF, 2006a).
      b. Adjust medication based on patient's response as discerned from current laboratory values.
      c. Order laboratory or diagnostic tests as indicated to rule out causes of hypo-response.
      d. Initiate a consult to hematology if cause of hyporesponse not easily identified.

D. Estimated dry weight/volume and fluid status.
   1. Assessment.
      a. Patient's response to therapy.
      b. Interpretation of current laboratory values.
      c. Assess fluid status as outlined in the initial determination of dry weight.
      d. Assess patient's understanding of fluid control to include the role of other factors such as sodium intake.
   2. Interventions.
      a. Adjust prescription to achieve the assessed goal.
      b. Educate patient in fluid control and benefits.
      c. Initiate a consult with interdisciplinary team if indicated.
      d. Order additional diagnostic and laboratory tests as indicated.

E. Hypertension.
   1. NKF/KODQI Guideline 12 of Clinical Practice Guidelines for Cardiovascular Disease in Dialysis Patients (NKF/KODQI, 2005).
      a. Factors implicated in the pathogenesis of hypertension in dialysis patients.
         (1) Sodium and volume excess.
         (2) Increased activity of vasoconstrictors.
            (a) The renin-angiotensin-aldosterone system.
            (b) The sympathetic nervous system.
            (c) Endothelin.
            (d) Ouabain-like substances.
         (3) Decreased activity of vasodilators.
            (a) Nitric oxide.
            (b) Kinins.
            (c) Atrial natriuretic peptides.
         (4) Erythropoietin use.
         (5) Divalent ions and parathyroid hormone.
         (6) Structural changes in the arteries.
         (7) Preexisting essential hypertension.
         (8) Renovascular disease.
         (9) Miscellaneous: anemia, AVF, vasopressin, serotonin, calcitonin gene-related peptide.
      b. Measurement of blood pressure (BP).
         (1) If patient had multiple vascular surgeries on upper extremities, then it is permissible to use the thigh or legs.
         (2) Must always make sure the right size cuff is being used and checked in supine position if other than arms.
      c. Prehemodialysis and posthemodialysis BP goals should be < 140/90 mmHg and < 130/80 mmHg respectively.
      d. Management of hypertension requires interventions in both fluid management and adjustments of antihypertensive medication therapy.
         (1) Fluid management.
            (a) Low sodium intake (2 to 3 gm/day).

(b) Increased ultrafiltration.
(c) Longer dialysis.
(d) More than three treatments a week.
(e) Assess patient's knowledge and understanding of the need to manage fluid and the consequences of not doing so.
(f) Referral to dietician for further education and counseling as needed.
         (2) Interventions with antihypertensive medications.
            (a) Drugs that inhibit the renin-angiotensin system.
            (b) Give at night to reduce the nocturnal surge of BP and minimize intradialytic hypotension.
            (c) Assess the dialyzability of the antihypertensive medications, using the guideline list when possible; the list is limited, as it is not comprehensive to all medications available.
               i. Angiotensin-converting enzyme inhibitors listed where partially removed, with lisinopril being at 50%.
               ii. Angiotensin-receptor-blockers listed where not removed with dialysis.
               iii. Beta blockers are removed with dialysis with exception of carvedilol.
               iv. Calcium channel blockers have a low removal profile.
               v. Vasodilators – minoxidil is removed but hydralazine is not.
   2. 2014 Evidence-Based Guidelines for the Management of High Blood Pressure in Adults (JNC8) does not address specifically the patient with CKD Stage 5 on hemodialysis but does include suggestions for therapy that are applicable, including drug therapy for different populations (e.g., persons with diabetes, African Americans) (James et al., 2014).
      a. Target for therapy for patients with CKD > 140/90.
      b. Assess for other identifiable causes of hypertension other than chronic kidney disease.
         (1) Sleep apnea.
         (2) Drug induced or related.
         (3) Primary aldosteronism.
         (4) Cushing syndrome or steroid therapy.
         (5) Pheochromocytoma.
         (6) Coaractation of the aorta.
         (7) Thyroid disease.
         (8) Review over-the-counter drugs that are being used.

c. Lifestyle modifications.
  (1) Weight reduction.
  (2) Aerobic physical activity as tolerated.
  (3) Moderation of alcohol consumption.
  (4) Dietary reduction in content of saturated and total fat.
  (5) Smoking cessation.

F. Mineral bone disease (Russell, 2008).
  1. Assessment.
     a. Interpret current laboratory values to include but not limited to: calcium, phosphorous, and intact PTH level.
     b. Assess patient's response to therapy.
     c. Assess patient's knowledge regarding the therapies prescribed.
     d. Assess patient's adherence to therapy.
     e. Monitor for financial considerations to adherence to therapy.
  2. Interventions.
     a. Adjust therapy to meet the goals set to NKF/KDOQI guidelines.
     b. Add or decrease phosphorous binder doses.
     c. Adjust Vitamin D analog doses.
     d. Add or adjust calcimemetic drug dose.
     e. Educate patient regarding bone metabolism and the expected results of therapy and benefits of the therapy.
     f. Initiate referrals to interdisciplinary team if needed.

G. Nutrition (Russell, 2008).
  1. Assessment.
     a. Interpret current laboratory values.
     b. Assess patient's response to current prescribed diet.
     c. Assess patient's knowledge regarding diet.
     d. Assess comorbid conditions that could influence nutritional status.
     e. Assess patient's functional status.
     f. Assess financial considerations that might impact nutrition.
  2. Intervention.
     a. Order further laboratory or diagnostic tests as indicated.
     b. Educate patient regarding nutritional needs.
     c. Initiate referrals to interdisciplinary team if indicated.
     d. Prescribe nutritional supplements as indicated.

H. Dyslipidemia and reduction of cardiovascular risk factors (Russell, 2008).
  1. Assessment.
     a. Interpret current laboratory values.
     b. Assess patient's cardiovascular risk status.
     c. Assess patient's knowledge of lipid control and other lifestyle changes to reduce cardiovascular risk, i.e., cigarette cessation, weight reduction, exercise.
  2. Intervention.
     a. Order further laboratory or diagnostic tests as indicated.
     b. Educate regarding lipid control and lifestyle changes.
     c. Refer to dietician as indicated.
     d. Prescribe therapies to achieve the Adult Treatment Panel III (ATP III)/NKF/KDOQI guidelines for dyslipidemia (National Cholesterol Education Program, 2004; NKF/KDOQI, 2003).
        (1) LDL < 100.
           (a) Therapeutic lifestyle changes (TLC).
           (b) HMG-Co A reductase inhibitors (statins).
        (2) Triglycerides < 180.
           (a) Fibrates.
           (b) Omega 3 fatty acids.
           (c) Niacin.

I. Diabetes mellitus (Russell, 2008).
  1. Assessment.
     a. Review related laboratory values, i.e., hemoglobin A1C and blood glucose levels.
     b. Response to prescribed therapy.
     c. Review patient's reported blood sugars.
     d. Assess for diabetic complications.
     e. Assess knowledge of disease and the patient's management of diabetes.
  2. Intervention.
     a. Educate patient regarding the disease and management and refer to diabetes educator if further education is indicated.
     b. Adjust medications to achieve the American Diabetes Association (ADA) goals for therapy: Hemoglobin A1C < 7% (ADA, 2013).
     c. Refer to endocrinologist, diabetologist, or primary care provider if management of patient's diabetes is provided by these practices.
     d. Order additional laboratory test or diagnostic tests as indicated.
     e. Initiate consults and referrals to assume care of diabetes if indicated or to treat complications.
     f. Prescribe therapies to alleviate or treat complications such as listed for neuropathy.
        (1) Tricyclic antidepressants.
        (2) Anti-seizure medications.
        (3) Anti-Parkinson's medications.

J. Transplantation (Russell, 2008).
  1. Assessment.
     a. Comprehensive history and physical.
     b. Determine if any absolute contraindications to transplant.
     c. Review patient's psychosocial status to include support.

2. Intervention – Refer to transplant center for further evaluation and determination of candidacy.

K. Cancer screening (Holley, 2013).
   1. Patients on dialysis are at risk for developing certain types of cancers such as renal cell carcinomas.
   2. Relatively rare cause of death among dialysis patients.
   3. Weigh the cost of large screenings and the survival benefit.
   4. Studies have shown net gain of life expectancy in patients with kidney failure via screening programs is low.
   5. Should be continued for those who are transplant candidates.

L. Functional status.
   1. Assessment: baseline functional status to current status.
   2. Intervention: initiate referrals to interdisciplinary team to ensure optimal status obtained.

M. Psychosocial.
   1. Assessment.
      a. Patient coping mechanisms.
      b. Family coping mechanisms.
   2. Intervention.
      a. Provide support.
      b. Initiate referrals to the interdisciplinary team as indicated.

SECTION C

Approaches to Care by the APRN in Hemodialysis Access

Donna Bednarski

I. Introduction.

The role of the advanced practice registered nurse in dialysis access is critical to the creation and maintenance of the ideal dialysis access. Ensuring a dialysis access that delivers adequate flow rates, long use life with low rate of complications (NKF/KDOQI, 2002) requires constant attention.

II. Preop evaluation for permanent hemodialysis access.

Adequate planning allows sufficient time for the creation of a functional permanent access at the time of initiation of dialysis.

A. Referral is recommended by KDOQI (NKF, 2006b) when the glomerular filtration rate (GFR) is less than 30 mL/min, chronic kidney disease (CKD) stage 4.
   1. Education of kidney replacement modalities with timely referral for access placement.
   2. Save-the-vein initiatives should be instituted for forearm and upper arm veins suitable for dialysis access limiting the use of the following.
      a. Venipuncture or placement of intravenous catheters.
         (1) Complications may limit the ability for fistula placement.
         (2) The dorsum of the hand should be the preferred site.
      b. Peripherally inserted central catheter (PICC) lines are associated with upper extremity thrombosis making the vein unusable.
      c. Subclavian catheters pose a risk for subclavian vein stenosis/occlusion and eliminate the ability to use the arm for dialysis access.
      d. Pacemaker/ICD wires should be avoided on side of future access placement.
   3. A fistula should be placed at least 6 months before dialysis is anticipated (NKF, 2006b).
   4. A graft should be placed at least 3 to 6 weeks before dialysis is anticipated (NKF, 2006b).

B. Health history.
   1. Complete health history: a thorough history and physical provide critical information in developing an individualized plan for each patient.
   2. Focus for dialysis access.
      a. Past medical history.
         (1) Disorders that may impact vasculature: diabetes, hypertension, systemic lupus erythematosus.
         (2) Disorders that may indicate generalized arterial disease: myocardial infarction, coronary artery bypass graft(s), peripheral bypass, cerebral vascular accident, or amputation(s)
         (3) Disorders that impact cardiac output: congestive heart failure, hypotension, decreased ejection fraction.
         (4) Coagulation disorders.
         (5) Disorders that may impact infection risks: those requiring immunosuppressants, heart valve disease, or prosthesis.
         (6) Disorders that may limit life expectancy: coronary artery disease, malignancy.
      b. Procedure and surgical history.
         (1) History of peripheral inserted central catheters.
         (2) History of central venous catheter and ports, including previous location of tunneled cuff catheters.

(3) Placement of pacemaker/ICD: associated with central venous stenosis.
(4) Previous arterial catheters.
(5) Previous surgeries to chest, neck, arms, and hands, including previous dialysis access.
  c. Social history.
    (1) Use of tobacco.
    (2) Use of alcohol.
    (3) Use of recreational drugs, including intravenous drug use.
  d. Medications.
    (1) Prescriptions.
      (a) Including anticoagulation therapy.
      (b) Including long-term steroid use.
    (2) Use of over-the-counter therapies.
    (3) Use of herbal therapies.
  e. Review of Systems.
  f. Determine the dominant arm.
    (1) Use of nondominant arm preferred.
    (2) Evaluate impact on quality of life.
    (3) Hemiparesis: may select side of paralysis to preserve functioning of opposite arm; however, may be limited with severe contractures and ability to cannulate.

C. Physical exam.
  1. Complete physical exam.
  2. Focus for dialysis access.
    a. Vital signs: bilateral upper extremity blood pressures.
      (1) Ensure adequacy to both arms.
      (2) Identify variances.
    b. General: alert and oriented, ability to educate.
    c. Cardiovascular.
      (1) Examination of arterial system: adequate arterial system is required for dialysis access, and the quality of the arterial system can influence the choice and placement of dialysis access (NKF, 2006b). Compare extremities noting differences (McCann et al., 2009).
        (a) Examination of pulses.
          i. Brachial, radial, ulnar.
          ii. Use a standardized scale to ensure ability to differentiate changes.
        (b) Allen's test.
          i. To determine palmar arch sufficiency.
          ii. Abnormal arterial flow may impact radial cephalic fistula placement.
        (c) Capillary refill.
      (2) Examination of venous system.
        (a) Edema: identification of venous outflow issues.
        (b) Arm size comparison.
          i. May indicate inadequate veins or venous obstruction.
          ii. Bilateral swelling may indicate central venous stenosis or occlusion that may be treated prior to dialysis access creation.
        (c) Collateral veins: indicates venous obstruction.
        (d) Evidence of previous central or peripheral vein catheters.
    d. Musculoskeletal: motor strength.
      (1) Arm.
        (a) Evaluate strength.
        (b) Determine if equal/unequal.
        (c) Use of a standardized scale allows for ease of identification of variances.
      (2) Hand grasps.
        (a) Evaluate strength.
        (b) Determine if equal/unequal.
        (c) Use of a standardized scale allows for ease.
    e. Integumentary: evidence of surgery and/or trauma to chest, shoulder, neck, arms, and hands and digits.
    f. Neurologic: hand and digits sensation. Evaluate bilaterally noting if equal or different in the following:
      (1) Temperature.
      (2) Functional ability, observe use.
      (3) Pain, tingling, or numbness.
      (4) Atrophy.
    g. Psychiatric: cooperative, mood including anxiety, depression, etc.

D. Vessel mapping.
  1. There is no generally accepted standard for vessel mapping (NKF, 2006b).
  2. The noninvasive duplex ultrasound of upper-extremity arteries is the preferred method, and it can evaluate both the arterial and venous systems (NKF, 2006b).
  3. Vessel mapping should be done bilaterally or, if unilaterally, to the nondominant arm (American College of Radiology, 2011a).
    a. Testing should include, bilateral:
      (1) Upper extremity arterial duplex: for arterial evaluation.
      (2) Upper extremity venous duplex: to evaluate veins including the central veins.
      (3) Physiologic upper extremity arterial study: to assess palmar arch patency and the identification of radial or ulnar dominance.
    b. Limitations to ultrasound scanning.
      (1) Situations that may impact vein size.
        (a) Hypotension.
        (b) Dialysis.
        (c) Dehydration.
        (d) Cold temperatures.
      (2) Arm size: evaluation of outflow vein may

be difficult with obesity or presence of edema.

    (3) Inability to maintain scanning position.

    (4) Situations that may limit access to superficial veins.

        (a) Intravenous lines.

        (b) Bandages.

        (c) Open areas on skin surface.

    (5) Central veins cannot be visualized (Breiterman-White, 2006).

E. Arteriography and venography: in patients for whom kidney function is no longer an issue (Breiterman-White, 2006), may be indicated when the following occurs.

    1. Diminished arterial pulses.

    2. Presence of extremity edema with or without collateral vein development.

    3. History of subclavian vein cannulation and pacemaker and ICD placement.

    4. Arm, neck, or chest surgery or trauma that may be associated with central vein stenosis or obliteration of central veins.

F. Education. Education and preparation of patients and their families is critical to the success of timely dialysis access creation and maintenance.

    1. Completion of modality counseling: hemodialysis, peritoneal dialysis, kidney transplantation, conservative management including palliative care (Fistula First, 2013c; Gomez, 2011).

    2. Preparation for dialysis access creation: allow patient participation in the development of their individualized plan of care (Fistula First, 2013c).

      a. Fistula maturation exercises: exercises that increase blood flow to the upper extremity may improve the chances of successful fistula development.

        (1) Ball squeezing. May include compression of bicep to increase fistula dilatation.

        (2) Bicep and hammer curls.

      b. Save-the-vein initiatives (Fistula First, 2013c; NKF, 2006b).

        (1) Use hand when possible for intravenous lines and blood draws.

        (2) Avoidance of peripherally inserted central catheters, central lines, and defibrillator wires on side of future access placement.

      c. Dialysis access. Advantages and disadvantages to fistulas, grafts, and catheters.

      d. Preoperative expectations.

        (1) NPO after midnight.

        (2) Early arrival for preparation and antibiotics.

      e. Intraoperative expectations.

        (1) Anesthesia options include axillary or regional block with sedation, local with sedation, or general.

        (2) Length of surgery and discharge expectations.

      f. Postoperative expectations.

        (1) Pain control.

        (2) When to follow up for postoperative visit.

        (3) When dressing can be removed and incision care.

        (4) Signs and symptoms to report.

          (a) Signs and symptoms of infection.

          (b) Wound opening.

          (c) Uncontrolled bleeding.

          (d) Development of fever.

          (e) Loss of thrill.

          (f) Signs and symptoms of ischemia: fingers cold, blue, numb, or painful.

    3. Care of dialysis access.

      a. Personal hygiene: keeping access clean and dry.

      b. Where and how to feel for the thrill.

      c. Use for hemodialysis only.

      d. Avoidance of scab picking.

      e. Avoidance of compression to access arm (Fistula First, 2013c).

        (1) Avoid carrying heavy items draped over the access arm.

        (2) Avoid jewelry and constrictive clothing.

        (3) Avoid sleeping on access arm.

        (4) No intravenous therapies or blood draws.

        (5) No blood pressures.

      f. How the dialysis unit is to care for dialysis access (Deaver, 2010).

        (1) Proper skin preparation prior to cannulation.

        (2) Each treatment:

          (a) Use of needle site rotation.

          (b) Use of buttonhole technique for AV fistulas.

        (3) General dialysis unit routines.

      g. Dialysis access maintenance expectations.

    3. When to contact a healthcare provider.

      a. Loss of thrill and need for early recognition to improve likelihood for salvaging access.

      b. Signs and symptoms of postop complications.

      c. Signs and symptoms of infection.

      d. Signs of malfunctioning access.

      e. In addition, for patients with catheters (Dinwiddie, 2010).

        (1) Exit site bleeding, drainage, pain.

        (2) Exit site or tunnel: bruising, swelling, pain.

G. Determining access site.

    1. Dialysis access should be placed only after resolution of local or systemic infection.

    2. Since the Fistula First Breakthrough Initiative in 2003, fistula placement has steadily increased to 60%. Shifting to fistulas first and catheters last to

continue the focus on decreased catheter use.
3. Should be placed in the most distal location of the upper extremity.
4. Fistulas.
   a. Requirements for AV fistula (NKF/KDOQI, 2006).
      (1) Start with nondominant hand.
      (2) Arterial diameter: 2.0 mm is recommended.
         (a) Calcified or atherosclerotic arteries may result in lower flow dialysis accesses.
         (b) When arterial flow is determined as healthy, then flow is determined by the vein characteristics.
      (3) Vein diameter of 2.5 mm is recommended.
         (a) Continuity of vein with proximal central veins, without evidence of obstruction.
         (b) Minimal or no scars in the veins.
         (c) No thrombi in the veins.
   b. Preferred location.
      (1) At the wrist: radial-cephalic.
      (2) At the elbow: brachial-cephalic.
      (3) Transposed brachial-basilic vein.
5. Grafts.
   a. The type of graft material should be based on surgeon experience and preference (NKF/KDOQI, 2006).
      (1) Polytetrafluoroethylene (PTFE) has been the material of choice for prosthetic bridge graft; however, other materials have been developed including biologic (bovine) and self-sealing.
      (2) New design developments including hybrids and hemodialysis reliable outflow (HeRO®) grafts have increased options for graft choice.
   b. Requirements for AV graft (Patel et al., 2011).
      (1) Lack of suitable vessels for fistula placement.
      (2) Immediate cannulation required.
      (3) Based on individual evaluation including life expectancy.
   c. Preferred location, starting most distal.
      (1) Forearm loop graft.
      (2) Upper arm graft.
      (3) Chest wall.
      (4) Thigh graft.
   d. Requirements for alternative access.
      (1) Self-sealing/immediate use graft materials (e.g., Vectra®, Flixene™) may be used when the following occurs.
         (a) Urgent initiation of dialysis is required.
         (b) Patients on dialysis who are experiencing significant tunneled

cuffed catheter concerns (e.g., repeated infections, repeated exchanges).
         (c) Limited access sites.
      (2) Hybrid grafts.
         (a) Does not require a venous anastomosis and may decrease intimal hyperplasia. The venous end is inserted and deployed into the vein.
         (b) Allows access to deeper and harder to reach vessels.
         (c) Criterion for placement.
            i. Check individual manufacturers' requirements.
            ii. Flexine™ IFG (Atrium, 2013).
               [a] Immediate use graft material.
               [b] Requires > 5.5 mm vein.
            iii. GORE® Hybrid (GORE, 2013).
               [a] Is an ePTFE graft with a nitinol-reinforced section.
               [b] Is selected to be 5–20% larger than vein.
      (1) HeRO® grafts (Atrium, 2013).
         (a) Candidates.
            i. Catheter dependence.
            ii. Failing fistulas or grafts due to central venous stenosis.
         (b) Target vein needs capacity to accommodate 19F outflow component.
         (c) Target artery size is 3 mm.
         (d) The outflow component of the HeRO® may be used to salvage current fistula or graft (Schuman & Ronfeld, 2011).
         (e) Immediate use graft material may be used (Schuman & Ronfeld, 2011).
            i. If the current tunneled cuff catheter site is used.
            ii. Prevent need for new catheter placement.
6. Catheters: to avoid whenever possible.
   a. Short-term, noncuffed catheters, should be used for acute dialysis of limited duration.
   b. Long-term, tunneled cuffed catheters (TCC), should be used in conjunction with a plan for permanent dialysis. Ideally, TCC should not be placed on the same side as the maturing fistula.
   c. Should be used in patients under the following conditions.
      (1) Assessed as ineligible for fistula or graft.
      (2) Temporary hemodialysis required (e.g., awaiting resolution of peritonitis from peritoneal dialysis).
      (3) Bridge gap waiting for permanent access placement and maturation.
      (4) Bridge gap due to fistula/graft repair and revisions.

III. Postoperative evaluation.

A. Postoperative physical exam.

B. Evaluation and treatment of complications.
1. Complete physical exam.
2. Focus for dialysis access.
   a. General: alert and oriented, ability to educate.
   b. Cardiovascular.
      (1) Examination of pulses, using standard scale: radial, ulnar.
      (2) Capillary refill.
      (3) Edema: identification of venous outflow issues.
      (4) Arm size comparison.
      (5) Access: type and inspection.
         (a) Discernable margins.
         (b) Edema.
            i. Swelling can be normal during the initial postoperative period and should be relieved within 1 to 2 weeks.
            ii. If present, institute use of arm elevation and arm rest.
            iii. Unrelieved swelling requires investigation for major outflow obstruction.
            iv. Ultrasound can be beneficial in determining cause of swelling including hematoma, seroma, infection, or outflow obstruction.
         (c) Pain: complete evaluation with onset, type, frequency, duration, and precipitating and alleviating events.
         (d) Aneurysm and pseudoaneurysm.
         (e) Incision description.
            i. Note if clean, dry, and intact.
            ii. Presence of erythema or fluctuance.
            iii. Signs and symptoms of infection: swelling, firm, may have drainage from incision, redness, warm/hot, possible fever.
         (f) Color changes.
            i. Bruising and ecchymosis.
               [a] Note swelling.
               [b] Soft or firm.
               [c] May have drainage from incision.
               [d] How it differentiates from infection: without temperature elevation or nonblanching.
            ii. Grafts: occasionally, within the first few weeks, a red flare will be present, overlying the course of the graft. Normal finding when restricted to overgraft, without swelling or other discoloration.
         (6) Palpation.
            (a) Thrill.
               i. Continuous, strongest at the arterial anastomosis, and should be felt throughout.
               ii. Indicate if strong, weak, discontinuous, or absent.
            (b) Pulse.
               i. Soft, continuous, compressible pulse.
               ii. Indicate if discontinuous, excessive pulsatile quality.
         (7) Auscultation.
            (a) Bruit
               i. Continuous low pitched.
               ii. Indicate if strong, weak, discontinuous, or absent.
            (b) Arm elevation: complete collapse or noncollapsible vein segment.
         (8) Fistula maturation.
            (a) Width: < 0.6 cm, > 0.6 cm.
            (b) Depth: < 0.6 cm, > 0.6 cm.
            (c) Length: < 0.6 cm, > 6 cm.
            (d) Outflow vein: soft/firm to touch.
            (e) Presence of collateral veins.
            (f) Occlusion of fistula outflow: augmentation of pulse, note location of lost augmentation.
   c. Musculoskeletal: motor strength.
      (1) Arm: strength, equal/unequal, using standard scale.
      (2) Hand grasps: strength, equal/unequal, using standard scale.
   d. Neurologic: hand/digits sensation. Evaluate bilaterally noting if equal or different in the following.
      (1) Temperature.
      (2) Loss of or full functional ability, observed use.
      (3) Pain.
      (4) Tingling or numbness: may indicate nerve damage or decreased blood flow.
      (5) Atrophy.
   e. Psychiatric: cooperative, mood including anxiety, depression, etc.

IV. Evaluating for readiness for hemodialysis access use.

A. AV Fistula.
1. Fistula maturation evaluation.
   a. Fistula maturation, by physical exam, should begin 4 weeks after fistula placement (Asif et al., 2006; Fistula First, 2013b).
   b. Interventions should be initiated at 4 weeks after placement to ensure fistula salvage. Prompt intervention for patients with catheters

will prevent prolonged use and minimize risk of complications (Asif et al., 2006).

c. A mature fistula needs to be ready for cannulation, with minimal risk for infiltration and the ability to achieve adequate blood flow (NKF/KDOQI, 2006).

d. Signs of mature fistula.

(1) Physical examination is about 80% accurate (Asif et al., 2006).

(2) The general rule of thumb used is the rule of 6's, which includes (NKF/DOQI, 2006):

  (a) Flow rate > 600 mL/min.

    i. Blood flow through the fistula should be strong and continuous on bruit and thrill.

    ii. A thrill that is palpated through the arterial end, middle, and venous end predicts flows greater than 450 mL/min. A thrill palpable through the axilla reflects a blood flow of at least 500 mL/min (Coentrao, 2013).

  (b) Diameter at least 0.6 cm.

  (c) Depth < 0.6 cm

  (d) Length > 6 cm

(3) In addition, the following is required (Asif et al., 2006; KDOQI, 2006).

  (a) Discernable margins: well developed and consistent in size.

  (b) Vessel collapse with arm elevation.

  (c) Outflow vein firm without prominent collateral veins.

  (d) Augmentation of pulse with occlusion of outflow, augmentation is weakened or lost at site of a tributary/accessory vein (Coentrao, 2013).

e. Use of duplex ultrasound (US) is indicated in patients with slow to mature fistulas (American College of Radiology, 2011b) and in determining fistula maturation. Evaluation should include:

(1) Venous outflow patency with identification of stenosis or thrombosis.

(2) Measure flow, depth, and width at three points.

  (a) Approximately 1 to 1.5 inches above anastomosis.

  (b) Midfistula.

  (c) Venous outflow.

(3) Identification and location of tributaries (American College of Radiology, 2011b).

(4) In addition, US can be used to identify the location of the anastomosis and for marking the functional portion of the fistula to indicate cannulation area.

(5) The limitation to US (NKF/KDOQI, 2006). Operator method with variation in the cross-sectional area as well as the angle and pressure used.

2. Interventions to assist in maturation. The need for intervention should be determined by the speed at which the access is required for use. If time allows, time for natural maturation of the fistula should be given. However, if the patient is on dialysis or initiation is imminent, then intervention may be required at 4 weeks.

a. Fistula exercises: should be continued to assist in maturation.

b. Fistulogram for evaluation and angioplasty.

c. Elimination of tributaries/accessory veins.

(1) Ligation is required if a single or multiple outflow veins limit fistula flow and the ability of a fistula to mature.

(2) Ligation can be done by one of three techniques: percutaneous ligation, venous cut down, coil (Asif et al., 2006).

(3) US can be used intraoperatively to assist in identification of tributary location to minimize dye use for patients not yet on dialysis.

d. Superficialization of the vein.

B. AV graft. Graft readiness includes the following.

1. No swelling.

2. Easily palpated with discernable margins.

3. Uniform graft size.

4. Soft compressible pulse.

5. Continuous thrill: strongest at the arterial anastomosis and should be felt throughout the graft.

6. Continuous bruit: low pitched.

7. Variants: manufacturers' guidelines should be used to determine the time required for tissue to graft incorporation.

a. Prosthetics (PTFE) generally should not be cannulated for at least 2 weeks after placement (NKF/KDOQI, 2006).

b. Biologic grafts(e.g., bovine material). Bovine carotid artery graft may be cannulated in 10 days (Artegraft, 2013).

c. Immediate-use/self-sealing grafts are designed for early cannulation and range from 24 to 72 hours for use.

d. Hybrid: dependent upon material used.

(1) PTFE: requires at least 2 weeks.

(2) Immediate-use/self-sealing: per manufacturer's guidelines.

8. To verify direction of flow through a graft.

a. Occlude midgraft.

(1) Arterial portion will continue to be pulsatile.

(2) Venous portion will be nonpulsatile.

V. Malfunctioning dialysis access.

A. When to refer.
1. An organized plan to monitor dialysis access with regular evaluation of dialysis access and dialysis adequacy should be implemented.
2. Trending of data vs. responding to an isolated abnormal value is required to recognition and initiate intervention of malfunctioning dialysis access. Persistent abnormalities in any of the monitoring or surveillance parameters should result in a prompt referral for further evaluation (KDQOI, 2006).
3. Continuous dialysis access monitoring and surveillance allows for the planning and coordination of elective interventions rather than urgent procedures to minimize under-dialysis and potential complications (Shah et al., 2013).
4. Blood flow through the access is directly related to blood pressure (Coentrao, 2013), therefore ensuring adequate blood pressure will rule out blood pressure as a risk factor for malfunctioning access.
5. Dysfunctional access.
   a. Any marked change in bruit/thrill may indicate a change in flow through the access and warrants an evaluation.
   b. Inspection, palpation, and auscultation are key tools in evaluating dialysis access (Coentrao, 2013; NKF/KDOQI 2006).
   c. According to the American College of Radiology (2014), US examination for evaluating postoperative dialysis access is designed to detect abnormalities that may cause the access to thrombose, or result in dysfunctional, nonfunctional, or negative arm symptomatology.
   d. Stenosis is the most common cause of malfunctioning access, and due to reduced access flow rate, can occur anywhere within access or through outflow vein.
   e. Changes in function, based on trend analysis, for further evaluation (Fistula First, 2013b; KDOQI, 2006).
      (1) Change in bruit or thrill.
      (2) Inability to achieve prescribed blood flows when needle size matches blood flow attempting to achieve.
      (3) Increases in venous pressures.
      (4) Excessive negative arterial pressures.
      (5) Difficult cannulation.
      (6) Prolonged bleeding postdialysis.
      (7) Frequent infiltrations.
      (8) Change in intra-access and direct flow measurements.
      (9) Downward trend in adequacy.
      (10) Access recirculation with properly cannulated access.
   f. Physical examination findings.
      (1) Incomplete maturation.
         (a) Irregular width.
         (b) Multiple tributaries and prominent collateral veins.
         (c) Lack of continued maturation to upper venous end.
      (2) Stenosis.
         (a) Visible narrowing along access.
         (b) Lack of vessel collapse (partial or full) with arm elevation (Ball, 2013; Gomez, 2011). The stenosis is located at area of engorgement.
         (c) Change in bruit.
            i. May be high pitched.
            ii. Discontinuous.
            iii. Weak with inflow stenosis.
         (d) Change in thrill.
            i. Increased at site of the stenosis.
            ii. Weak with inflow stenosis.
         (e) Change in pulse over the access.
            i. Presence of a strong pulse suggests an increase in the downstream resistance.
            ii. The intensity of the pulse is proportional to the severity of the stenosis. Eventually becomes pounding in character or water hammer pulse.
            iii. Diminished pulse beyond stenosis.
         (f) Edema.
   g. KDOQI (2006) preferred surveillance is based on access type.
      (1) Fistulas.
         (a) Direct access flow measurements.
         (b) Physical exam.
         (c) Duplex US.
      (2) Grafts.
         (a) Intra-access flow measurements.
         (b) Directly measured or derived static venous dialysis pressure.
         (c) Duplex US.
   h. Interventions.
      (1) Treatment of stenosis is required with diameter reduction of > 50% and signs of malfunctioning access (Beathard, 2009; KDOQI, 2006; McCann et al., 2009).
      (2) Most common cause of stenosis in grafts is neointimal hyperplasia, particularly at venous anastomosis and venous valves (Beathard, 2013).
      (3) US is a noninvasive, diagnostic step (American College of Radiology, 2011b) and can confirm presence of stenosis, including location and diameter (McCann et al., 2009).
         (a) Venous evaluation.

i. Can determine venous diameter, patency, and continuity.
ii. Identify tributaries.
iii. Evaluate venous outflow path.
(b) Arterial evaluation.
i. Determine arterial diameter.
ii. Calculate arterial flow.
iii. Identify stenotic segments and/or calcifications.
(4) Fistulogram is the gold standard for evaluating dialysis access (Beathard, 2009; KDOQI, 2006). A fistulogram can be used in conjunction with percutaneous transluminal angioplasty, and stent placement may be considered for unresolved or recurrent stenosis.
(a) Radiographic contrast is used to define arterial and venous portions of the access to the level of the superior vena cava.
(b) Minimally invasive.
(c) May not result in a permanent solution.
(5) Surgical revision is used for unsuccessful resolution of the lesion after several attempts with fistulogram.
6. Swelling to access extremity without improvement to arm elevation.
a. Differential diagnosis includes hematoma, seroma, infection, and venous hypertension.
b. US examination is indicated in the development of arm swelling (American College of Radiology, 2011b) and can assist in differentiation diagnosis. US can also demonstrate dilated central veins and possible reversal of flow.
c. Interventions.
(1) Fistulogram to evaluate patency of the central veins with angioplasty for identified stenosis.
(2) Stenting may be considered for unresolved or recurrent stenosis.
7. Hematoma or infiltration can be the result of poor cannulation technique.
a. Initial use of dialysis access: established break in protocols can assist in increasing needle gauge and blood flow rates at a pace to prevent or minimize risk of infiltrations (NKF/KDOQI, 2006).
b. Physical examination findings.
(1) Discoloration or bruising.
(2) Localized swelling.
(3) May have pain and/or tenderness to site.
c. Interventions.
(1) Use of ice, intermittently, for first 24 hours then use of warm compresses.
(2) Arm elevation.

(3) The dialysis access needs to be rested if the access is without discernable margins unable to be cannulated.
8. Thrombosis: leading cause of access loss.
a. Treatment should start as early as possible.
(1) Delays can result in further thrombus growth.
(2) The goal is to resume regular dialysis and prevent need for catheter placement.
b. Physical examination findings.
(1) Undetectable flow.
(2) Without bruit/thrill.
(3) Without pulse or may have slight pulse at the arterial anastomosis.
c. Interventions.
(1) Fistulogram.
(a) Allows for mechanical (dilatation and aspiration) or chemical (thrombolytic) thrombectomy or a combination of both.
(b) In addition, allows for angioplasty of underlying condition (Allon & Maya, 2013).
(2) Surgical revision and open thrombectomy (Allon & Maya, 2013).
(a) Requires a small incision.
(b) Uses a Fogarty embolectomy catheter.
(c) If successful, a fistulogram can be completed to detect and treat stenosis (Allon & Maya, 2013).
9. Infection.
a. More common in graft than fistulas. The most common infection in fistulas is local, occurring at cannulation sites.
b. Assessing the dialysis access every treatment is a primary intervention in identifying for signs and symptoms of access infection (Deaver, 2010).
c. Physical examination findings (Gomez, 2011; NKF/KDOQI, 2006).
(1) Warm to touch.
(2) Change in skin: erythema, fluctuance, denuded.
(3) Swelling.
(4) Pain or tenderness.
(5) Drainage from previous cannulation sites, including buttonholes.
(6) US: can be used to differentiate superficial/extensive infection vs. infiltration, seroma or hematoma.
d. Interventions begin with the determination of the type of infection and extent of involvement (Deaver, 2010).
(1) Fistulas.
(a) Superficial infections: avoid cannulation to area and treat with topical or oral antibiotics.
(b) Extensive infections are rare and

should be treated with 6 weeks of antibiotic therapy, based on culture and sensitivities (NKF/KDOQI, 2006).

   (c) AV anastomosis infections: surgery is required to resect the infected tissue with use of an interposition graft or with the creation of a new, more proximal, AV anastomosis (NKF/KDOQI, 2006).

  (2) Grafts.

   (a) Superficial infections: Do not involve the graft itself.

     i. Attempt graft savage through the use of antibiotic therapy, based on cultures and sensitivities.

     ii. Incision and drainage of infected areas with avoidance of cannulation to area.

   (b) Extensive infections: involves the graft, and resection of the infected graft material combined with antibiotic therapy is required.

   (c) Subclinical infections can develop from retained graft material. Diagnosis based on presenting symptoms and may require white blood cell scan.

10. Aneurysms/pseudoaneurysms.
  a. Definitions.
   (1) Fistulas: Aneurysms are localized dilatations of vessels caused by high pressures or excessive blood turbulence.
   (2) Grafts: Pseudoaneurysms can be localized dilatations due to high pressure in the graft or caused by subcutaneous bleeding outside the access wall (McCann et al., 2009).
  b. Causes (Shah et al., 2013).
   (1) Lack of needle-site rotation.
   (2) Proximal stenosis.
  c. Progressive enlargement of aneurysms/pseudoaneurysms.
   (1) Can compromise the skin leading to risk of rupture.
   (2) Result in thrombotic material within aneurysms and pseudoaneurysms.
   (3) Result in increased turbulence within aneurysms/pseudoaneurysms.
  d. Physical examination findings (Ball, 2013; Shah et al., 2013).
   (1) May be asymptomatic or have pain and throbbing.
   (2) Pulse: usually hyperpulsatile/excessive pulsatile quality.
   (3) Bruit: high-pitched, discontinuous.
   (4) Thrill: minimal.
   (5) Considered stable aneurysm/pseudoaneurysm.
    (a) Unchanged over time.

    (b) Soft with thick walls.
   (6) Considered unstable aneurysm/pseudoaneurysm.
    (a) Rapidly enlarging.
    (b) Firmness around aneurysm.
    (c) Thin, shiny appearance with or without break in skin covering.
    (d) Spontaneous bleeding.
    (e) Size restricts cannulation sites, and cannulation is difficult.
  e. Interventions.
   (1) Avoidance of cannulation to aneurysms/pseudoaneurysms.
   (2) Patient education (Ball, 2013).
    (a) Signs of imminent access rupture.
    (b) What to do in case of access rupture.
   (3) Timely referral may prevent rupture and may increase opportunity for access salvage. Indications for surgical evaluation referral include (Shah et al., 2013):
    (a) Signs of unstable aneurysm/pseudoaneurysm.
    (b) Evidence of infection.
    (c) Limited segment for cannulation.
    (d) Unsightly appearance.
   (4) US is indicated for patients with aneurysms/pseudoaneurysms (American College of Radiology, 2011b). US can obtain baseline size, evaluate for outflow stenosis, and identify intra-aneurysmal thrombus formation.
  f. Surgical interventions.
   (1) Stable aneurysm or pseudoaneurysm: consider fistulogram to evaluate and treat for outflow stenosis.
   (2) Fistula (Shah et al., 2013).
    (a) Plication (Hong-Yee & Seck-Guan, 2009).
     i. Multiple aneurysms may require completion in stages to prevent need for catheter placement.
     ii. Plicated area may be cannulated after surgical clearance and complete wound healing in 3 weeks.
    (b) Dissection and ligation of aneurysmal segment with placement of interposition saphenous vein segment or interposition graft. Use of immediate-use graft material may prevent need for catheter placement.
   (3) Graft (Shah et al., 2013).
    (a) Covered stenting within the pseudoaneurysm.
    (b) Resection and placement of interposition graft. Use of immediate-use graft material may prevent need for catheter placement.

11. Ischemia/steal syndrome.
  a. Definition of ischemia/steal syndrome is when the arterial supply to the access hand becomes insufficient (Coentrao, 2013).
  b. Patients should be evaluated on a regular basis for possible ischemia. Ischemic symptoms can occur early after surgery, but they can also develop months to years after access placement.
  c. Any new findings of ischemia should be referred immediately to the dialysis access surgeon.
  d. Mild cases, without loss of sensation or function, can be observed closely. Many will reverse in a few weeks. Severe cases require immediate intervention to prevent ischemic complications (Mickley, 2008; Zamani et al., 2009).
  e. Risk factors include (Zamani et al., 2009):
    (1) Diabetes mellitus.
    (2) Peripheral artery disease.
    (3) > 60 years of age.
    (4) Women.
    (5) Multiple surgeries/access to arm.
    (6) Type of access.
      (a) Upper arm fistula more than lower arm fistula.
      (b) Grafts.
  f. Physical examination findings: compare hand of the access arm to opposite side (Coentrao, 2013; Gomez, 2011; KDOQI, 2006; Zamani et al., 2009).
    (1) Diminished or absent radial and/or ulnar pulses.
    (2) Coolness of hand/digits.
    (3) Discolored, pale, or cyanotic.
    (4) Pain, paresthesia, or weakness.
    (5) Prolonged capillary refill.
    (6) Change in function to hand and fingers.
    (7) Muscle wasting.
    (8) Ulceration or gangrene in late cases.
    (9) Symptoms may become more pronounced while on dialysis or in cold temperatures.
    (10) Compressing of access may result in improvement in symptoms.
  g. Additional evaluation.
    (1) US evaluation (Zamani et al., 2009).
      (a) Can confirm the diagnosis.
      (b) Assist in determining the cause and therefore intervention required to improve ischemia.
      (c) Physiologic upper extremity arterial study: measures distal limb perfusion (Zamani et al., 2009).
        i. Digital plethysmography and pulse volume recordings.
          [a] Nonischemia demonstrates a phasic waveform that is augmented with access compression.
          [b] Ischemia demonstrates flat waveform with return to pulsatile waveform with access compression.
        ii. The digital pressure index (ratio of digital to brachial pressure) measures usually indicate steal syndrome (Mickley, 2008).
          [a] A digital pressure of < 50 mmHg.
          [b] A digital pressure index of < 0.6.
        iii. The systolic pressure index (ratio of the access forearm to contralateral forearm pressure).
        iv. Measures are then reevaluated with access compression and demonstrate marked improvement.
      (d) Additional US evaluation needs to include arterial inflow and venous flow measurements.
    (2) If US does not reveal significant ischemia, referral to neurology or neurosurgery for evaluation and EMG or nerve conduction studies.
      (a) Differentiate from other neuropathies or nerve damage postsurgical access placement (Talebi et al., 2011).
      (b) Differentiate from carpal tunnel, which involves entrapment of the median nerve. Signs and symptoms include dull pain, paresthesias, weakness, clumsiness of hand and/or hand atrophy (Dains et al., 2012).
  h. Interventions.
    (1) Avoidance of hypotension during dialysis.
    (2) Surgical intervention: dependent upon cause of steal syndrome.
      (a) US can also be used intraoperatively to assist in identification of return of blood flow to digits (digital pressure > 50 mmHg and digital pressure index > 0.69) (Zamani et al., 2009).
      (b) If signs of severe ischemic manifestations threaten the ability to salvage the limb, the access should be ligated (Mickley, 2008).
      (c) Arterial stenosis and obstruction of arterial inflow, not caused by arterial calcification; a fistulogram may be used to dilate by angioplasty (Zamani et al., 2009).
      (d) High flow induced requires a decrease in flow through the access (Mickley, 2008; Zamani et al., 2009).
        i. Banding procedures of the postanastomotic vein segment

diverting blood flow down through the native artery.

   ii. Modified banding procedure: minimally invasive limited ligation endoluminal-assisted revision (MILLER). A balloon is introduced into the fistula and a nonabsorbable suture is tied around the inflated balloon/vein to reduce balloon diameter.

   iii. Decrease the diameter of the anastomosis.

   iv. Create a new AV anastomosis distally. Revision using distal inflow (RUDI) requires ligating the original anastomosis and using the more distal portion of the artery.

(e) Normal flow to low flow induced requires distal revascularization interval ligation (DRIL). The arterial anastomosis is bridged by a venous bypass after which the artery is ligated (Mickley, 2008; Zamani et al., 2009).

(f) Low flow induced can benefit from proximal AV anastomosis (PAVA) technique. The current anastomosis is ligated and a new arterial anastomosis is created closer to the subclavian artery. Blood flow is carried to the vein through an interposition graft (Mickley, 2008; Zamina et al., 2009). Cannulation of the access can be completed immediately.

12. Ischemic monomelic neuropathy (IMN).
  a. Acute neuropathy with pain and weakness to distal muscle groups with the hand appearing well profused (Coentrao, 2013).
  b. Results from damage to a peripheral nerve due to compromise of blood supply. The findings may be located in the distribution of one or more of the median, ulnar, or radial nerves.
  c. Usually begins within hours of access placement (Coentrao, 2013).
  d. Physical examination findings.
    (1) Palpable pulses.
    (2) Severe pain.
    (3) Wrist drop.
    (4) Loss of hand or finger function.
  e. Interventions: mandatory ligation of the access.

13. Malfunctioning catheter: The catheter is associated with the greatest risk of infection and all-cause mortality compared with the fistula or graft (Deaver, 2010).
  a. Dysfunctional catheter (Dinwiddie, 2010; NKF/KDOQI, 2006).
    (1) Failure to attain prescribed blood flow (< 300 mL/min).

(2) Arterial pressures <-250 mmHg.
(3) Venous pressure > 250 mmHg.
(4) Dialysis adequacy trending downward.
(5) Unable to aspirate blood freely.
(6) Frequent pressure alarms without resolution to patient repositioning or catheter flushing.
(7) Requires reversal of lines to achieve blood flow.
    (a) Due to increased recirculation.
    (b) Should only be used as a temporary intervention.
(8) Interventions: early identification and prompt intervention ensures adequate dialysis.
    (a) Repositioning of catheter.
    (b) Thrombolytics/other modalities (endoluminal brushing).
    (c) Catheter exchange.

b. Infected catheter.
  (1) Exit-site infection: inflammation in the area surrounding the catheter exit site does not extend past the cuff, with confirmed positive exudates culture (NKF/KDOQI, 2006).
  (2) Tunnel infection: the tunnel past the cuff is inflamed, painful, and may have drainage through the exit site that has confirmed positive cultures (NKF/KDOQI, 2006). Evaluate for (Gomez, 2011):
    (a) Redness.
    (b) Induration or swelling.
    (c) Pain or tenderness along the tunnel.
    (d) Drainage or bleeding.
    (e) Evidence of catheter migration or exposed cuff.
  (3) Catheter-related bacteremia: blood culture positive for bacteria with or without fever (NKF/KDOQI, 2006).
  (4) Treatment.
    (a) Exit-site infections: catheters can usually be salvaged with topical or oral antibiotics (NKF/KDOQI, 2006).
    (b) Tunnel infection and bacteremia: parental antibiotic therapy should be initiated for suspected organism with definitive therapy initiated when culture and sensitivities are determined. Follow-up blood cultures should be completed at least 1 week after antibiotics are completed.
    (c) Catheter exchange, ideally by guide wire to save site, as soon as possible. Bacteremia with tunnel track involvement requires removal (NKF/KDOQI, 2006).

VI. Ensuring success.

A. Ensure a comprehensive quality improvement process (Fistula First, 2013a).
   1. Requires assessment by the interdisciplinary team (Coentrao, 2013; Dinwiddie, 2010; Fistula First, 2013a). The interdisciplinary team, described as the vascular access team by KDOQI (2006), includes the patient and professionals who participate in the care, monitoring, detection, and repair of dialysis access (nurse practitioner, nephrologist, nephrology nurse, patient care technician, physician assistant, interventionalist, and surgeon) (Fistula First, 2013a).
   2. Development of access monitoring protocols.
      a. Standard for predialysis and postdialysis evaluations.
      b. Flow measurements and static pressure measurements; frequency is based on what method is used (Gomez, 2011; KDOQI, 2006).
         (1) Intra-access flow measure monthly.
         (2) Static venous dialysis pressures every 2 weeks.
         (3) Computer-derived static pressures.
      c. Diagnostic testing.
      d. Computer design programs to monitor access trending.
   3. Development of a comprehensive database to track patients and data on dialysis access to include such items as current status of functioning dialysis access, access failure rates, and access complications and performance (Breiterman White, 2006).
   4. Establish break-in protocols for new dialysis access.
      a. Cannulation protocols.
         (1) Who initiates cannulation orders.
         (2) Identification of qualified staff to cannulated new access.
         (3) Needle size and specific flow rates and when to advance needle size.
      b. Tunneled cuffed catheter removal standards.

B. Skill set of staff.
   1. Access teams for new access cannulation.
   2. Physical exam of dialysis access (Coentrao, 2013).
   3. Cannulation techniques.
   4. Aseptic techniques.

C. Developing collaborative relationships between dialysis units, dialysis access centers, and surgical teams will allow for ease of transition for patients and improved communication.

D. When the patient refuses dialysis access or refuses use of a placed dialysis access.
   1. To facilitate self-care, develop partnerships with patients and recognize that patients do know their bodies while on and off dialysis (Richard, 2010). Fistula First (2013c) identifies the understanding of self-management through the use of ensuring dignity and respect, information sharing, participation, collaboration, and empowerment.
   2. Develop protocol for formal patient discussions, including frequency.
   3. Continue to reinforce risk factors of catheter use.
   4. Consider use of an informed refusal form so the patient is accountable for refusal.
      a. Develop protocols for frequency of review and re-signing.
      b. Should contain pertinent information of the benefits of permanent dialysis access and risks of continued catheter use.

VII. Planning for future access should be considered for all patients. However, initiate evaluations for patients with the following.

A. Access dysfunction/malfunction requiring repeated interventions.

B. Aneurysms/pseudoaneurysms.

C. Grafts. Consider secondary fistula in patients with grafts (Fistula First, 2008).
   1. Evaluation of patients with forearm grafts for upper arm fistula candidacy.
   2. Evaluation of suitable outflow vein. Vessel mapping may still be required.
   3. Expedited evaluation should begin with the first signs of graft dysfunction as loss of the graft may result in loss of ability to create secondary fistula.
   4. Sleeves Up protocol for evaluating patients is available on the Fistula First website at http://www.fistulafirst.org/

   Prompt placement, ensuring adequate dialysis through maintenance of dialysis access function and patency, requires a multidisciplinary team approach. The advanced practice nurse plays a pivotal role in proactively monitoring and promptly responding to changes in dialysis access.

SECTION D

Approaches to Care by the APRN in Peritoneal Dialysis

Mary M. Zorzanello

I. Introduction.

A. Peritoneal dialysis is a kidney replacement modality that has developed from being most often used as an acute treatment in the 1950s and 1960s to a well-established home-based therapy. Patients, families, and skilled nursing facilities (SNF) are trained to perform the procedure at home or in the SNF, and thus become active participants in their care.

B. Clinic visits are important to assess overall effectiveness of the PD prescription and medication regimen. Hospitalized PD patients require special attention and prescription management while they are inpatient, and follow-up evaluation in the outpatient clinic after discharge.

C. The use of PD varies throughout the world, being highest in Hong Kong (80%) and Mexico (65%). In 2011, PD patients accounted for 6.6% of dialysis patients in the United States (Vardhan & Hutchison, 2014).

II. Peritoneal dialysis.

A. Definition.
1. Transport of solutes and water from the bloodstream across the peritoneal membrane when it is exposed to a specially formulated, physiologically balanced solution (dialysate) in the peritoneal cavity. Figure 3.4 portrays a PD exchange.

B. Principles of peritoneal dialysis.
1. The peritoneal membrane. Figure 3.5 depicts the anatomy of the peritoneal cavity.
a. Visceral and parietal surfaces; visceral covers the intestine and other viscera; parietal lines the abdominal cavity wall.
b. Membrane is largest serosal surface in the body, 1 to 2 m² in an adult; indirect estimates put blood flow at 50 to 100 mL/min.
c. In the membrane, blood and lymphatic vessels are below a single layer of mesothelial cells. Microvilli cover those cells and increase surface area.
d. In females, the membrane is discontinuous because the ovaries and fallopian tubes open into the peritoneal cavity, while the male

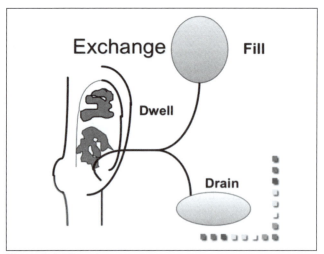

Figure 3.4. PD exchange.
Courtesy Mary M. Zorzanello.

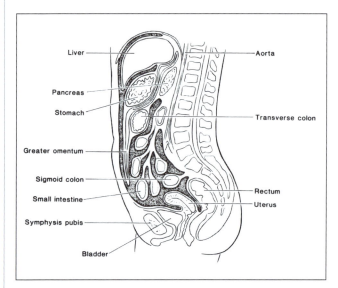

Figure 3.5. Anatomy of the peritoneal cavity (shaded) in an adult female.

membrane is closed.
e. Parietal peritoneum blood supply is from lumbar, intercostal, and epigastric arteries and then drains into the inferior vena cava.
f. Visceral peritoneum blood supply from superior mesenteric artery.
g. Lymphatic drainage into openings in the sub-diaphragmatic peritoneum accounts for some fluid reabsorption (Vardhan & Hutchison, 2014).

C. Fluid and solute transport. Figure 3.6 demonstrates the process of osmosis and diffusion.
1. Solute transport.
a. Solutes move from peritoneal capillaries to the

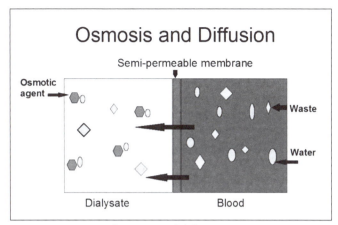

Figure 3.6. Process of osmosis and diffusion.
Courtesy Mary M. Zorzanello.

dialysate solution and from the solution into peritoneal capillaries as a result of diffusion and convection.
b. The concentration gradient between areas of higher and lower concentration influences the direction of solute movement.
c. Potassium, creatinine, magnesium, urea, and other solutes cross from the capillaries through the membrane and into the peritoneal cavity.
d. Solutes such as bicarbonate will move from the solution in the cavity into the peritoneal capillaries.
2. Fluid transport.
a. Affected by types of pores (aquaporins) in peritoneal capillary walls.
b. Hydrostatic and colloid osmotic forces affect water transport.
c. Osmosis is movement of water molecules from an area of lower solute concentration to one of higher solute concentration.
d. Dialysate contains dextrose or icodextrin in high concentrations; water concentration is low in relation to serum, causing movement of water out of peritoneal capillaries, through membrane pores and into peritoneal cavity.
e. Excess water removed is called ultrafiltration.
3. Factors that influence solute removal.
a. Membrane permeability – may increase with infection or inflammation.
b. Scars and adhesions may reduce membrane surface area.
c. Volume of dialysate – more dialysate results in more solute removal.
d. Solute size – smaller molecules move faster.
e. Solutes bound to proteins – move more slowly.
f. Concentration gradient – high gradient leads to faster initial solute removal.
g. Dialysate temperature – better diffusion at body temperature.
h. Solute drag – solutes pulled into peritoneal

cavity along with water from ultrafiltration.
i. Dwell time and equilibrium between dialysate and serum: As concentration gradient decreases, so does rate of solute removal over time.
j. Membrane classification – composition of membrane determines rate at which solutes cross membrane.
4. Factors that influence fluid removal.
a. Membrane permeability and classification. A more permeable membrane loses water more quickly.
b. Amount of dextrose in dialysate fluid affects transport because of the osmotic concentration gradient. It is highest at the start of a dwell because the gradient is also highest at that point.
c. Icodextrin is a long chain, glucose polymer that exerts colloid oncotic rather than osmotic pressure to pull fluid into the peritoneal cavity.
d. Dwell time.
(1) Osmotic equilibrium occurs over time as more water moves into the peritoneal cavity and thus dilutes the dextrose concentration.
(2) Dextrose can then be absorbed back into the blood and ultrafiltration will be greatly reduced (Vardhan & Hutchison, 2014).
5. Table 3.4 details the composition of various dialysate solutions.

D. Modality choice.
1. Ideally, patients are educated about kidney replacement therapies well before time to start dialysis. It is important to emphasize that for

Table 3.4

Composition of Peritoneal Dialysis Solutions

	Standard Solution	Low Calcium Solutions	Icodextrin Solution
Sodium (mEq/L)	132.0	132.0	132.0
Calcium (mEq/L)	3.5	2.5	3.5
Magnesium (mEq/L)	0.5	0.5	0.5
Chloride (mEq/L)	96.0	95.0	96.0
Lactate (mEq/L)	40.0	40.0	40.0
pH	5.2–5.5	4.0–6.5	5.0–6.0
Osmolarity (mOsm/L)			
1.5% Dextrose	346	344	
2.5% Dextrose	396	395	
3.5% Dextrose	447	445	
4.25% Dextrose	485	483	
Icodextrin			282–286

many patients, it is physically possible to switch between hemodialysis and peritoneal dialysis, and vice versa, if the need arises.

2. Good candidates include:
   a. Patients who work or whose lifestyles prevent them from attending hemodialysis treatments three times per week.
   b. Homebound patients with good support systems and partners to help.
   c. Skilled nursing facility (SNF) patients where the nursing staff is trained and regularly retrained in their care.
   d. Patients who refuse to consider hemodialysis.
   e. Patients who do poorly on hemodialysis, such as those with poor vascular access, congestive heart failure, and extensive vascular disease.

3. A home visit will be done by dialysis unit nurses to verify that the environment is appropriate. Access to a bathroom and space to store supplies are important.

4. Before a choice is finalized, it is a good idea to have the patient and any significant others visit the program where they will receive training and follow-up care.

5. Some absolute contraindications to PD include:
   a. History of extensive abdominal surgery with scarring and adhesions.
   b. Lack of support system if a patient is unable to perform PD due to physical or mental disabilities.
   c. Patent fistula between pleural and peritoneal cavities.

6. Relative contraindications to PD: Malnutrition, severe inflammatory bowel diseases, abdominal malignancies, severe diabetic gastroparesis, morbid obesity, abdominal skin conditions that predispose to infection, severe chronic back pain, or presence of an ostomy (Diaz-Buxo, 1996).

E. Peritoneal dialysis modalities.

1. The basic procedure of infusing dialysate into the peritoneal cavity, allowing it to dwell in contact with the membrane, draining it out, and replacing with fresh solution is called an exchange. A peritoneal dialysis catheter is surgically implanted for access to the peritoneal cavity.

2. This process can take place either manually, called continuous ambulatory peritoneal dialysis (CAPD) or automatically via a machine, called automated peritoneal dialysis (APD). Other common abbreviations used are CCPD (continuous ambulatory cycling peritoneal dialysis) or IPD (intermittent peritoneal dialysis). Continuous means dialysate fluid is always in the peritoneal cavity. Intermittent denotes that there are periods of time when the cavity is empty.

3. CAPD (continuous ambulatory cycling peritoneal dialysis).
   a. A closed system that contains an empty bag for draining the contents of the peritoneal cavity (effluent), a sterile port for connecting to the patient's access catheter, and a bag that contains the dialysate solution.
   b. Typical inflow volumes for an adult are 1.5, 2.0, 2.5, and 3.0 liters.

4. APD (automated peritoneal dialysis) systems rely on a machine that will cycle fluid in and out of the abdomen; for that reason they are known as *cyclers*.

5. Both systems require a training period.
   a. Most often this is one-to-one training by the same nurse in the dialysis unit.
   b. SNF staff are trained by arrangement with individual dialysis units either in the unit, at the SNF, or some combination of both.

6. See Table 3.5 for a comparison of the chronic PD therapies. Figures 3.7 and 3.8 show available cyclers for PD.

F. The peritoneal catheter.

1. Various catheter designs exist, but the basic configuration includes an external segment, a tunneled segment, and an internal segment. They are made of silicone rubber material with a radiopaque stripe. Catheters may be placed surgically by open dissection or laparoscopic technique, or via fluoroscopic guidance in Interventional Radiology.
   a. The external segment is the visible portion of the PD catheter. It is only functional when attached via a small plastic or titanium adapter to a piece of tubing called a transfer set. The transfer sets have sterile ends that can connect to CAPD or APD tubing, and clamping systems to open and close so that fluid can either enter or exit the peritoneal cavity. The transfer set should be compatible with the CAPD and APD manufacturer's equipment. Universal converters can be used to connect incompatible equipment in emergencies or if a patient is hospitalized in a setting that uses a different system. The length of the external portion is not standardized, and may be shortened to accommodate a smaller patient.
   b. The tunneled segment of the catheter is created by passing the catheter from the peritoneal membrane, through the rectus muscle, the subcutaneous fat, and finally through the skin. The opening is called the exit site. The catheter may have a single or a double Dacron cuff that allows fibrous tissue ingrowth, anchors it in position and makes accidental dislodgement

Table 3.5

Comparison of Chronic Peritoneal Dialysis Therapies

CAPD (continuous ambulatory peritoneal dialysis)	CCPD (continuous cycling peritoneal dialysis)	NIPD (nightly intermittent peritoneal dialysis)
4–5 manual exchanges during the day; may use assist device for extra nighttime exchange(s).	Automatic cycling of exchanges overnight with a long daytime dwell.	Automatic cycling of exchanges overnight.
Solution in peritoneal cavity continuously, except for drain and fill times.	Solution in peritoneal cavity continuously, except for drain and fill times.	Dialysate is drained completely at end of dialysis; no solution in the peritoneal cavity between dialyses.
Some techniques require portable equipment, e.g., an exchange assist device.	Requires cycler; typically uses 5 liter bags.	Requires cycler; typically uses 5-liter bags.
Closed system is opened for each exchange.	Closed system opened for setup and on/off procedures.	Closed system opened for setup and on/off procedures.
Requires 20–40 minutes per exchange.	Requires ~ 45 minutes for setup and on/off procedures.	Requires ~ 45 minutes for setup and on/off procedures.
Blood chemistries stable.	Small diurnal biochemical fluctuations.	Biochemical fluctuations.
Fluid balance stable.	Diurnal fluctuations in fluid balance.	Fluid balance fluctuations.
Daytime interruptions for exchanges; sleep uninterrupted.	Sleep may be disturbed; may require an additional daytime exchange.	Sleep may be disturbed; no interruption of daytime routine.

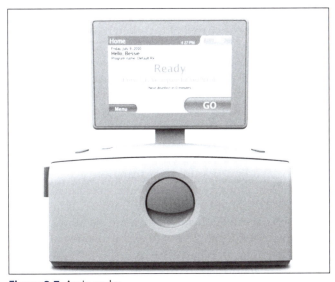

Figure 3.7. Amia cycler.
Courtesy of Baxter Healthcare. Used with permission.

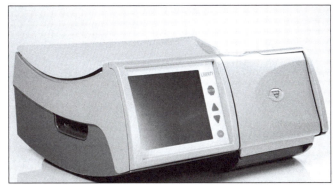

Figure 3.8. Liberty cycler.
Courtesy of Fresenius Medical Care. Used with permission.

almost impossible. A double cuff catheter will have one cuff about 2 cm in from the exit site and another in the rectus muscle, anterior to the posterior rectus sheath. A single cuff catheter will only have the deeper, preperitoneal cuff. There is some consensus that having two cuffs is safer in terms of securing the catheter in position, preventing dialysate leaks, and preventing infection. (Eklund et al., 1997). Tunneled segments are usually from 5 to 7 cm in length, though presternal segments are much longer.

c. This portion of the catheter may be straight or arched. The arched shape, also called swan neck, should prevent the catheter tip from flipping out of position from the lower portion of the peritoneal cavity to a level where fluid

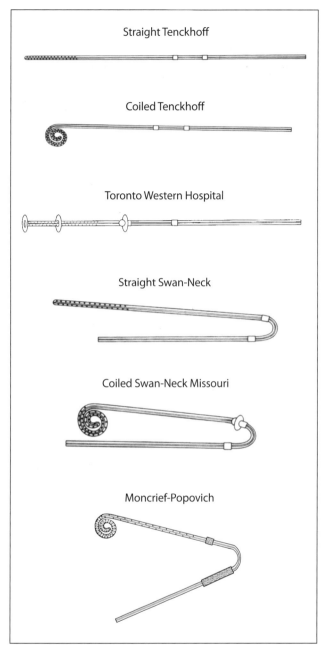

Figure 3.9. Chronic peritoneal dialysis catheters. From top: Double-cuff Tenckhoff catheter with straight intraperitoneal segment; double-cuff Tenckhoff catheter with coiled intraperitoneal segment; Toronto Western Hospital catheter with preperitoneal flange and bead and intraperitoneal discs; swan-neck catheter with straight intraperitoneal segment; swan-neck Missouri catheter with preperitoneal flange and bead and coiled intraperitoneal segment; Moncrief-Popovich catheter with wider tunnel angle and longer subcutaneous cuff.

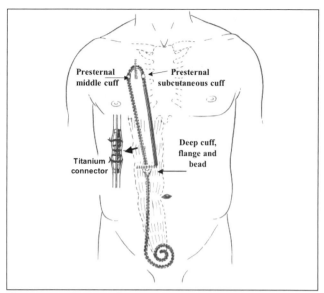

Figure 3.10. Swan-neck Missouri presternal peritoneal dialysis catheter.

Source: Twardowski, Z.J., Prowant, B.F., Pickett, B., Nichols, W.K., Nolph, K.D., & Khanna, R. (1996). Four-year experience with swan neck presternal peritoneal dialysis catheter. *American Journal of Kidney Diseases, 27*(1), 99-105. Used with permission. Reprinted from C.S. Counts (Ed.). (2008). *Core curriculum for nephrology nursing* (5th ed.). Pitman, NJ: American Nephrology Nurses' Association.

outflow is compromised (Eklund et al., 1995).
d. The internal catheter segment may be straight or coiled and is about 11 to 15 cm in length. To facilitate fluid flow, there are numerous side holes in addition to the open tip. Straight internal segments may cause discomfort with inflow of solution because they direct the stream to one location instead of dispersing throughout the lower abdomen. Coiled segments have more weight and thus may prevent catheter tip migration (Di Paolo, 2004; Prowant et al., 2008a).
e. Figures 3.9 and 3.10 will help in visualizing a variety of chronic PD catheters.

G. Catheter placement. Patient preparation includes planning for catheter placement to occur at least 2 weeks prior to training and usage.
1. Examine the abdomen for presence of scars, hernias, and the general shape and architecture of the belly.
2. Place a mark on the skin for the exit site. Avoid the belt line, skin folds, or scars, and evaluate patient in both supine and sitting positions. The exit site should not be underneath a pannus to prevent infection and to increase visibility.
3. Instruct the patient not to allow anyone but peritoneal dialysis nurses to remove the initial surgical dressing. By keeping the dressing in place and the catheter immobilized for as long as possible, tissue ingrowth into the cuff can proceed undisturbed and the tunnel can begin to heal as tightly as possible. If the dressing is grossly soiled or bloody, a PD nurse will change it under sterile conditions, taking care to move the catheter as little as possible (Gokal, 1998).
4. Instruct the patient not to shower until cleared by nurses in the PD unit. Explain that water is not sterile, and if exposed to healing tissue, can cause

an early exit-site or tunnel infection.

5. The PD unit nurses will ensure that the patient has a follow-up appointment with them within a day or two of catheter implantation. The catheter will be irrigated, the dressing checked, and plans made for training.

H. Catheter break-in and care.
1. Goals are to assure that the catheter is patent and in correct position in the lower pelvis, prevent complications such as leaks and infections, and assure that healing is proceeding.
2. If dialysis can be delayed for at least 10 days to 2 weeks, the risk of such complications are minimized. The site of entry into the peritoneal cavity will heal, forming a seal that prevents leakage.
3. Catheter irrigation to assess patency.
   a. May be done within the first few days postimplantation. Usually, the lowest dextrose concentration (1.5%) is used because the object is not to promote ultrafiltration. The solution is heparinized with 500 to 1000 units per liter.
   b. Exchanges of 500 mL to 1000 mL are infused and immediately drained.
   c. This procedure gives the nurse information about patency, residual bleeding, possible dialysate leaks, and appearance of the effluent.
   d. This is done per unit policy in a new patient, often weekly until training begins, but more often if there are concerns with catheter performance.
   e. Volume is increased incrementally as tolerated by the patient. For most patients, 2 liters is the goal for initial dialysis. This is often modified when the full PD prescription is developed.

I. Exit-site care.
1. Postplacement. Goals are to prevent bacterial colonization, immobilize the catheter to promote tunnel healing and tissue ingrowth into the cuffs, and identify early complications.
2. First dressing change under sterile conditions, subsequent ones are aseptic. Masks should be worn by anyone in the room.
3. Dressing change frequency can be weekly at the beginning unless very soiled; this will aid the healing process by minimizing catheter movement and possible trauma.
4. Skin should be cleaned with a nonirritating cleanser. Avoid oxidizing agents such as hydrogen peroxide or povidone iodine as they can interfere with healing by damaging new epithelial cells. Rinse with sterile water or saline.
5. Site should be dried and a nonocclusive dressing applied followed by immobilizing the catheter.
6. No showers until healed, and no immersion in a

tub, due to high bacterial content in bath water. After healing is complete, patients may swim in chlorinated pools and salt water providing exit-site care is done as soon as they leave the water. When swimming in the ocean, consideration should be given to proximity of the water to sewage outlets and to highly populated areas (Luong & Prowant, 2009). Lake and river swimming is discouraged due to high bacteria counts in fresh water.
7. During healing, some tenderness and pink color is normal. There will usually be a scab and some serous to serosanguineous drainage. Sinus tissue will appear to be white.
8. The healed site should have no drainage, and granulation tissue should convert to epithelium. Color will depend on the patient's ethnicity. Healing should be complete in 4 to 6 weeks.
9. Chronic exit-site care can take place in the shower, but patients should be reminded to use a clean washcloth each time that has not touched other body areas. Site is dried with a clean towel, used only once, and not on other body parts. Liquid antibacterial soap is recommended because bar soap is a reservoir for bacterial growth.
10. Topical agents such as mupirocin cream and gentamicin cream may be applied after exit-site care as bacterial prophylaxis. Avoid any petroleum-based ointments as they damage the silicone catheters. Some units may use a 0.9% or 3% saline soak to soften exit-site crusting.
11. Dressings may be optional but are often recommended by programs to cushion the site and help secure the catheter. Absorbent gauze dressings are often used; each PD program will have specific recommendations (Crabtree, 2006; Prowant et al., 2008a).

J. The training process.
1. Schedule is dependent on the dialysis unit. A brand new patient on dialysis will already have been seen for postop catheter care, and a schedule that meets the patient's needs will have been developed. Ideally, daily visits for the first week should prepare a patient to do basic CAPD. It is most important to customize training to accommodate a particular patient or caregiver's learning style, social situation, disabilities, or language barriers. The length of a training session is also very much dependent on patient circumstances.
2. If the patient needs hemodialysis or is transitioning from HD to PD, training will have to be scheduled to accommodate HD treatments.
3. Usual training curriculum includes basic principles of PD, asepsis and hand washing, fluid management, nutrition, supply management,

exit-site care, troubleshooting, and practice doing procedures repeatedly until they become automatic.

4. Many dialysis units train first in CAPD, and if the patient desires APD, they are retrained in a few weeks or as soon as the unit can accommodate. A home visit is usually done before releasing the patient to perform either PD modality independently. A safe and clean home environment is essential for the patient to be successful. The dialysis unit should provide a 24-hour on-call service to deal with questions and emergencies.

5. If a patient with a new catheter needs to start dialysis but is unable to do hemodialysis, training can still take place. Low volume, frequent exchanges with the patient supine will reduce chances of leakage and provide some ultrafiltration and solute clearance while training proceeds. The exchanges may be performed manually or by a cycler.

K. Peritoneal membrane classification.
1. Prescription regimens are individualized to each patient depending on body size, residual kidney function, and membrane classification.
2. Membrane classification: fluid and solute transport is measured to determine membrane transport characteristics.
   a. Low molecular weight solutes such as potassium, creatinine, and urea pass easily from peritoneal capillaries, across the membrane, and into dialysate solution.
   b. As dwell time increases, the ratio of dialysate to serum solute levels (D/P) gets close to 1.0.
   c. Large molecules such as albumin cross over more slowly, and negatively charged molecules such as phosphate also move slowly because the membrane's net charge is negative.
   d. As dwell time progresses, glucose is absorbed from dialysate into the bloodstream, thus decreasing the osmotic gradient across the membrane. After a while, fluid ends up being reabsorbed back into circulation because oncotic pressure rises intravascularly.
   e. Each patient's membrane is different, resulting in a different rate of solute movement between blood and dialysate (Vardhan & Hutchison, 2014).

L. The peritoneal equilibration test (PET).
1. The PET assesses the rate of transport of glucose from dialysate into plasma and creatinine from plasma into dialysate.
2. The test is standardized as a 4-hour, 2-liter, 2.5% dextrose exchange, preceded by an overnight dwell, also 2 liters, 2.5% dextrose. The patient is

instructed to collect a 24-hour urine sample and bring it in on the day of the PET.

3. The overnight dwell is drained and the 2-liter, 2.5% dextrose exchange is infused; infusion time is noted as is the time the 4-hour dwell begins. A dialysate sample is removed from the abdomen immediately on completion of infusion. This is the 0-hour dialysate sample. It will be tested for glucose, urea, and creatinine, as will all subsequent samples and the blood draw at hour 2.

4. At exactly 2 hours from 0 hour, another dialysate sample is withdrawn and blood is drawn.

5. At 4 hours, the entire exchange is drained. Another dialysate sample is collected and note is made of the amount drained and how long it took to drain completely. Infusion and drain times are important in the discussion of prescription development.

6. Most dialysis companies work with labs that are set up to analyze the dialysate, 24-hour urine, and blood samples. They report them to the unit in such a way that membrane characteristic and residual kidney function are easily noted. It is also possible to manually analyze PET data.

7. Membrane classification is based on the dialysate to plasma creatinine ratio (D/PCr) at the end of 4 hours. A D/PCr > .81 is classified as a high transport membrane; 0.65 to 0.81 is high average; 0.5 to 0.65 is low average; and below 0.5 is a low transport membrane (NKF, 2006). Figure 3.11 displays the PET curves.

M. Evaluating PET results and implications for prescription development.
1. A high transporter will quickly clear small molecules. At the same time, glucose is rapidly absorbed and the osmotic gradient between blood and dialysate is reduced. The most efficient dialysis regimens for these patients are built around short dwells. APD serves this group well.
2. Conversely, a low transporter clears solutes slowly and will benefit from longer dwells with more volume to achieve adequate clearance. Ultrafiltration is usually preserved because of slower glucose absorption and maintenance of an osmotic gradient. CAPD may be a better choice for these patients.
3. The majority of patients fall somewhere in the high average and low average category and will do well on either APD or CAPD.
4. Prescription modeling software is very common. It accounts for PET data, residual kidney function, infusion and drain times, dialysate dextrose percentage or icodextrin, and body surface area when formulating a regimen that will provide adequate dialysis. It can also predict fluid removal and amount of calories absorbed from the

dialysate – important considerations for diabetics. By having a variety of prescription options, the patient can truly have a regimen that suits lifestyle and gives adequate solute clearances and fluid removal. In order to increase the accuracy of the prescription-modeling program, it is critical that the patient receive explicit instructions on timing the overnight dwell and on the 24-hour urine sample collection. PET samples must be obtained at the proper time with meticulous attention to the procedure.

5. Once the patient's transport characteristic is known, a prescription can be built based either on CAPD or APD. The programs allow flexibility to individualize volume and dwell time for either modality. CAPD volumes range from 1.5 L in a small adult to 3 L; average is either 2 L or 2.5 L. The number of exchanges per day is also dependent on adequacy targets and may be as few as 3 per day to 5 or even 6. APD treatments are often started at 8 hours on the cycler, but the programs are quite versatile and can be developed to accommodate almost any lifestyle. Normally there is an overnight treatment with a number of exchanges and volumes that suit the patient's membrane and clearance needs. A last fill of 100 mL to over 2 L completes treatment in the morning, leaving fluid in the peritoneal cavity throughout the day. This makes it a true continuous therapy. Often, patients need an additional daytime exchange or exchanges either to meet the adequacy target or because they reabsorb fluid during the day. This type of APD treatment can also be programmed into the cycler. Another choice, tidal APD, retains a designated percentage of the initial exchange. Theoretically, by doing this, the concentration gradient is maintained in a high transporter if about 50% of dialysate is retained. Tidal is also used to help allay pain at the end of drain. Typical tidal percentages for this are 80–90%. A small pool of dialysate is left behind with each drain, and the cycler must be programmed to plan for a fixed amount of ultrafiltration per cycle so the abdomen does not become overfilled by the end of the treatment. A full drain will take place when the treatment is finished. Pain at the end of a drain cycle is more common with a new catheter that is still healing, so this type of tidal program might only be needed for a short time.

6. PET testing is done a month after training is completed and may be repeated at intervals established by dialysis unit protocol. Membranes

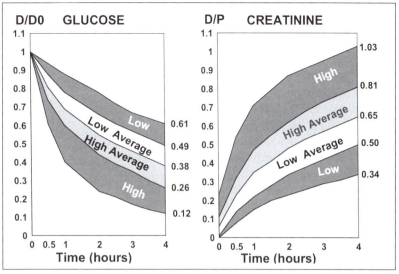

Figure 3.11. Peritoneal equilibration test curves for dialysate glucose to dialysis solution glucose at time 0 (D/D0) ratios (left) and corrected creatinine dialysate to plasma (D/P) ratios (right); determined from 103 equilibration studies in 86 patients.

can slowly change over time, especially if the patient has frequent bouts of peritonitis, so it is important to develop a standard of when to reassess the membrane (Li et al., 2010).

N. Adequacy of dialysis.
1. Clinical assessment and solute clearance measurements define peritoneal dialysis adequacy.
   a. Clinically, a patient feels well, has minimal fatigue, no nausea, and reports a good appetite.
   b. Regarding solute clearance, measurements of urea and creatinine clearances are used. Urea clearance is expressed as Kt/V. Urea clearance (K) is multiplied by time (t) and divided by body water volume (V). The calculation involves multiplication of the ratio of dialysate effluent to plasma urea nitrogen by the 24-hour effluent amount. Residual kidney urea clearance is added which gives a total daily body clearance. That value is multiplied by 7, yielding a weekly value. Sixty percent is used as the estimate of body water volume in males, 55% in females. Most dialysis company labs provide the Kt/V without unit staff having to do the calculation themselves.
   c. Creatinine clearance (CrCl) also combines both residual kidney function and peritoneal clearance. Residual kidney function in this calculation is an estimate of glomerular filtration rate (GFR), which is an average of both urea and creatinine clearances, adjusted for body surface area. Again, the dialysis lab company usually reports the result.

2. Kt/V and creatinine clearance are the accepted methods of estimating adequate dialysis, though over the years there have been changes to the standards.
   a. In 2006, the NKF's KDOQI Practice Guidelines for PD established a weekly Kt/V of 1.7 and creatinine clearance of 50 L/week as minimum targets for adequate dialysis.
   b. These values are based on a large, randomized prospective study (ADEMEX) reported in 2002 that found no difference in patient survival with dialysis targets higher than Kt/V of 1.7 and creatinine clearance of 50 L/week (Paniagua et al., 2002). Other international organizations such as the United Kingdom Renal Association Guidelines, the International Society for Peritoneal Dialysis Guidelines, and the European Best Practice group all produced similar recommendations. It is important to remember that these are minimum standards, and clinical evaluation remains equally important.
3. Adequacy testing is determined per unit policy but usually measured quarterly.
4. Patients bring in a 24-hour urine and a representative sample of 24-hour effluent. Important teaching points emphasize a true 24-hour urine collection and ensuring that the dialysis treatment for which the fluid is collected also represents a 24-hour period. Results will not be accurate if timing is incorrect. A blood sample is also sent to the lab, and results usually return with all calculations done. A good lab will also separate out the effect of residual function as part of the total.

O. Complications and troubleshooting.
1. Catheter-related issues.
   a. Dialysate will not flow into or out of the peritoneal cavity.
   b. Assess for any closed clamps or kinks in the system.
   c. Question patient about constipation. A full bowel can obstruct the catheter and interfere with inflow and outflow. If the patient is indeed constipated, prescribe a laxative to promote immediate bowel evacuation, and institute a bowel regimen of stool softeners and an osmotic laxative such as polyethylene glycol oral powder daily. Commercially prepared enemas and soapsuds enemas are not used due to high phosphate content (McCormick, 2007).
   d. Try irrigating the catheter with a large syringe with either heparinized saline or dialysate solution. If able to inject solution, try only gentle aspiration and if not successful, stop immediately to prevent aspiration of tissue into the catheter.

e. Abdominal x-rays, A/P and lateral views, can diagnose constipation, internal kinks, or catheter migration.
f. Fibrin clots may be obstructing the catheter, especially a new catheter, due to residual postinsertion inflammation or bleeding or during and after an episode of peritonitis. Tissue plasminogen activator (tPA) may be infused, 1 mg/mL in sterile water, volume sufficient to fill the catheter; dwell for 1 to 2 hours. After the tPA has been in the catheter for the prescribed time, try to drain by gravity. If successful, flush the catheter in and out with a small volume of heparinized dialysate, then proceed with routine dialysis. Some patients normally produce more fibrin than others and will need to be taught how to inject heparin daily into their dialysate (Zorzanello, 2004).
g. A migrated catheter can be seen on x-ray. Sometimes it can be brought back into place by inducing peristalsis through administration of a strong laxative. If that does not work, the catheter may be repositioned by the surgeon or interventional radiologist using a guidewire before taking the patient back to the operating room (see Figure 3.12)
h. Omental wrapping can also obstruct catheter flow and is suspected if none of the interventions listed above are successful. It is relieved in the operating room by partial or more extensive omentectomy. Sometimes adhesions are also identified and lysed during surgery to correct catheter obstruction (Vardan & Hutchison, 2014). Depending on the extent of internal manipulation and surgery, the patient may need to rest the abdomen for a few weeks, necessitating a bridge on hemodialysis. If the surgery is relatively uncomplicated and the patient has enough residual function, he/she may resume low volume (500 to 1000 mL) PD exchanges while supine for about 2 weeks. The abdomen remains empty when the patient is out of bed. Exchange volume may be increased slowly and a day dwell re-introduced once all surgical incisions look well healed and there is no evidence of dialysate leakage into subcutaneous tissue or exiting the tunnel. They will be followed closely in the PD unit to make sure uremic symptoms do not develop while on the reduced PD prescription.
2. Hernias.
   a. Any abdominal wall hernias should be repaired prior to starting PD. The presence of 2 to 3 liters of fluid in the abdomen will increase intraabdominal pressure and can worsen an existing hernia. New hernias can also form once PD is established, most commonly

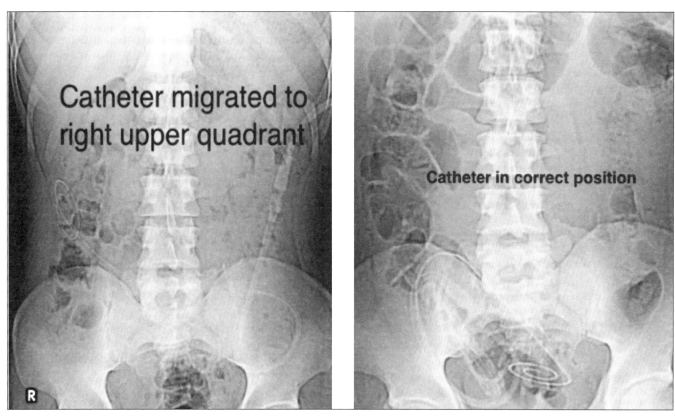

Figure 3.12. Catheter migrated to right upper quadrant (left). Catheter in correct position (right).

umbilical, inguinal, and incisional. The hernia should be evaluated frequently and repaired when it starts to enlarge.

b. Postoperatively, the patient may need a short time on hemodialysis or continue with reduced volume inflows as noted above (Shah, 2006).

3. Dialysate leaks.
   a. Dialysate leaks may be noted shortly after catheter implantation after dialysate is infused and dwelling in the abdomen. It appears as clear fluid at the exit site or suture sites. Dialysate can be identified by checking for glucose, by dipstick or glucometer. All dialysate, even 1.5% dextrose, will read HIGH.
   b. A late leak can occur at the site of entry into the peritoneal cavity or at any suture line. Dialysate will leak into subcutaneous tissue and is noted as swelling that may give the abdomen an asymmetric appearance. It may also leak into the scrotum or the labia and be very uncomfortable. An abdominal CT scan can identify the location and extent of leakage after infusion of dialysate containing radiocontrast material. Treatment is usually a period of resting the abdomen and temporary hemodialysis, followed by IPD, then incremental volume increases until full prescription reached. A recurrent leak will need surgical repair (Leblanc, 2001).

4. Cuff extrusion.
   a. The external cuff should be palpable about 2 cm from the exit site and should not be visible. In cuff extrusion, a portion of the cuff is visible at the exit site. This may be the result of poor placement or from placing a straight catheter in a curved tunnel. The silicone attempts to return to its straight configuration and may push the cuff toward the exit site. Pulling on the catheter may also result in cuff extrusion.
   b. Chronic inflammation and exit-site infections almost always accompany cuff extrusion. The cuff irritates the exit site, thus meticulous daily care must become routine. An attempt can be made to remove the Dacron cuff by shaving it with a surgical blade. Extreme care must be taken not to nick the catheter during this procedure (Crabtree et al., 2012; Guest, 2012).

5. Damage to the catheter.
   a. The most obvious evidence of a damaged catheter is leakage from the catheter that wets the patient's clothing or bedclothes.
   b. A hole in the catheter can be the result of accidental puncture, acute bending at the junction of the adaptor and the catheter, erosion from topical agents that damage silicone, or use of a metal, toothed hemostat. Patients may also accidentally slice the catheter if using a scissors to remove a dressing.

c. Close inspection will reveal a crack or opening in the catheter, a small segment of silicone that is worn or no longer elastic, or even an area that is brittle and crumbles easily. Occasionally, the adapter will become separated from the catheter, either because the catheter has lost elasticity, the adapter was too small, or the catheter was pulled forcefully.

d. In all cases of catheter damage, the patient is instructed to place a plastic clamp between the exit site and the damaged area and to stop dialysis. They must get into clinic as soon as possible to assess and repair the damage and to receive prophylactic intraperitoneal antibiotics.

e. If there is a long enough undamaged segment, the catheter can be trimmed and a new adapter and transfer set placed. The catheter will first be disinfected; then a sterile scissors is used to cut away the damaged area. Many units are replacing plastic with titanium adapters because they have all rounded edges and are less likely to cause a break at the catheter/adaptor junction.

f. If the damaged area is close but at least 15mm from the exit site, a repair kit can be used to extend the catheter before adding the new adaptor and transfer set. There are different manufacturers of these kits, and each unit should have some available.

g. Prophylactic intraperitoneal antibiotics are always administered for any catheter break or leak. Usually, a one-time dose of coverage for both gram-positive and gram-negative organisms is sufficient to prevent peritonitis (Crabtree et al., 2012).

P. Infection: identification and treatment.
1. The major infections in peritoneal dialysis are peritonitis, exit-site, or tunnel infections.
2. Peritonitis is a major cause of hospitalizations and may lead to catheter loss and technique failure. Bacteria gain entry to the peritoneal cavity most often through touch contamination. Bacteria can also move into the abdomen along the tunnel tract or migrate across an inflamed bowel wall or from a ruptured diverticulum. Fortunately, thanks to improved connection technology that reduces risk of touch contamination, the peritonitis rates have been reduced to less than one in every 2 to 3 dialysis years. This is a fact that should be conveyed to patients considering PD, as there is still mythology surrounding a "high infection rate" in PD, and patients are reluctant to consider it for this reason. Healthcare providers and hemodialysis nurses should also be made aware of this fact because they often unwittingly convey it to patients who are making a modality decision.
3. Presenting symptoms include abdominal pain,

sometimes accompanied by nausea or diarrhea, fever, or chills. Occasionally, the symptoms are nonspecific or vague. Drained effluent will be cloudy and often contain fibrin.
4. Diagnosis of peritonitis is confirmed by fluid white blood cell count (WBC) > 100/mm³ with > 50% neutrophils, and PD fluid culture positive for bacteria.
5. Gram stain may or may not be helpful in bacterial infections, though fungus can usually be detected (Tzamaloukas et al., 1993).
6. Sampling technique is important to prevent cultures that show no growth despite presence of cloudy fluid, abdominal pain, and elevated fluid WBCs. Positive culture yield is best after a minimum dwell of 2 hours (Li et al., 2010).
7. Most commonly identified gram-positive organisms are: *Staphylococcus epidermidis* (*S. epi*) 30–40%; *Staphylococcus aureus* (*S.aureus*) 15–20%; *Streptococcus* (strep) 10–15%, other gram-positive 2–5%.
8. Most commonly identified gram-negative organisms are as follows.
   a. *Pseudomonas aeruginosa* 5–10%.
   b. *Enterobacter cloacae* 5–20%.
   c. Other gram-negative 5–7%.
9. Fungus is identified in 2–10% of cases of peritonitis, all other organisms in 2–5% of cases, and culture negative 10–30%.
10. Polymicrobial peritonitis should be dealt with urgently as it may indicate intraabdominal pathology.
11. International Society of Peritoneal Dialysis (Piraino et al., 2005) Guidelines recommend that each dialysis unit develop protocols for empiric antibiotic therapy based on local history of identified organisms and sensitivities.
12. Antibiotics are given immediately. Many centers have a high rate of methicillin resistant staph aureus (MRSA) and need to start gram-positive coverage with Vancomycin. Gram-negative coverage is usually an aminoglycoside or a third generation cephalosporin (Piraino et al., 2005).
13. Antibiotics for continued treatment are then adjusted based on organism and sensitivities.
14. Antibiotics are preferentially given intraperitoneally, for a 6-hour dwell. CAPD is also preferred over APD to offer uniform dosage and peritoneal exposure around the clock. For this reason, APD patients should convert to CAPD while treating peritonitis.
15. Length of treatment depends on severity and organism. Effluent should be observed daily if possible and improvement both in symptoms and cell count seen by 48 hours. *S. epi* and strep infections usually require 2 weeks of treatment. Three weeks are required for most others (such as

S. aureus and *Enterococcus*), or if a concurrent tunnel or exit-site infection is present. A single gram-negative such as *E.coli*, proteus, or klebsiella can respond in 2 weeks but may require 3 weeks treatment. *Stenotrophomonas* will require a longer course, 3 to 4 weeks and treatment with two drugs. Fungal prophylaxis with either fluconazole 100 mg/day or nystatin 500,000u tablets three times a day for the duration of antibiotic therapy is believed to prevent fungal peritonitis that may be promoted by reducing natural gut bacteria with antibiotics.

16. Catheter removal is likely if effluent does not clear within 4 to 5 days of appropriate antibiotics, or in *S. aureus* or *Pseudomonas* peritonitis accompanied by tunnel infection. Antibiotics should be given an additional 2 weeks after the patient is switched to HD.

17. Fungal peritonitis always indicates catheter removal, as cure by medical management is extremely rare. Antifungal agents should be continued at least 10 days after the catheter is removed (Piraino et al., 2005).

18. During peritonitis, the membrane is inflamed, accompanied by increased protein loss, temporary decrease in ultrafiltration, and increased fibrin production. All exchanged should be heparinized and dialysate dextrose percentage adjusted accordingly. Multiple episodes of peritonitis may cause scarring and membrane changes.

19. Relapsing peritonitis is defined as peritonitis with the same organism that recurs within 4 weeks of therapy completion. Recurrent peritonitis is an infection within 4 weeks of therapy completion with a different organism, and reinfection is peritonitis with the same organism that occurs more than 4 weeks after therapy completion (Li et al., 2010).

20. Some common risk factors for peritonitis include *S. aureus* nasal carriage, chronic exit-site or tunnel infections, PD systems that require multiple connections, malnutrition, diabetes, bacteremia, immunosuppressive therapy, HIV positivity, and catheter biofilms (Prowant et al., 2008b; Vardhan & Hutchison, 2014).

21. Prophylactic antibiotic therapy should be given before colonoscopy, dental procedures, and pap smear/pelvic exam. Here are some examples, often modified by unit protocol.
    a. Colonoscopy: peritoneal cavity should be emptied just before the patient leaves for the procedure. Give ampicillin, 1 to 2 grams orally; ciprofloxacin, 750 mg PO; fluconazole, 100 mg PO; or metronidazole, 500 mg PO; 1 to 2 hours prior to the procedure. If allergic to ampicillin, use vancomycin 1 gm, IP x a 6 hour dwell prior to procedure. If allergic to ciprofloxacin,

substitute either ceftazidime 1 gm or gentamycin, 0.6 mg/kg in a 6-hour dwell prior.
    b. Dental prophylaxis: amoxicillin 2 grams orally 1 hour preprocedure; if allergic, erythromycin 2 gm or zithromax 500 mg 1 hour before.
    c. Pap smear: drain the abdomen; may consider fluconazole 100 mg PO preprocedure (Fleming, 2013).

22. Exit-site and tunnel infections.
    a. Exit-site infection presents with erythema, purulent drainage, and crust.
    b. Tunnel infection will present with localized erythema and tenderness over the tunnel tract.
    c. Often, both the exit site and tunnel are simultaneously infected.
    d. Common organisms are *S. aureus* and *Pseudomonas*. Also seen are *S. epi* exit-site infections, and corynebacterium.
    e. *S. aureus* exit-site infections can be difficult to treat and may progress to a tunnel infection that requires catheter removal. If the patient's nares test positive for *S. aureus*, treatment is intranasal mupirocin twice daily for 5 days per month. Also effective is application of mupirocin daily to the exit site and some prescribers add oral rifampin, 600 mg/day for 5 days every 12 weeks. Daily mupirocin application to the exit site has reduced *S. aureus* exit-site infections and peritonitis. Gentamicin cream has a broader spectrum and is now used in place of mupirocin in many programs.
    f. *Pseudomonas* exit-site and tunnel infections are treated according to sensitivities, but often relapse and lead to catheter replacement (Prowant et al., 2008b) (Crabtree et al., 2012).
    g. Figure 3.13 shows a healthy PD catheter exit site while Figure 3.14 demonstrates an infected exit site.

Q. Other complications of peritoneal dialysis.
    1. Hemoperitoneum: bloody effluent.
        a. Usually noted postoperatively for the first few exchanges/flushes.
        b. Ovulation and/or menstruation may result in bloody appearance in the effluent due to the anatomical position of ovaries within the peritoneal cavity. It is transient and should clear up in a day or two. Instruct patient to heparinize solution to prevent catheter obstruction by blood clots.
        c. Other reasons such as a bowel source or malignancy should be assessed and worked up according to degree of acuity, other systemic symptoms, and length of time blood is present.
    2. Hydrothorax.
        a. Peritoneal fluid enters the thoracic cavity via a

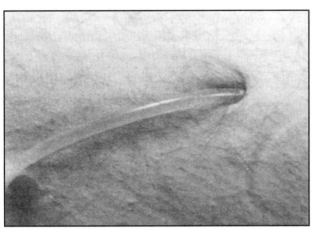

Figure 3.13. Healthy peritoneal dialysis catheter exit site.

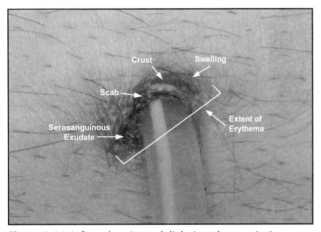

Figure 3.14. Infected peritoneal dialysis catheter exit site.

defect in the diaphragm. This usually occurs acutely, is more common in females, and causes dyspnea and increasing shortness of breath. Drain volumes diminish despite increasing dextrose concentrations. It will progress to acute respiratory distress. Pleural effusions are seen on x-ray, and a thoracentesis will show a very high glucose level.

    b. PD is usually discontinued for 2 to 4 weeks to see if the defect will seal itself. Some procedures that are tried to close the defect include pleurodesis with an agent such as talc or tetracycline, fibrin glue, or surgical repair. PD can be reintroduced slowly, but if the defect recurs, the patient should switch to hemodialysis.

  3. Shoulder pain from air infusion.

    a. Occurs when dialysis solution lines are not fully primed with dialysate prior to a dialysis session.

    b. Pain is referred from the diaphragm to the shoulder and may mimic a cardiac event.

    c. After discovering air infusion, air may be

removed by draining patient in knee-chest or Trendelenburg positions. This forces the air to float up to the catheter tip. Air bubbles will be seen as fluid drains.

  4. Pain on infusion or drain.

    a. Usually noted with initial exchanges. May be due to incomplete internal healing or as catheter finds its best location. A straight catheter may cause more infusion pain due to the stream being directed in one area rather than dispersed as with a coiled catheter.

    b. Rectal or suprapubic pain may be from a catheter that is too long and thus irritates local tissues.

    c. If pain does not resolve after a few weeks, a tidal program on the cycler will help because the abdomen is never completely emptied until the last exchange and the reservoir left behind acts as a cushion (Maaz, 2004).

  5. An abdominal x-ray, anterior/posterior and lateral will be obtained if pain does not resolve. Sometimes catheter replacement is the only fix.

  6. Back pain.

    a. Preexisting back pain can worsen when carrying fluid daily.

    b. The center of gravity moves forward and lumbar lordosis increases.

    c. Physical therapy can help by teaching body mechanics and muscle strengthening exercises.

    d. The prescription may need to be adjusted to APD with reduced daytime volumes.

  7. Noninfectious peritonitis.

    a. Cloudy effluent seen without abdominal pain or symptoms of bacterial peritonitis. Dialysate WBC count will be low, with < 50% neutrophils but eosinophils > 10%.

    b. Is likely to be allergy to either a new PD catheter or a newly used IP medication. It usually resolves after discontinuing the presumed provoking factor, but should still be cultured and closely monitored.

    c. Chylous peritonitis.

      (1) A rare presentation resulting from disruption of peritoneal lymphatics.

      (2) Effluent appears milky and is notable for high triglycerides.

      (3) It is a sign of intraabdominal or hepatic pathology and warrants diagnostic work up (Prowant et al., 2008b; Roodhooft, 1987).

  8. Peritoneal membrane changes.

    a. Dialysate solutions containing dextrose are not physiologic and over time, the interstitium and basement membrane of the peritoneum thicken. Implicated in this change are glucose degradation products (GDPs) and advanced glycation end products (AGEs). The microvessels change and neovascularization is seen along with collagen deposition. Peritoneal thickening is hastened by recurrent peritonitis.

b. Most patients will show varying degrees of peritoneal change after 5 years, especially if using higher dextrose dialysate or if peritonitis is frequent. PET testing will show trend toward high transport. It is important to be alert to ultrafiltration changes and to ensure that the lowest percent of dextrose is used. Icodextrin use can be helpful as it is not reabsorbed, and thus maintains ultrafiltration (Finkelstein et al., 2005).

c. If the ultrafiltration is less than 400 mL after a 4-hour, 2-L dwell using 4.25% dextrose, the patient has ultrafiltration failure and should be converted to hemodialysis.

d. Encapsulation peritoneal sclerosis (EPS) is a rare condition that results when the peritoneum becomes dense, fibrous, and thickened. The bowel develops adhesions and areas of encapsulation. The incidence is highest after 5 years on PD. Bowel obstruction and ileus are seen, with progressive reduction in motility as areas of fibrosis bind intestinal loops. Vague abdominal pain and diarrhea can be early signs that progress to more debilitating pain. Surgery is tricky but may be necessary in some cases to resect the bowel and relieve obstruction. Mortality rate is dependent on patient status at diagnosis. If the process is already severe and advanced, survival rate is lower. Patients will convert to hemodialysis, and their abdominal symptoms should be closely monitored as bowel obstruction can repeatedly occur. EPS may also occur in a previously undiagnosed patient who switches from PD to HD. The major risk factor for developing EPS is duration on peritoneal dialysis, but peritonitis and glucose exposure have been postulated as causes (Vardhan & Hutchison, 2014).

9. Pregnancy.

a. Though rare and not technically a complication of PD, pregnancy presents a management challenge.

b. High risk pregnancy specialists in collaboration with the nephrology team will follow the patient.

c. Residual kidney function increases the chance of live birth.

d. Medications need to be changed if the patient is on anything teratogenic such as angiotensin converting enzyme inhibitors (ACEIs). Erythropoietin supplements will increase as pregnancy progresses.

e. Fill volume will decrease as the uterus enlarges. There is no universal agreement on a Kt/V value; instead the patient is monitored for uremic symptoms.

f. Often the woman is hospitalized by the 20th week and may be converted to hemodialysis as the gravid uterus occupies the abdominal cavity (Reddy, 2007).

R. The routine monthly clinic visit.

1. History and physical exam.
   a. Changes since last visit, hospitalizations, and interventions by other specialty providers or PCP.
   b. General appearance and review of systems.
   c. Vital signs and weight, lungs, heart, exit-site/tunnel examination, and extremities for edema.

2. Flow sheet review. Look for blood pressure and weight trends, type of dialysate being used, and adherence with prescription. Some APD cyclers have the ability to download treatment information. This can help if the patient has honestly entered treatment details such as weight, blood pressure, and type of dialysate.

3. Medication review. Check for adherence, side effects, need for any renewals.

4. Anemia management. Check trends in hemoglobin, hematocrit, iron stores, and erythropoietin or iron supplementation. Erythropoietin doses are usually lower than with HD patients and are administered weekly or less often. Oral iron supplements are poorly tolerated; IV iron can be infused during the clinic visit.

5. Bone mineral management. Check trends in calcium, phosphorus, intact PTH, and alkaline phosphatase. Vitamin D analogs for management of secondary hyperparathyroidism are given orally. Cinacalcet may also be used to control elevated iPTH levels. Assess need for parathyroidectomy if iPTH is unable to be medically controlled, and monitor patient carefully after surgery as calcium levels tend to fall and oral calcium supplements will be necessary.

6. Adequacy of dialysis. Ensure that adequacy is being assessed per unit protocol. Review all PET and adequacy data, and monitor changes in residual kidney function. Adjust the PD prescription if needed.

7. Nutrition evaluation. Collaborate with dietitian. PD patients lose some protein in the effluent so this is a constant challenge. PD does not clear phosphate well, and a review of diet and binder use is essential. Potassium does not present a major problem for PD patients as it is readily removed from blood.

8. Fluid balance and hypertension. PD patients typically retain residual kidney function longer than hemodialysis patients, probably because the hemodynamics of the kidneys are not challenged as in an HD treatment. It is important to ensure that the patient still controls sodium intake to

prevent edema and elevations in blood pressure. As always, make sure the patient adheres to the antihypertensive regimen before making changes.

9. Diabetes. Patients with diabetes and on PD expose themselves to extra glucose from the dialysate and will often need to increase insulin doses or may need to start insulin if previously managed on an oral hypoglycemic. Weight gain can result from both the extra sugar and insulin. Insulin regimens often include injecting a long-acting preparation daily and short-acting injections with meals. Injecting insulin into the dialysate bags is only rarely used as it can cling to the plastic, thus making delivery unreliable and requiring a much higher dosage. It can also increase risk of introducing bacteria if excellent technique is not used (Dasgupta, 2004). Another important consideration for the patient with diabetes who may use icodextrin solutions is glucometer choice. Maltose is a metabolite of icodextrin and may interfere with glucose test strips or glucometers that use glucose dehydrogenase-pyrroloquinolinequinone (GDH-PDQ) as a testing reagent. This can lead to falsely elevated blood glucose readings, leading to overdosing insulin. True hypoglycemia may also be hidden by the false readings. Dialysis units have been taught to check each individual's glucometer to ensure safe use with icodextrin (Tsai, 2010 #43).

10. Transplant referral and candidacy. Patients should be referred to the transplant center of their choice. If they meet criteria established by that center, the dialysis unit can collaborate by collecting a monthly sample for antibody screen. They can also assist with ordering any tests the transplant center needs to maintain the patient as active on their list. It is also important that the transplant center be notified if the patient has any infection or change in medical status that would prevent transplantation.

11. Routine immunizations. The clinic visit can also be time to review status of annual flu shots, periodic pneumococcal vaccination, hepatitis B immunity, and any other vaccines such as herpes zoster or a tetanus/pertussis booster. PPD is also checked annually.

S. When the PD patient is hospitalized.
1. For elective procedures, patients are reminded to drain the abdomen prior to the procedure.
2. For emergencies, patients should always have a copy of their prescription and relevant information, especially if they are traveling in an unfamiliar location.
3. In cases of peritonitis, patients who cannot be seen in their unit should be told to bring the cloudy bag with them. Effluent samples should

always be obtained from a port on the dialysate bag after disinfecting the port. It is never acceptable to remove the catheter cap and allow fluid to run freely into a culture cup. Culture and cell count should be obtained immediately and empiric antibiotics administered. Collaboration with the patient's nephrology care provider must take place as well. An APD patient will be converted to CAPD to ensure uniform IP antibiotic coverage. On discharge, communication with the patient's home unit is essential to describe details of the hospitalization.

T. Transition to hemodialysis.
1. Reasons for temporary transition to HD include catheter complications that interfere with function such as dialysate leaks, catheter migration, omental wrap repair, hernia repair, chronic tunnel infection, unresponsive peritonitis, relapsing peritonitis or peritonitis accompanied by tunnel infection, fungal peritonitis, or other catheter damage that cannot be repaired.
2. Permanent transition to HD should be made if: the patient has ultrafiltration or clearance failure, internal abdominal catastrophes or presence of too many adhesions or scars to allow catheter placement. Some patients with polycystic kidneys may have enlarging cysts that, although retroperitoneal, can reduce the amount of volume that is comfortable for the patient and make adequate dialysis impossible.
3. Sometimes the patient simply can no longer tolerate doing PD for physical or psychosocial reasons (Prowant et al., 2008b).

Y. Palliative care.
1. The option of "no dialysis" should have been presented when the patient and significant others were choosing a modality. Choices should be reviewed on a regular basis. It is important to explore patients' value systems in regard to withdrawal of treatment well in advance of the need to make such a decision and to have their advance directives on file.
2. There are many reasons that patients may withdraw from dialysis therapy, such as incurable malignancies, chronic severe pain, perception of poor quality of life, and failure to thrive.
3. When the decision to stop dialysis is made, the patient can be referred to a hospice program. Hospice is covered by Medicare and requires physician referral. An APRN cannot yet make the referral ("Medicare Update: Attending in Home Health Care and Hospice," 2014). A life expectancy of less than 6 months must be certified.
4. Hospice teams may care for the patient in the

home or in a dedicated facility. Stopping dialysis is not necessary if the patient is being admitted for a terminal process other than kidney failure, such as end-stage cancer.

5. Patient and family should know that uremic symptoms will bring on increased fatigue and somnolence, and that pain will be expertly managed in the hospice setting.

6. Grief counseling should be available to all the patient's family, friends, and caregivers as well.

V. Special situations.

1. Hearing impairment. Assistive devices can be obtained and set up to detect audible alarms from the cycler that the patient cannot hear. The patient would be alerted via a flashing light or vibration. Special accommodations are needed during training, and a sign language interpreter or lip reader should always be present. The patient's home phone system will also need to have a text feature. The patient may already have such assistive devices in the home.

2. Visual impairment. The visually impaired patient may need something simple, such as a magnifier to read instructions. Other helpful aids are use of contrast and texture on equipment and supplies. Recorded instructions are also helpful.

3. Travel. It is much easier for patients on PD to travel. Unlike hemodialysis, they do not depend on availability of a dialysis chair. They must coordinate with their home unit to find a backup unit at their destination. The supply companies require sufficient notice to ship supplies to the travel address. They should check with the unit social worker to help coordinate payment for dialysis outside of the USA. When flying with a cycler, a letter will be given explaining that it is medical equipment and must not be checked baggage.

4. Cirrhosis and ascites. These patients are a challenge in that they have potential problems with both PD and HD. Coagulopathy may make HD difficult, and in PD, ascites can lead to catheter leakage if used early or if catheter implantation is not preceded by large volume paracentesis. Ascites can be managed in the initial period by attaching an empty drain bag and allowing ascitic fluid to be removed in that manner rather than leaking out through the tunnel. When PD is the chosen modality, fluid and nutritional management require active and ongoing collaboration with the multidisciplinary team. Risk of spontaneous bacterial peritonitis (SBP) is real, and the role of antibiotic prophylaxis has yet to be clarified (Guest, 2010).

SECTION E
Approaches to Care by the APRN in Home Dialysis
Elaine Go, Katherine Houle

I. Introduction.

Home hemodialysis started in 1964 in the United States and was the most common type of kidney replacement therapy until the early 1970s. End-stage renal disease (ESRD) Medicare entitlement was signed into law in 1972 and payment for dialysis was secured by Medicare. This event caused the rise in in-center hemodialysis units and the decline of home hemodialysis use.

More than 20 million (10%) of adults in the United States are estimated to have chronic kidney disease (CKD) and most are undiagnosed. According to the 2014 USRDS report, there are 449,342 prevalent dialysis patients. Broken down into modalities, 402,514 patients receive hemodialysis and 40,605 patients are on PD. Home dialysis accounts for 49,000 patients. Of those, 16.3% are treated with hemodialysis and 83.7% with PD (USRDS, 2014).

In its final ruling released in November 2013, the Centers for Medicare and Medicaid Services (CMS), among others, finalized an increase of 50% for home dialysis training for both peritoneal and hemodialysis. It is projected that there will be an increase in home hemodialysis use due to evidence-based studies showing improved patient outcomes and CMS's final policy affecting home hemodialysis.

II. Overview of home hemodialysis.

A. History of home hemodialysis.

1. In 1960, the Teflon arteriovenous shunt was introduced by Belding Scribner and colleagues at the University of Washington. This device enabled long-term hemodialysis in the treatment of ESRD.

2. In 1961, Scribner met with a Norwegian urologist who had developed a flat plate dialyzer. Scribner, seeing the potential of this flat plate dialyzer, brought one back with him to Seattle. Together with a friend, they were able to produce Kiil boards with flat plates and uniform blood film thickness from polypropylene slabs. For over 10 years, Kiil dialyzers were the dialyzers used in the Seattle dialysis program.

3. In 1962, Quinton developed a softer tip for shunts using silastic tubing with Teflon tips (Blagg, 2007). In the same year, Cimino and Brescia led the development of what is now known as the arteriovenous fistula.

4. In 1965, there were two home hemodialysis programs in the United States: one in Boston led by John Merrill and one in Seattle led by Belding Scribner (Twardowski, 1997).

5. In 1966, Dr. Kolff from Cleveland Clinic started a successful home hemodialysis program. It was thus proven that home hemodialysis was a safe, effective, and inexpensive kidney replacement modality for treating chronic kidney insufficiency (Nose, 2000).

6. Proportioning pumps were used to make dialysate from concentrates containing sodium acetate. At the same time came the development of the prototype for single patient dialysis machines.

7. Frequency and length of home hemodialysis treatments varied from center to center. The Boston group was dialyzing patients 5 hours twice a week using twin coil dialyzers. The Seattle patients dialyzed once every 5 to 7 days when symptoms of uremia redeveloped and was noted. Treatment time was further increased to 12 to 20 hours twice a week due to the development of severe hypertension and symptoms of peripheral neuropathy (Blagg, 2007).

8. Numerous scientific and technical innovations have continued to improve home hemodialysis through the years. The number of home hemodialysis patients continued to increase until 1972, when President Richard Nixon signed and enacted the Medicare ESRD program. Home hemodialysis became unaffordable, and the number of home hemodialysis patients gradually declined. The dialysis industry mushroomed into more than 5,500 Medicare-certified hemodialysis units that offered outpatient, in-center hemodialysis (MedPAC, 2012).

B. Types of home hemodialysis (see Table 3.6).
1. Daily hemodialysis allows for increased clearance of middle molecules because of less rebound of β 2 microglobulin.
2. Nocturnal hemodialysis increases middle molecule removal as a result of higher frequency and longer duration of hemodialysis treatments.
3. Greater convective removal is also seen as a result of higher weekly ultrafiltration (Perl & Chan, 2009).

C. Benefits of home hemodialysis.
1. Increasing evidence supports the benefits of home hemodialysis. Numerous randomized control trials have shown better blood pressure control with fewer to no antihypertensive medications used. This leads to a decrease in cardiovascular morbidity and regression of left ventricular hypertrophy.
2. Increased phosphate removal is evident in short

Table 3.6

Types of Home Hemodialysis

Types	Frequency	Length of Time
Intermittent	3 to 4 tx/wk	3 to 4 hr/day
Short daily	> 3 tx/wk (average 6)	2 to 4 hr/day
Nocturnal/extended	Any combination	> 6 hr/day

Source: ANNA Home Hemodialysis Fact Sheet.

daily home hemodialysis. Phosphate binders are usually not required for patients doing nocturnal dialysis. Dietary phosphate restriction is also seldom required.
   a. In many cases, intradialytic phosphate supplementation is used to prevent hypophosphatemia (Perl & Chan, 2009).
   b. Mineral bone disorders in kidney failure (e.g., abnormalities of calcium, phosphorus, parathyroid hormone, and vitamin D metabolism; bone turnover and vascular and soft tissue calcification commonly seen in conventional hemodialysis) are less evident in home hemodialysis patients due to better calcium and phosphorus homeostasis.
3. Daily hemodialysis and nocturnal hemodialysis allow for increased removal of middle molecules due to increased frequency and duration of dialysis and higher weekly ultrafiltration.
4. Less fluctuation in volume status even with liberalization of fluid intake is made possible due to increased frequency and/or time on dialysis.
5. Because of more frequent hemodialysis, patients are encouraged to maintain a higher protein and phosphorus intake. Potassium intake is more liberal than it is on conventional dialysis. Malnutrition is decreased and appetite improved in most patients on home hemodialysis due to the liberalization of their diet.
6. Some studies have shown that patients on nocturnal dialysis are more functional and enjoy a better quality of life (Jassal et al., 2006).
7. Home hemodialysis provides opportunity for rehabilitation and employment. Patients are able to maintain their independence and they tend to know more about their illness. They feel "in charge" of their own treatment and often have better outcomes (Blagg & Mailloux, 2013).
8. Home hemodialysis is a viable option for kidney replacement therapy due to concerns over costs, ESRD Medicare spending, and shortage of nephrologists, nurses, and other staff taking care

of an increasing population of chronic kidney disease (CKD) patients.

D. Barriers to home hemodialysis. Literature has shown evidence of adopting home hemodialysis for its benefits. However, there are barriers that may preclude one from opting for home hemodialysis.
   1. Systems barriers may exist due to lack of experience with home hemodialysis by nephrologists and nurses. This in part may be due to bias and lack of incentive. It remains to be seen if the Medicare changes in the Prospective Payment System (ESRD Bundle 2011) will result in an increase in home hemodialysis patients.
   2. Patient-related barriers may preclude patients from doing home hemodialysis. Some of these are related to fear of cannulation by both patient and/or care partner. Some patients may have a perceived fear of causing more burdens by bringing dialysis to the home setting. Education level of both the patient and caregiver may make training a challenge.
   3. The patient's medical condition and comorbidity make home hemodialysis an unsuitable option. Impaired left ventricular heart function and/or congestive heart failure may cause hemodynamic instability thus making home hemodialysis an unsafe option (Perl & Chan, 2009).
   4. A poorly functioning vascular access will make the patient a poor candidate for home hemodialysis. Both patient and caregiver must be comfortable in cannulation. Buttonhole cannulation may alleviate the patient's fear of pain.

E. Regulatory requirements in home hemodialysis programs. There are special requirements and recommendations in setting up a home hemodialysis program.
   1. The ESRD Conditions for Coverage detail regulatory standards for home hemodialysis programs to provide safe and quality care. It addresses home dialysis training and support, environment, water quality, equipment maintenance record, personnel record review, and Quality Assurance and Performance Improvement (QAPI) review. A medical record review is done to look at the patient's adherence with therapy and to address other issues that may preclude the patient from doing home hemodialysis (Federal Register, 2008).
   2. The Association for the Advancement of Medical Instrumentation (AAMI) has guidelines that focus on patient safety as a priority. There are set standards for dialysis water quality monitoring, dialysate, bacteria and endotoxin testing, medical electrical equipment, chemical sampling, and home environment, to name a few.

3. The home hemodialysis program must have written policies and procedures that cover:
   a. Training of staff, patients, and caregivers.
   b. The patient's monthly clinic visits with the multidisciplinary team.
   c. Monthly lab draws and reviewing of results.
   d. Monthly treatment monitoring.
   e. Treatment adherence.
   f. Patient responsibilities and expectations.
4. Policies and procedures must also be in place to address the technical and biotechnical aspects of the program, ensuring safe operation of water systems and all other medical equipment in the home.

F. Patient selection for home hemodialysis.
   1. It has been shown that predialysis education provides the patient with a more complete understanding of dialysis options. Schiller et al. (2011) have shown that 46% of patients who received predialysis education opted for home therapy with 20% of those patients choosing home hemodialysis.
   2. An assessment by the home dialysis nurse is important to determine patient's suitability for home hemodialysis. Chow and Tran (2012) have developed a validated tool to assess suitability for home hemodialysis. This tool assesses the patient's suitability for home hemodialysis, addressing communication, nutritional status, ability to maintain care, and psychosocial and social support aspects (Chow & Tran, 2012). Motivation and compliance are important factors in patient selection. Most home dialysis programs require a care partner to help the patient with every hemodialysis treatment. The partner can be a family member or a friend. Thus it is equally important to include family members and potential caregivers in this initial interview.
   3. Factors involved that may influence patient selection for home hemodialysis include general medical condition and hemodynamic stability during hemodialysis, living accommodations and circumstance, learning ability and motivation of patient, family and care partner, and patient and family level of anxiety. Adherence is an important factor.

G. Vascular access.
   1. Arteriovenous fistulae (AVF), arteriovenous grafts, and tunneled dialysis catheters have all been used successfully in home hemodialysis programs, though the AVF is the preferred vascular access.
   2. AV fistulae should tolerate blood flow rates from 150 mL/min for slow nocturnal dialysis to 400 mL/min for intermittent hemodialysis 3 to 4 times

per week. AV fistulae have a low rate of infection. A rotating site method or buttonhole technique may be used for cannulation of the fistula. For daily hemodialysis treatments, buttonhole technique may be preferred. Use of the buttonhole technique can have lower complication rates and reduce pain. The buttonhole technique is not recommended for the AV graft.

3. The use of aseptic technique is crucial in the prevention of vascular access infection. NKF K/DOQI 2006 recommendations outline the basic principles of vascular access infection. Hand washing is the first step in the prevention of infection. During training, guidelines for access management should be provided for the patient, care partner, and other family members. The patient should be instructed to recognize signs and symptoms of infection and immediately report any of these symptoms. When using the buttonhole technique, patients should be instructed on meticulous scab removal and aseptic technique to prevent infection.

4. Safety related to vascular access should be addressed. Needle dislodgement is a very serious accident that can happen during hemodialysis. Use of a moisture sensor patch or enuresis alarm will alert the patient of needle dislodgment.

H. Home physical setup and utility considerations.
1. During the patient selection process, home assessment is done to determine if renovations of the home need to be done to achieve regulatory compliance.
   a. Technical support staff will do an initial home visit to determine the location for dialysis and water treatment equipment. There should be easy accessibility to equipment.
   b. Storage space should be adequate to accommodate supply delivery.
   c. Electrical supply, plumbing drains and vents, and water supply must meet city codes (Harwood & Leitch, 2006).
2. Water quality is a very important component of hemodialysis. The standards for safe water for hemodialysis are set by the Association for the Advancement of Medical Instrumentation (AAMI). The CMS Conditions for Coverage require that home hemodialysis programs ensure that water used for dialysis meets AAMI standards.

I. Patient and partner education and training.
1. It is important to consider the patient's level of education. Education materials provided to the patients should be in short and easy-to-read materials. Education is aimed at giving the patient an understanding of the disease process. An

informed patient is empowered to be competent and confident in self-care.
2. One objective of training is to assist the patient in performing safe dialysis and achieving good outcomes. The training period gives the nurse the opportunity to assess the patient's suitability for home hemodialysis. During this period it may be necessary to provide emotional support to the patient and family as they adjust to the change in lifestyle and the stress of home hemodialysis.
3. A training checklist should reflect a satisfactory return demonstration and recall of all aspects of training.

J. Components of home hemodialysis training.
1. Standard precautions.
   a. Infection control practices are designed to protect patients, healthcare providers, and the general public. These practices include hand hygiene, use of personal protective equipment such as face shields, masks, gloves, and fluid resistant gowns to provide a barrier to contamination with body fluids, blood, mucous membranes, and nonintact skin.
   b. Standard precautions also include vaccination of patients and immunization of healthcare workers.
   c. Aseptic technique is used to reduce exposure to microorganisms.
   d. Patients and caregivers are also trained on the management of sharps, blood spills, soiled linens, disposal of medical waste, and environmental cleaning to maintain a safe environment.
2. Infection control precautions are designed to prevent the transmission of bloodborne viruses and bacterial pathogens. These practices include routine serological testing and surveillance for Hepatitis B infection. Patients are taught to recognize symptoms of infections and report them immediately to the home dialysis staff.
3. Hemodialysis equipment.
   a. Hemodialysis equipment includes the dialysis machines, all the disposables used in the hemodialysis procedure, water treatment, and instruments such as blood pressure equipment, stethoscope, and clamps. Patients should have a basic understanding of how the hemodialysis delivery system works and demonstrate how to troubleshoot problems.
   b. Cleaning and disinfection of all equipment and handling of other disposable supplies is critical for the safety of patients.
   c. Dialysis machines are disinfected internally and externally cleaned according to CDC and manufacturer's recommendations.
4. Hemodialysis procedures.

a. Review of normal and altered kidney function provides patient with a better understanding of dialysis as a kidney replacement therapy. Based on the patient's learning ability and style, patients are taught the principles of dialysis such as osmosis, diffusion, and ultrafiltration. This will also enable the patient to better understand the hemodialysis process and manage complications.

b. Patients are shown the benefits of home hemodialysis as compared to other kidney replacement therapies for a better appreciation of the modality they have chosen.

c. Patients are trained in medical recordkeeping of their treatment logs, medication administration, and equipment monitor logs. A good functioning vascular access is the key to the success for a home hemodialysis patient. It should be able to provide the prescribed blood flow. Patients are taught routine assessment and should report any complications such as absence of a thrill or bruit, and signs of infection immediately to the home dialysis nurse.

d. Routine predialysis and postdialysis care of the vascular access is crucial for the long-term survival of the access.

5. Preparation and administration of medications.

a. Patients are taught how to name and identify their medications, state their purpose, and know the dosage and administration route.

b. Patients should be educated on side effects, drug-to-drug interactions, and what foods to avoid when taking certain classes of medications.

c. Patients should be instructed to let the home dialysis nurse know if they are regularly taking over-the-counter medications and use of alternative medicine.

d. Proper storage of medication is addressed, especially injectables. Proper disposal of unused injectables and used needles and syringes is also addressed.

6. Complications during hemodialysis. Home hemodialysis is generally very safe, especially with the advancement of technology. More frequent and longer hemodialysis treatments have reduced the risk of hemodynamic instability.

a. Complications during hemodialysis may occur either due to technical or clinical issues. Policy and procedures should address prevention of these complications.

b. Patients and caregivers are instructed to recognize signs and symptoms of complications and actions to be taken to rectify the problem.

c. The home dialysis staff is available 24/7 and, in the event of life-threatening complications, patients and caregivers are taught to seek emergency medical treatment via paramedics.

7. Troubleshooting technical problems.

a. Issues with alarms, air in line, and clotting are some technical problems that may occur during hemodialysis. During training, patients and caregiver are taught how to prevent these issues and to strictly follow manufacturer's recommendations in the setting up of the hemodialysis machine.

b. Patients need to know how to call for technical help.

c. Patients should also be taught emergency discontinuation of treatment prior to a technical issue turning into a clinical event.

8. Laboratory specimen collection and handling.

a. Proper specimen collection, identification, and handling are essential in obtaining valid laboratory results. Patients should be able to show how specimens are collected for adequacy, routine monthly draws, and blood culture. Correct blood tubes and filling out of requisition forms are essential to timely acquisition of results. Specimens should be packed properly for transport.

b. In addition, patients are taught normal and acceptable laboratory ranges and significance of tests done. Test results are reviewed during monthly clinic visits with the multidisciplinary team.

K. Home hemodialysis equipment and systems.

1. NxStage® System One – portable hemodialysis system that uses 4 to 6 L bags of ultrapure dialysate. It has a highly automated system design with a drop-in cartridge that makes training and use easy.

2. Fresenius 2008K@home™ hemodialysis machine – has the same functionality as machines that are used in dialysis centers.

L. Clinical management of home hemodialysis patients.

1. Initial home visit is made at the completion of training when the patient is doing the first treatment at home. Home visits allow for the healthcare team to ensure continuity of care during transition from the in center hemodialysis unit and home hemodialysis. At the home visit, the nurse makes an assessment of the home situation and the comfort level of the patient and caregiver. Emergency procedures are also reviewed at this time. Inspection of medication storage should also be performed at this time.

2. A 6-month visit will allow the nurse to address any concerns, looking for signs of burnout.

3. The annual home visit allows the nurse to review

infection control practices, emergency management, and treatment and equipment logs.

4. Monthly clinic visits with the nephrologist or the Advanced Practice Registered Nurse (APRN) is required by ESRD Federal Regulations. The patient will also be visiting with the interdisciplinary team at this time. Review of treatment logs is done during these monthly visits.

5. During an ESRD core survey, hemodialysis treatment logs are reviewed for staff monitoring of the patient's adherence to treatment and medication orders, machine safety checks, blood pressure/fluid management, and recognizing and addressing issues (CMS ESRD Core Survey Version 1.3).

M. Future of home hemodialysis.

1. There is much work to be done to increase home hemodialysis use. The Advanced Practice Registered Nurse is in a good position to do early identification of potential patients in CKD clinics and in the primary care setting. Early education on dialysis modality options will provide patients the opportunity to select the modality of their choice. More time should be devoted to emphasize the benefits of home hemodialysis.

2. A change in the reimbursement policy by CMS to pay for frequent dialysis and training days, as well as the development of new technology to make home dialysis machines simpler and safer, may encourage greater use of home hemodialysis.

References

Alleman, K., & Longton, S. (2008). Kidney transplantation. In C.S. Counts (Ed.), *Core curriculum for nephrology nursing* (5th ed., pp. 608–623) Pitman, New Jersey: American Nephrology Nurses' Association.

Allon, M., & Maya, I.D. (2013). *Overview of the treatment of stenosis and thrombotic complications of hemodialysis arteriovenous grafts and fistulas.* Retrieved from http://www.uptodate.com/contents/overview-of-the-treatment-of-stenosis-and-thrombotic-complications-of-hemodialysis-arteriovenous-grafts-and-fistulas?detectedLanguage=en&source=search_result&search=overview+of+the+treatment+of+stenosis+and+thrombotic+complications+of+hemodialysis&selectedTitle=1%7E150&provider=noProvider

American Association of Nurse Practitioners (AANP). (2013). *Main page.* Retrieved from https://www.aanp.org

American Diabetes Association. (2013). Standard of medical care in diabetes. *Diabetes Care, 26*(Suppl. 1), S11-S66. Retrieved from http://www.care.diabetesjournals.org

American College of Radiology (2011a). *ACR–AIUM–SRU practice guideline for the performance of ultrasound vascular mapping for preoperative planning of dialysis access.* Retrieved from http://www.acr.org/~/media/ACR/Documents/PGTS/guidelines/US_Preoperative_Dialysis.pdf

American College of Radiology. (2011b). *ACR–AIUM–SRU practice parameter for the performance of vascular ultrasound for postoperative assessment of dialysis access.* Retrieved from

http://www.acr.org/~/media/ACR/Documents/PGTS/guidelines/US_Postoperative_Dialysis.pdf

Artegraft Inc. (2013). *Artegraft® bovine carotid artery graft.* Retrieved ofrom http://artegraft.com/Home

Asif, A., Roy-Chaudhury, P., & Beathard, G.A. (2006). Early arteriovenous fistula failure: A logical proposal for when and how to intervene. *Clinical Journal of the American Society of Nephrology, 1*(2), 332-339.

Atrium medical corporation. (n.d). *Flixene™ graft.* Retrieved from http://www.atriummed.com/EN/Vascular/flixene.asp

Ball, L.K (2013). Fatal vascular access hemorrhage: Reducing the odds. *Nephrology Nursing Journal, 40*(4), 297-303.

Bander, S.J & Schwab, S.J. (2012). *Overview of central catheters for acute and chronic hemodialysis access.* Retrieved from http://www.uptodate.com.

Bartucci, M. (2006). Kidney transplantation. In D. LaPoint, L. Ohler, & T. Shafer (Eds.), *A clinician's guide to donation and transplantation* (pp. 393-410). Lenexa, KS: NATCO.

Beathard, G.A. (2009). *Percutaneous angioplasty for the treatment of venous stenosis affecting hemodialysis access grafts.* Retrieved from http://www.uptodate.com/contents/percutaneous-angioplasty-for-the-treatment-of-venous-stenosis-affecting-hemodialysis-access-grafts.

Blagg, C.R. (2007). The early history of dialysis for chronic renal failure in the United States: A view from Seattle. *American Journal of Kidney Disease, 49*(3), 482-496.

Blagg, C.R., & Mailloux, L.U. (2013). Home hemodialysis. *Up-To-Date 2013.* Retrieved from http://www.uptodate.com

Bolton, W. (1998) Nephrology nurse practitioners in a collaborative care model. *American Journal Kidney Disease, 31*(5), 786-793.

Breiterman White, R. (2006). Vascular access for hemodialysis. In A.E. Malzahn, & E. Butera (Eds.), *Contemporary nephrology nursing: Principles and practice* (2nd ed., pp. 559-580). Pitman, NJ: American Nephrology Nurses' Association.

Chow, J., & Tran, D.T. (2012). Health professionals' perceptions of the JPAT – An assessment tool for home hemodialysis suitability. *Renal Society of Australasia Journal, 8*(3), 126-131.

Centers for Medicare and Medicaid Services (CMS). *CMS ESRD core survey versions 1.3 (p 14).* Retrieved from http://www.cms.gov/Medicare/Provider-Enrollment-and-Certification/GuidanceforLawsAndRegulations/Downloads/ESRD-Core-Survey-Field-Manual.pdf

Coentrao, L., & Turmel-Rodrigues, L. (2013). Monitoring dialysis interventions fistulae: It's in our hands. *The Journal of Vascular Access, 14*(3), 209-215.

Russell, T. (Section editor). (2008). APN role in chronic kidney disease stage 5 and hemodialysis. In C.S. Counts (Ed.), *Core curriculum for nephrology nursing* (5th ed., pp. 426-430). Pitman, NJ: American Nephrology Nurses' Association.

Crabtree, J. (2006). Selected best demonstrated practices in peritoneal dialysis access. *Kidney International, 70*, S27.

Crabtree, J.F., Firanek, C.A., Piraino, B., Abu-Alfa, A.K., & Guest, S. (Eds.). (2012). *Access care and complications: Management update.* Baxter Healthcare: Renal Division. Retrieved from http://www.homebybaxter.com/Documents/AL06058C%20AFP%20Access%20Guide%20.pdf

Daily Med. (2014a). *Everolimus.* Retrieved from http://dailymed.nlm.nih.gov.

Daily Med. (2014b) *Tacrolimus.* Retrieved from http://dailymed.nlm.nih.gov

Dains, J.E., Bauman, L. & Scheible, P. (2012). *Advanced health assessment and clinical diagnosis in primary care* (4th ed.). St. Louis: Elsevier Mosby.

Dasgupta, M.K. (2004). Strategies for managing diabetic patients on peritoneal dialysis. *Advances in Peritoneal Dialysis, 20*, 200-202.

Deaver, K. (2010). Preventing infections in hemodialysis fistula and graft vascular access. *Nephrology Nursing Journal, 37*(5), 503-505.

Di Paolo, N.C., Capotondo, L., Sansoni, E., Romolini, V., Simola, M, Gaggiotti, E., … Tessarin, M.C. (2004). The self-locating catheter: Clinical experience and follow-up. *Peritoneal Dialysis International, 24*, 359. Retrieved from http://www.pdiconnect.com/content/24/4/359.full.pdf

Diaz-Buxo, J. (1996). Patient selection and the success of peritoneal dialysis. *Nephrology News and Issues, 3*, 7-19.

Dinwiddie, L.C., & Bhola, C. (2010). Hemodialysis catheter care: Current recommendations for nursing practice in North America. *Nephrology Nursing Journal, 37*(5), 507–528.

Eklund, B.H., Honkanen, E.O., Kala, A.R., & Kyllönen, L.E. (1995). Peritoneal dialysis access: Prospective randomized comparison of the Swan neck and Tenckhoff catheters. *Peritoneal Dialysis International, 15*(8), 353-356.

Eklund, B.H., Honkanen, E.O., Kyllönen, L.E., Salmela, K, & Kala, A.R. (1997). Peritoneal dialysis: Prospective randomized comparison of single cuff and double cuff straight Tenckhoff catheters. *Nephrology Dialysis Transplantation, 12*(2), 2664-2666.

Federal Register. (2008, April 15). Vol. 73, No. 73, Rules and Regulations.

Ferrari, P., & Klerk, M. (2009). Paired kidney donations to expand the living door pool. *Journal of Nephrology, 22*(6) 699–707.

Fine, R.N., Becker, Y., De Geest, S., Eisen, H., Ettenger, R., Evans, R., … Dobbels, F. (2009). Nonadherence Consensus Conference summary report. *American Journal of Transplantation; 9*, 35–41.

Finkelstein, F., Healy, H., Abu-Alfa, A., Ahmad, S., Brown, F., Gehr, T., . . . Mujais, S. (2005). Superiority of icodextrin compared with 4.25% dextrose for peritoneal ultrafiltration. *Journal of the American Society of Nephrology, 16*(2), 546–554. doi:10.1681/ASN.2004090793

Fistula First Breakthrough Initiative (FFBI). (2009). *Fistula First Breakthrough Initiative strategic plan.* Mary Teresa Casey, RD, LD, Government Task Leader, Edwin Huff, PhD, Project Officer. Submitted by Mid-Atlantic Renal Coalition.

Fistula First Catheter Last (FFCL) Workgroup. (2008). *Arteriovenous Fistula First: Secondary AV fistula in patients with A-V grafts.* Retrieved on August 20, 2013, from http://fistula.memberpath.com/LinkClick.aspx?fileticket=114e0dJlPZg%3d&tabid=125

Fistula First Catheter Last (FFCL) Workgroup. (2013b). *Arteriovenous Fistula First: Change concept 9. Monitoring and maintenance to ensure adequate access function.* Retrieved from http://fistula.memberpath.com/HealthcareProfessionals/FFBIChangeConcepts/ChangeConcept9.aspx

Fistula First Catheter Last (FFCL) Workgroup. (2013a). *Arteriovenous Fistula First: Change concept 1. Routine CQI review of vascular access.* Retrieved from http://fistula.memberpath.com/HealthcareProfessionals/FFBIChangeConcepts/ChangeConcept1.aspx

Fistula First Catheter Last (FFCL) Workgroup. (2013c). *Arteriovenous Fistula First. Change concept 13. Support patient efforts to live the best possible quality of life through self-management.* Retrieved from http://www.fistulafirst.org/HealthcareProfessionals/FFBIChangeConcepts/ChangeConcept13.aspx

Fleming, W.J. (2013). Standing orders for peritoneal dialysis. DaVita New Haven-Yale Nephrology. Not published.

Gokal, R., Alexander, S; Ash., S., Chen, T.W., Danielson, A., Holmes, P., … Vas, S. (1998). Peritoneal catheters and exit-site practices toward optimum peritoneal access: 1998 updates. (Official report from the International Society for Peritoneal Dialysis). *Peritoneal Dialysis International, 18*(1), 11-33.

Gomez, N.J. (Ed.). (2011). *Nephrology nursing scope and standards of practice* (7th ed.). Pitman, NJ: American Nephrology Nurses' Association.

GORE® hybrid vascular graft. Retrieved from http://www.goremedical.com/hybrid/

Guest, S. (2010). Peritoneal dialysis in patients with cirrhosis and ascites. *Advances in Peritoneal Dialysis, 26*, 82-87.

Gupta, G., Unruh, M., Thomas, D., & Hasley, P. (2010). *Primary care of the renal transplant patient. Journal of General Internal Medicine, 25*(7), 731-740.

Harwood. L., & Leitch. R. (2006) Home dialysis therapies. In A.E. Molzahn & E. Butera (Eds.), *Contemporary nephrology nursing* (pp. 607-623.) Pitman, NJ: American Nephrology Nurses' Association.

Henrich, W.L. (2013). *Hemodynamic instability during hemodialysis.* Retrieved from http://www.uptodate.com

Henrich, W.L. (Ed). (2009). *Principles and practices of dialysis,* (4th ed.). Philadelphia: Lippincott Williams & Wilkins.

Holechek, M., & Armtrong, G. (2013) Kidney transplantation in core curriculum for transplant nurses. In L. Ohler & S. Cupples (Eds.), *Core curriculum for transplant nurses* (pp. 512-555). Chicago: International Society of Transplant Nurses.

Holley, J.L. (2013). *Acute complications during hemodialysis.* Retrieved from http://www.uptodate.com

Holley, J.L. (2013). *Cancer screening in patients with end-stage renal disease.* Retrieved from http://www.uptodate.com

Hong-Yee, L., & Seck-Guan, T. (2007). Arteriovenous fistula aneurysm – Plicate, not ligate. *Annals, Academy of Medicine, Singapore, 36*(10), 851–853.

Horn, J., & Hansen, P. (2008). *Get to know an enzyme: CYP34A.* Retrieved from http://www.pharmacytimes.com

James, P.A., Oparil, S., Carter, B.L., Cushman, W.C., Dennison-Himmelfarb, C., Handler, J., … Ortiz, E. (2014). 2014 evidence-based guideline for the management of high blood pressure in adults. Report from the panel members appointed to the Eighth Joint National Committee (JNC 8). *Journal of the American Medical Association, 311*(5), 507-520. doi:10.1001/jama.2013.284427

Jassal S.V., Devins, G.M., Chan, C.T., Bozanovic, R., & Rourke, S. (2006). Improvements in cognition in patients converting from thrice weekly hemodialysis to nocturnal hemodialysis: A longitudinal pilot study. *Kidney International, 70*(5), 956-962.

Kidney Disease: Improving Global Outcomes (KDIGO). (2006). KDOQI clinical practice guidelines and clinical practice recommendations for 2006 updates: Hemodialysis adequacy, peritoneal dialysis adequacy and vascular access. *American Journal of Kidney Diseases, 48*, S1–S322.

Kidney Disease: Improving Global Outcomes (KDIGO). (2009). KDIGO clinical practice guideline for the care of kidney transplant recipients. *American Journal of Transplantation, 9*(3).

Kidney Disease: Improving Global Outcomes (KDIGO). (2012). KDIGO 2012 clinical practice guidelines for the evaluation and management of chronic kidney disease. *Kidney International, 3*(1). Retrieved from http://kidney-international.org

Kovalik, E.C. (2013). *Hemodialysis anticoagulation.* Retrieved from http://www.uptodate.com.

Leblanc, M., Ouimet, D., & Pichette, V. (2001). Dialysate leaks in peritoneal dialysis. *Seminars in Dialysis, 14*(1), 50-54.

Li, P.K., Szeto, C.C., Piraino, B., Bernardini, J., Figueiredo, A.E., Gupta, A., . . . International Society for Peritoneal, D. (2010). Peritoneal dialysis-related infections recommendations: 2010 update. *Peritoneal Dialysis International, 30*(4), 393-423. doi:10.3747/pdi.2010.00049

Luongo, M., & Prowant, B. (2009). Peritoneal dialysis program organization and management, the nurses's role. In R. Khanna & R.T. Kredict (Eds.), *Nolph and Gokal's textbook of peritoneal dialysis* (3rd ed., pp. 335-370). New York: Springer Science and Business Media.

Maaz, D.E. (2004). Troubleshooting non-infectious peritoneal dialysis issues. *Nephrology Nursing Journal, 31*(5), 521-532, 545.

Marcen, R. (2009) Immunosuppresive drugs in kidney transplantation: Impact on patient survival, and incidence of cardiovascular disease, malignancy and infection. *Drugs, 69*(16) 2227-2243.

Martin, S., Tichy, E., & Gabardi, S. (2011). Belatacept: A novel biologic for maintenance immunosuppression after renal transplantation. *Pharmacotherapy, 31*(4), 394-407.

McCann, M., Einarsdottir, H., Van Waeleghem, J.P. Murphy, F., & Sedgwick, J. (2009). Vascular access management II: AVF/AVG cannulation techniques and complications. *Journal of Renal Care, 35*(2), 90-98.

McCormick, B.B., & Bargman, J.M. (2007). Noninfectious complications of peritoneal dialysis: Implications for patient and technique survival. *Journal of the American Society of Nephrology, 18*(12), 3023–3025.

Mickley, V. (2008). Steal syndrome – Strategies to preserve vascular access and extremity. *Nephrology Dialysis Transplantation, 23,* 19-24.

National Cholesterol Education Program (NCEP). (2004). *Third report of the expert panel on detection, evaluation, and treatment of high blood cholesterol in adults (Adult Treatment Panel III).* Retrieved from http://www.nhlbi.nih.gov/files/docs/resources/ heart/atp3full.pdf

National Kidney and Urologic Diseases Information Clearinghouse (NKUDIC). *Main page.* (2014). Retrieved from kidney.niddk.nih.gov

National Kidney Foundation (NKF). (2002). *KDOQI clinical practice guidelines for chronic kidney disease: Evaluation, classification, and stratification.* Retrieved from http://www.kidney.org .professionals/kdoqi/guidelines.

National Kidney Foundation (NKF). (2003). KDOQI *clinical practice guidelines for bone metabolism and disease in chronic kidney disease.* Retrieved from http://www.kidney.org.professionals/ kdoqi/guidelines

National Kidney Foundation (NKF). (2005a). *KDOQI clinical practice guidelines for cardiovascular disease in dialysis patients.* Retrieved from http://www.kidney.org.professionals/kdoqi/ guidelines

National Kidney Foundation (NKF). (2005b). *KDOQI clinical practice guidelines for managing dyslipidemias in chronic kidney disease.* Retrieved from http://www.kidney.org.professionals/ kdoqi/guidelines

National Kidney Foundation (NKF). (2006a). *KDOQI clinical practice guidelines and clinical practice recommendations for anemia in chronic kidney disease: 2007 update of hemoglobin target.* Retrieved from https://www.kidney.org/professionals/ KDOQI/guidelines_commentaries

National Kidney Foundation (NKF). (2006b). *KDOQI clinical practice guidelines for hemodialysis adequacy, update 2006.* Retrieved from https://www.kidney.org/professionals/KDOQI/ guidelines_commentaries

National Kidney Registry (NKR). (2014). Retrieved from http://www.kidneyregistry.org

Nose, Y. (2000). Home hemodialysis: A crazy idea in 1963: A memoir. *American Society for Artificial Internal Organs, 46*(1), 13-7.

Oliver, M.J. (2012). *Arteriovenous fistulas and grafts for chronic hemodialysis access.* Retrieved from http://www.uptodate.com.

Organ Procurement and Transplantation Network. (2012, December 19). *OPTN/SRTR 2012 annual data report: Kidney.* Retrieved from http://srtr.transplant.hrsa.gov/annual_reports/2012/flash/01 _kidney_13/index.html

Paniagua, R., Amato, D., Vonesh, E., Correa-Rotter, R., Ramos, A., Moran, J., … Mexican Nephrology Collaborative Study, G. (2002).

Effects of increased peritoneal clearances on mortality rates in peritoneal dialysis: ADEMEX, a prospective, randomized, controlled trial. *Journal of the American Society of Nephrology, 13*(5), 1307–1320.

Patel, P.P., Altieri, M., Jindal, T.R., Guy, S.R., Falta, E.M., Elster, E.A., … Jindal, R.M. (2011). Current status of synthetic and biological grafts for hemodialysis. In M.G. Penido (Ed.), *Hemodialysis – different aspects.* Intech. Published online. doi:10.5772/21814

Perl, J., & Chan, C.T. (2009). Home hemodialysis, daily hemodialysis, and nocturnal hemodialysis: Core curriculum 2009. A*merican Journal of Kidney Disease. 54*(6), 1171-1184.

Piraino, B., Bailie, G.R., Bernardini, J., Boeschoten, E., Gupta, A., Holmes, C., … ISPD Ad Hoc Advisory Committee. (2005). Peritoneal dialysis-related infections recommendations: 2005 update. *Peritoneal Dialysis International, 25*(2), 107-131.

Ponferrada, L.P., Prowant, B.F., & Satalowich, R.J. (2008). Peritoneal dialysis access. In C.S. Counts (Ed.), *Core curriculum for nephrology nursing,* (5th ed., pp. 768-794). Pitman, N.J.: American Nephrology Nurses' Association.

Prowant, B.F., Ponferrada, L.P., & Satalowich, R.J. (2008a). Peritoneal dialysis access. In C. Counts (Ed.), *Core curriculum for nephrology nursing* (5th ed., pp. 768-794). Pitman, NJ: American Nephrology Nurses' Association.

Prowant, B.F., Ponferrada, L.P., & Satalowich, R.J. (2008b). Peritoneal dialysis complications. In C. Counts (Ed.), *Core curriculum for nephrology nursing* (5th ed., pp. 824-852). Pitman, NJ: American Nephrology Nurses' Association.

Reddy, S.S., & Holley, J.L. (2007). Management of the pregnant chronic dialysis patient. *Advanced in Chronic Kidney Disease, 14*(2), 146-155.

Richard, C.J., & Engebretson, J. (2010). Negotiating living with an arteriovenous fistula for hemodialysis. *Nephrology Nursing Journal, 37*(4), 363-374.

Roodhooft, A.M., Van Acker, K.J., & De Broe, M.E. (1987). Chylous peritonitis: An infrequent complication of peritoneal dialysis. *Peritoneal Dialysis International, 7*(3), 195-196.

Schiller, B., Munroe, H., & Neitzer, A. (2011). Thinking outside the box – Identifying patients for home dialysis. *Clinical Kidney Journal, 4*(Suppl. 3), iii11–iii13. Retrieved from http://ckj.oxfordjournals.org/content/4/suppl_3/iii11.full

Schmidt, R.J., & Holley, J.L. (2012). *Overview of the hemodialysis apparatus.* Retrieved from http://www.uptodate.com/ contents/overview-of-the-hemodialysis-apparatus

Schuman, R., & Ronfeld, A. (2011). Early use conversion of the HeRO dialysis graft. *Journal of Vascular Surgery, 53*(17), 42-44.

Shah, H., Chu, M., & Bargman, J.M. (2006). Perioperative management of peritoneal dialysis patients undergoing hernia surgery without the use of interim hemodialysis. *Peritoneal Dialysis International, 26*(6).

Shah, R., Vachharajani, T.J., & Agarwal, A.K. (2013). Aneurysmal dilatation of dialysis arteriovenous access. *The Open Urology and Nephrology Journal, 6,* 1–5

Sherry, D., Simmons, B., Wung, S.F., & Zerwic, J. (2003). Noncompliance in heart transplantation: A role for the Advanced Practice Nurse. *Progress in Cardiovascular Nursing, 18*(3), 141-146.

Talebi, M., Salari, B., Ghannadan, H. Kakaei, F., & Azar, S.A. (2011). Nerve conduction changes following arteriovenous fistula construction in hemodialysis patients. *International Urology and Nephrology, 43*(3), 849-853.

The Renal Association. (2011, January 12). *Assessment of the potential kidney transplant recipient.* (Clinical guideline). (Authors: Dudley, C., Bright, R., & Harden, P.) Retrieved from http://www.renal .org/guidelines/modules/assessment-of-the-potential-kidney-transplant-recipient#sthash.JL5dxAaW.dpbs

Twardowski, Z.J. (1997). *Third International Home Hemodialysis Symposium 1997.* 17th Annual Conference on Peritoneal Dialysis. Retrieved from http://www.hdcn.com/symphome.htm

Twardowski, Z.J., Nolph, K.O., Khanna, R., Prowant, B.F., Ryan, L.P., Moore, H.L, & Nielsen, M.P. (1987). Peritoneal equilibration test. *Peritoneal Dialysis Bulletin, 7,* 138.

Tzamaloukas, A.H., Obermiller, L. E., Gibel, L.J., Murata, G.H., Wood, B., Simon, D., ... Kanig, S.P. (1993). Peritonitis associated with intra-abdominal pathology in continuous ambulatory peritoneal dialysis patients. *Peritoneal Dialysis International, 13*(Suppl. 2), S335–337.

United Network for Organ Sharing. (n.d.). *Main page.* Retrieved from OPTN.Transplant.HRSA.gov

United States Renal Data System (USRDS). (2014). *USRDS 2014 annual data report: An overview of the epidemiology of kidney disease in the United States.* National Institutes of Health, National Institute of Diabetes and Digestive and Kidney Diseases, Bethesda, MD. Retrieved from http://www.usrds.org/adr.aspx

Van Gelder, F., & Ohler, L. (2013). Basics in transplant immunology. In L. Ohler & S. Cupples (Eds.), *Core curriculum for transplant nurses* (pp. 27-49). Chicago: International Society of Transplant Nurses.

Vardhan, A.H., & Hutchison, A.J. (2014). Peritoneal dialysis. In S.J. Gilbert, D.E. Weiner, D.S. Gipson, M.A. Perazella, & M. Tonelli (Eds.), *National Kidney Foundation's primer on kidney diseases* (6th ed., pp. 520-533). Philadelphia: Elsevier Saunders.

Watson, C.J., & Dark, J.H. (2012). Organ transplantation: Historical perspective and current practice. *British Journal of Anaesthesia, 108*(1), 29–42. doi: 10.1093/bja/aer384

Watts, S., Gee, J., Schaub, K., Lawrence, R., Aron, D., & Kirsh, S. (2009). Nurse practitioner-led multidisciplinary teams to improve chronic illness care: The unique strengths of nurse practitioners applied to shared medial appointments/group visits. *Journal of the American Academy of Nurse Practitioners, 21*(3), 167-172.

Zamani, P., Kaufman, J., & Kinlay, S. (2009). Ischemic steal syndrome following arm arteriovenous fistula for hemodialysis. *Vascular Medicine, 14,* 371–376.

Zorzanello, M.M., Fleming, W.J., & Prowant, B. E. (2004). Use of tissue plasminogen activator in peritoneal dialysis catheters: a literature review and one center's experience. *Nephrology Nursing Journal, 31*(5), 534-537.

Overview of Acute Care for the APRN

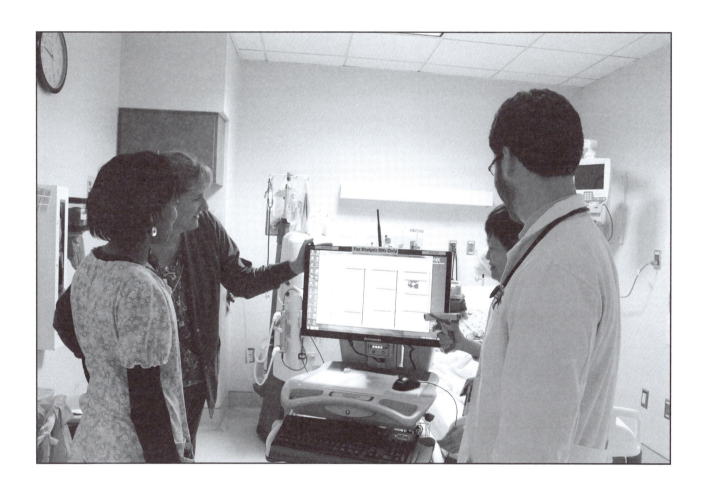

Chapter Editors
Kim Alleman, MS, APRN, FNP-BC, CNN-NP
Katherine Houle, MSN, APRN, CFNP, CNN-NP

Author
Timothy Ray, DNP, CNP, CNN-NP

CHAPTER **4**

Overview of Acute Care for the APRN

This offering for **1.6 contact hours with .75 contact hour of pharmacology content** is provided by the American Nephrology Nurses' Association (ANNA).

American Nephrology Nurses' Association is accredited as a provider of continuing nursing education by the American Nurses Credentialing Center Commission on Accreditation.

ANNA is a provider approved by the California Board of Registered Nursing, provider number CEP 00910.

This CNE offering meets the continuing nursing education requirements for certification and recertification by the Nephrology Nursing Certification Commission (NNCC).

To be awarded contact hours for this activity, read this chapter in its entirety. Then complete the CNE evaluation found at **www.annanurse.org/corecne** and submit it; or print it, complete it, and mail it in. Contact hours are not awarded until the evaluation for the activity is complete.

Example of reference for Chapter 4 in APA format. One author for entire chapter.

Ray, T. (2015). Overview of acute care for the APRN. In C.S. Counts (Ed.), *Core curriculum for nephrology nursing: Module 6. The APRN's approaches to care in nephrology* (6th ed., pp. 111-152). Pitman, NJ: American Nephrology Nurses' Association.

Interpreted: Chapter author. (Date). Title of chapter. In ...

Cover photo by Counts/Morganello.

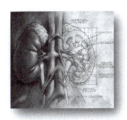

Overview of Acute Care for the APRN

Purpose

The purpose of this chapter is to discuss the evaluation and management of hospitalized patients diagnosed with kidney disease from the perspective of the advanced practice registered nurse (APRN).

Objectives

Upon completion of this chapter, the learner will be able to:
1. Identify roles of the nephrology APRN in the inpatient setting.
2. Describe management strategies of the hospitalized patient diagnosed with acute kidney injury (AKI).
3. Describe management strategies of the hospitalized patient diagnosed with chronic kidney disease not on dialysis.
4. Describe management strategies of the hospitalized patient diagnosed with general nephrology disorders.
5. Discuss components of the acute hemodialysis, acute peritoneal dialysis, and continuous kidney replacement therapy prescriptions.
6. Highlight complications of kidney replacement therapy in the inpatient arena.
7. Identify the components and documentation needed for a consult with a nephrologist.

I. The role of the nephrology APRN in acute care.

A. Background information.
1. Over the last several years, the role of the nephrology APRN has evolved from the traditional role of rounding in the out-patient/community dialysis center, to a more inclusive role that encompasses acute care and inpatient/hospital work.
   a. While the healthcare community as a whole has been moving toward a more multidisciplinary team approach, the APRN role within nephrology has been doing the same.
   b. The APRN practicing in nephrology is now viewed as an integral part of the entire nephrology team.
2. A transition in clinical focus has taken place. The APRN provides care to the patient with chronic kidney disease (CKD) and kidney failure and within general practice of nephrology provides a collaborative approach to patient care.
   a. The duties of a nephrology APRN are quite extensive, depending upon the needs of the nephrologist and practice setting at which he/she works.

   b. Collaborative agreements, mutually developed with nephrologists, afford the APRN a great deal of independence and autonomy, yet also provide the support and clinical backing needed when a situation is outside the APRN's scope of practice.
3. Both patients and nephrologists value the APRN's input.
   a. The unique nursing background possessed by an APRN allows that practitioner to view a clinical situation from both a nursing and a medical standpoint.
   b. APRNs continue to be patient and family advocates, while at the same time focusing on complex, detailed clinical problems, working out solutions, and coming up with appropriate plans of action for patients with kidney disease.

B. Roles of the nephrology advanced practice registered nurse in the inpatient setting.
1. Assess, diagnose, and manage hospitalized patients with kidney disease in collaboration with the nephrologist.
2. Communicate clinical condition and changes with primary care physician and other consultants.

3. Communicate hospital course and update dialysis – both hemodialysis (HD) and peritoneal dialysis (PD) – orders upon discharge with the outpatient dialysis clinic or extended care facility.
4. Coordinate posthospital care of CKD patients, including arranging CKD clinic follow-up.
5. Counsel and educate patients and their family regarding disease process and treatment options.
6. Serve as a resource, consultant, and mentor to the healthcare team.
7. Initiate and revise hospital protocols to reflect evidence-based practice.
8. Integrate current scientific knowledge into advanced nursing practice.
9. Promote nursing research at the bedside level.

II. Acute care evaluation.

A. Overview.
1. Due to the complexity of the renal system, patients can often present with a wide range of signs and symptoms from subtle to overt, affecting all body systems.
   a. Critical changes can occur rapidly so the APRN must be knowledgeable with the pathophysiology of not only the renal system, but also all other body systems.
   b. Understanding how these systems interact when a patient is healthy gives great insight into what to look for when the patient is ill.
2. Agreements with the nephrologist with whom they collaborate should include a formal understanding concerning what role the APRN will be undertaking.
   a. Specific discussions about the levels of care should be reviewed ahead of time, such as whether an APRN will be allowed to see new consults and how much autonomy the APRN will have with direct patient care.
   b. Discussion concerning when to consult other disciplines should also be reviewed.

B. The reason for consultation should include why you were asked to see the patient, such as acute kidney injury or hyperkalemia.

C. History of present illness.
1. Obtain information from patients about the onset, duration, and character of the present illness. Also discuss anything that may aggravate or ameliorate the symptoms.
2. Asking patients what they feel caused the problem may also bring out helpful information concerning their present condition.

D. Patient assessment. It is important to give a thorough inspection of any documentation provided,

electronic or paper, that would give insight into the patient's medical history. Often a comprehensive review of the information and discussion with the patient will provide valuable clues as to what clinical problem needs to be addressed and how best to go about it.
1. Past medical history.
   a. Document all pertinent medical problems known.
   b. Ask specifically about any prior kidney and urinary problems or if they've ever seen a nephrologist ("kidney doctor") or been told that they have kidney problems before.
2. Surgical history.
   a. Document all pertinent surgical procedures done, including date.
   b. If a kidney biopsy was done in the past, ask when and where and if the results of the biopsy are known.
3. Family history.
   a. Ask about biologic relatives and what crucial medical problems they may have had.
   b. Specifically ask about any kidney and urinary problems.
   c. If a relative has CKD or is on dialysis, ask if it is known what caused their kidneys to fail (e.g., diabetes, hypertension).
4. Social history.
   a. Document prior and current tobacco use, alcohol, or drug use: what kind and how long the exposure occurred.
   b. An occupational history and review of possible hazards and toxins often can give insight into what stressors or substances may contribute to kidney dysfunction.
   c. Document social support and family life.
5. Medications.
   a. An area of particular importance to review with the patient, family, or institution (nursing home and assisted living facility) that they were in prior to the hospitalization.
   b. Many nephrology imbalances or problems can be triggered or exacerbated by pharmaceutical agents.
   c. It is important to take the time to document timelines of when medications were started or stopped, especially if the presenting problem may have been caused by one or more medications.
   d. Talking to the patient's outpatient pharmacy is a good way to obtain accurate medication information as well.
   e. Outpatient medications.
      (1) Encouraging all patients to keep an accurate and up-to-date list of their medications with them is helpful.
      (2) Prescriptive.

(a) All prescriptive medications should be reviewed and documented.

(b) Confirm which practitioners and pharmacies are used for their medications.

(c) Be aware of potential duplicate medications if generic and trade names are both used on the prescriptions.

(d) Reviewing medications is a good way to pick up what other medical problems the patient may have that were not previously listed.

(e) Understanding the different renal dosing of medications as it pertains to the patient's current estimated glomerular filtration rate (eGFR) may also help provide a clue to what may be a presenting problem.

(3) Over-the-counter (OTC).

(a) Many patients do not view nonprescriptive medications as a potential problem so may not volunteer the information unless asked directly.

(b) As it relates to nephrology, asking specifically about nonsteroidal anti-inflammatory (NSAID) medication is of particular importance as it can cause many kidney problems.

(c) Asking about specific brand names may trigger their memory as well.

(d) Inquiring about herbal medications is also important as some are well known to have nephrotoxic effects (Blowey, 2005; Dugo et al., 2010; Perazella, 2009).

f. Inpatient medications.

(1) As many nephrology consults may be initiated after the hospital admission, a thorough review of medications given from the time of admission is helpful.

(2) This is important not only during the initial consult but every day that an APRN sees the patient.

(3) Many practitioners are often involved in patient care in the hospital and with the use of electronic medical records (EMRs), medications can be added or changed quickly, unknowingly by the nurse, as well as remotely.

(4) Understanding medications and how they act at all levels of GFR is essential since many are excreted by the kidneys; as the kidney function changes, the medications need to be correspondingly adjusted as well. This is especially true of antibiotic therapy.

(5) Use of reference databases and

collaboration with infectious disease (ID) staff and pharmacists can provide guidelines as to what doses to give as the kidney function changes (Aronoff et al., 2007).

(6) Review medications given by EMS as well as in the emergency room.

(7) Review all medications given since admittance.

6. A review of the patient's allergies, and if known detailing the resulting effect of the allergy, is important to document.

7. Review of systems (ROS).

a. A detailed assessment of the subjective symptoms as perceived by the patient.

b. There are 14 systems recognized by the Centers for Medicare and Medicaid Services (CMS) (CMS, 2010).

c. The acuity of the patient may determine how detailed you need to be during your consult evaluation, which will then influence your level of billing.

(1) Constitutional (e.g., fever, weight loss).

(2) Eyes.

(3) Ears, nose, mouth, throat.

(4) Cardiovascular.

(5) Respiratory.

(6) Gastrointestinal.

(7) Genitourinary.

(8) Musculoskeletal.

(9) Integumentary.

(10) Neurologic.

(11) Psychiatric.

(12) Endocrine.

(13) Hematologic/lymphatic.

(14) Allergic/immunologic.

8. Physical exam.

a. Examination of the patient using a systematic approach is helpful in assuring that any important presenting findings are not missed.

b. As with the ROS, the extent of the physical exam will be based upon the acuity of the patient and guided by the information already obtained through the history and other discussion with the patient.

c. CMS recognizes 12 organ systems that can be addressed depending upon the clinical judgment and nature of the presenting problem (CMS, 2010).

(1) Constitutional (e.g., vital signs, general appearance).

(2) Eyes.

(3) Ears, nose, mouth, and throat.

(4) Cardiovascular.

(5) Respiratory.

(6) Gastrointestinal.

(7) Genitourinary.

(8) Musculoskeletal.

(9) Skin.

(10) Neurologic.

(11) Psychiatric.

(12) Hematologic/lymphatic/immunologic.

d. When evaluating a nephrology patient, the areas of interest related to body and organ systems can be quite broad and detailed given the complexity of the renal system and its pathophysiologic effects throughout the body.

e. Understanding how these systems interact and react to changing kidney function is essential so it is important not to become too target-focused and limit what you evaluate with the patient.

E. Diagnostic data.

1. Much of the determination of what is wrong with a patient with kidney disease falls to evaluating laboratory and radiologic data.

2. Selecting the right set of tests to order is essential in making an accurate diagnosis.

3. Management and treatment then rely on subsequent data to provide trends showing changes in the patient's clinical condition.

4. Laboratory

a. Reviewing the patient's laboratory data is a crucial part of any nephrology evaluation.

b. Often the presenting lab data will provide the essential clue to determining what is wrong with the patient.

c. Obtaining old data and comparing it to the current information helps determine how acute or chronic a presenting problem is.

d. Often you need to gather data from multiple sources, including multiple hospital systems, private physician practices, dialysis units, or freestanding community laboratories.

e. Establishing a timeline once this information is obtained can often pinpoint when the problem started.

f. Of the hundreds of lab tests available to choose from, the initial workup for a patient with problems related to the kidneys often involves just a few basic tests. Once obtained and reviewed, and the diagnosis is narrowed further, more specific tests can be ordered. The initial tests for a renal patient should include the following.

(1) Chemistry panel (one of the following).

(a) Basic metabolic panel (BMP).

(b) Comprehensive metabolic panel (CMP).

(c) Renal function panel (RFP).

(2) Complete blood count (CBC) with differential.

(3) Urinalysis with microscopic exam.

5. Radiologic.

a. Use of simple noninvasive studies should be used first as long as they provide the information needed.

b. Further and more involved studies may need to be done if the diagnostic yield of the initial imaging study is low.

c. What you are diagnostically looking for, the accuracy and reliability of the study, cost, degree of invasiveness, and use of potential nephrotoxic dye all need to be taken into account when choosing which study to order.

(1) Kidney ultrasound is an effective, noninvasive approach to determine the size of the kidneys and if there are any urinary blockage, mass, or stones.

(2) Computed tomography (CT) scan.

(a) Can be used with or without intravenous dye to evaluate solid masses and stones and trauma to the kidney.

i. If any degree of kidney failure is present, one must weigh the risk of potential dye-induced nephrotoxicity to the data needed if IV dye is used. Close monitoring is essential.

ii. To minimize nephrotoxicity if IV contrast dye is planned, the patient's diuretics, ACE/ARB, and Metformin® should be held and IV hydration given before the dye procedure is started.

(b) Correlation to ultrasound is often used to confirm and stage degree of urological abnormalities and treatments, such as hydronephrosis and ureteral stent placement.

(c) Less effective than ultrasound to determining the size of the kidney.

(3) Other radiologic studies are often second line and are usually done after other procedures yield some type of abnormality that needs clarification. Consultation with an interventional radiologist can be helpful in deciding the preferred study given a specific clinical situation.

(a) Magnetic resonance imaging (MRI) and angiography (MRA) can be used to help further detect and stage renal cell carcinoma.

(b) Retrograde pyelography.

i. Is used to evaluate the urethral structures and to look for possible filling defects or obstruction.

ii. The need for contrast dye for this study as well as other options (ultrasound) has made it a less appealing choice.

iii. Used more often by urology than the nephrology team.

(c) Radionuclide kidney imaging.
  i. Is used most commonly for evaluating "split" kidney function to determine the degree of function (often listed as a percentage) of each individual kidney.
  ii. May be done to determine if a nephrectomy is warranted or safe.
(d) Kidney angiography is used to evaluate kidney vasculature for stenosis or patency, or to help establish the diagnosis of renal vein thrombosis.

F. Impression and plan of current illness.
  1. Develop an impression of what the diagnosis is, and present a plan of action to manage the clinical condition.
    a. Each diagnosis should be listed and broken down separately to make it easier to follow your overall plan.
    b. Document what labs and studies you plan to order.
    c. Discuss what the next course of action and plan will be as well as possible outcomes.
  2. Clarify the plan of action with the attending practitioner, as well as other consultants.
  3. Collaborate with all members of the clinical team.

III. Evaluation of clinical findings.

A. Calculation of estimated glomerular filtration rate (eGFR).
  1. As kidney function declines, the filtration and clearance of many substances/fluids are affected.
    a. Measurement of these substances is helpful in determining the degree of kidney failure the patient is experiencing.
    b. It is important to understand that the percentage of kidney function is in flux all the time.
    c. While whatever measurement that is used will only be accurate for that moment, it at least offers some sense of where the patient's kidney function is when establishing a plan of care.
    d. It is most accurate when the patient is clinically stable and not ill, which is usually not the case within the hospital.
    e. Comparing the current blood work to earlier results will help determine the degree of acute vs. chronic dysfunction.
  2. The glomerular filtration rate is a measurement of how much fluid and solute is filtered by the glomeruli within the kidneys.
    a. Since a measurement of each glomerulus is not realistic, an estimated filtration rate is used instead.
    b. There are many ways to measure filtration and

all have their advantages and disadvantages.
  (1) Spot checks and calculations vs. 24-hour collections each have their own advantages and disadvantages. During an acute hospitalization, the patient's kidney function is often quite variable, and the use of a spot check/calculation is preferable.
  (2) The 24-hour collections are used more when the patient's kidney function is stable or when clarification of the spot or calculation results is needed.
  (3) The calculations are also not as accurate for patients who fall outside the norm, such as the very young or old patients and those who are quite lean or obese.
  (4) Formulas include:
    (a) Modification of diet in renal disease (MDRD) formula.
    (b) Chronic kidney disease epidemiology collaboration (CKD-EPI) formula.
    (c) Cockcroft-Gault (CG) formula.
    (d) 24-hour creatinine clearance.

B. Urinalysis (UA) assessment.
  1. The UA is a very important noninvasive evaluation that can provide important clues about the patient's clinical condition.
    a. If an acute condition change is suspected, comparing current and prior urinalysis is important.
    b. Volume status, glomerular dysfunction, urinary tract infections, and poor glycemic control can be evaluated.
    c. Systemic abnormalities, such as gout, rhabdomyolysis, and others, can be suspected with an abnormal urine (Fischbach, 2000). (See Table 4.1.)
  2. Color.
    a. Yellow, straw colored.
    b. Clear.
      (1) Indicates a more dilutional urine, which can be seen during normal volume diuresis or postdiuretic therapy.
      (2) Clinical conditions such as diabetes insipidus can also cause clear urine.
    c. Dark indicates a more concentrated urine often seen in dehydration.
    d. Cloudy often indicates infection.
    e. Red indicates hematuria or myoglobulinuria.
  3. Specific gravity measures the concentration of dissolved solutes and gives a gross measurement of the osmolality of the urine.
  4. pH.
    a. Average urine pH is 6.0, with the range varying widely.
    b. Acidotic: diabetic ketoacidosis (DKA), diarrhea, metabolic acidosis, *E. coli* UTI.

Table 4.1

Urinalysis Findings in Rhabdomyolysis

Color	Dark (cola-colored)
pH	Acidic

Blood
  Benzidine reagent
  Microscopy
	3+ to 4+
	Less than 5 RBCs per high power field

Sediment	Pigmented brown granular casts Renal tubular epithelial cells
Urinary sodium concentration	> 20 mEq/L
FE$_{NA}$	> 1%

FE$_{NA}$ = fractional excretion of sodium

Source: Russell, T.A. (2005). Acute renal failure related to rhabdomyolysis: pathophysiology, diagnosis, and collaborative management. *Nephrology Nursing Journal, 32*, 409-417. Used with permission.

c. Alkalotic: renal tubular acidosis, CKD, *Proteus mirabilis* UTI.

5. Glucose.
   a. Should be none.
   b. Serum glucose is actively filtered by the glomeruli and usually reabsorbed, unless the blood glucose levels exceed the reabsorption capacity of the tubules.
   c. When the serum glucose is over 160 to 180 mg/dL, glucose will be seen in the urine. This may indicate poor glycemic control, but also needs to be taken into account when evaluating postprandial measurements.

6. Ketones.
   a. Should be none.
   b. Most commonly seen in DKA, but can also be seen in severe malnutrition, septic conditions, and strenuous exercise.

7. Blood.
   a. Should be none.
   b. An indication of damage to the kidneys or urinary tract, which can range from benign (strenuous exercise) to significant disease processes.
   c. When the urine is positive for "blood" but microscopically no red blood cells (RBC) are visible, myoglobinuria can be suspected, as seen in rhabdomyolysis.
   d. Microscopic examination of the RBCs is important to see if they are intact or damaged, which can yield clues to the origin of where they entered the urinary system. Irregularly shaped RBCs are often damaged while passing through abnormal glomeruli indicating a possible glomerulonephritis.

8. Leukocytes and nitrates.
   a. Should be none.
   b. When a urinary tract infection is present, often positive, but not always.

9. WBC and RBC.
   a. Should be none.
   b. White blood cells (WBC) are an indication of infection.
   c. Red blood cells (RBC) are seen during damage to the urinary system.

10. Protein.
    a. Should be none to trace amounts.
    b. Positive proteinuria is an indication of some type of kidney disease, as the glomeruli normally prevent protein from passing into the urine.
    c. Proteinuria.
       (1) A combination of albuminuria and other globulins.
       (2) If present, needs to be quantified (spot or 24-hour collection).
       (3) Evaluate further for any pathologic processes.
       (4) Diabetes mellitus is the most prevalent cause of proteinuria; a host of kidney diseases also cause proteinuria. Proteinuria can range from trace to significant nephrotic range and results in the loss of grams of protein a day.
       (5) Trending multiple proteinuria samples is an effective way to monitor disease processes that are causing the kidney disease, as well as being able to document if a particular course of treatment is being successful.

11. Sediment.
    a. Usually trace amounts of normal epithelial cells are present.
    b. In an unhealthy state, a multitude of sediment can be seen, often providing clues to the cause of the kidney impairment.
    c. Bacteria are an indication of infection. If present, check a urine culture to clarify what type of infection is present before antibiotics are started, if the patient's clinical condition allows.
    d. Casts.
       (1) Fatty: nephrotic syndrome.
       (2) Granular/waxy.
          (a) Renal parenchymal disease.
          (b) Acute tubular necrosis (ATN).
       (3) Hyaline.
          (a) Acidic urine.
          (b) Dehydration.
       (4) Red blood cells (RBC): acute glomerulonephritis.

(5) White blood cells (WBC).
    (a) Infection.
    (b) Acute interstitial nephritis (AIN).
    (c) Inflammatory state.
  e. Crystals.
    (1) Urinary tract calculi.
    (2) Systemic gout.
12. Eosinophils: acute interstitial nephritis (AIN).
13. Other urinary evaluation.
  a. Osmolality.
    (1) A more exact measurement of urine concentration than specific gravity.
    (2) Often used to evaluate a systemic disease state.
    (3) Increased.
      (a) Prerenal/dehydration state.
      (b) Congestive heart failure.
      (c) Syndrome of inappropriate anti-diuretic hormone (SIADH).
      (d) Hyponatremia.
    (4) Decreased.
      (a) AKI.
      (b) Diabetes insipidus.
      (c) Hypernatremia.
      (d) Polydipsia.
  b. Fractional secretion.
    (1) Usually measured as a fractional secretion of sodium ($FeNa^+$).
      (a) Can be an effective measurement to provide objective data to determine the intravascular volume status of a patient.
      (b) For example, is the patient volume overloaded or volume depleted?
    (2) However, $FeNa^+$ is abnormally affected by diuretic therapy, making results difficult to interpret and possibly inaccurate.
    (3) If a diuretic has been recently given, a fractionated secretion of urea (FeUrea) or fractionated secretion of uric acid (FeUric) may be calculated instead. These tests are less likely to be diuretic sensitive.

C. Kidney imaging. As noted in the diagnostic data section, choosing the appropriate imaging test(s) is critical when seeking valuable information to evaluate a patient.
  1. Ultrasound.
  2. CT scan.
  3. Magnetic resonance imaging (MRI) and angiography (MRA).
  4. X-ray.
  5. Retrograde pyelogram.
  6. Radionuclide studies.
  7. Kidney angiography.

D. Laboratory data (Fischbach, 2000). These panels can determine what current kidney impairment is present as well as the severity of dysfunction. Serial testing and comparing results is essential in establishing the course of treatment, determining whether or not the treatment is effective, and if the patient is improving clinically.
  1. Chemistries. Listed below are the three most commonly used chemistry panels.
    a. Basic metabolic panel (BMP).
    b. Comprehensive metabolic panel (CMP). BMP components plus basic liver tests (bilirubin, AST/ALT) and albumin levels.
    c. Renal panel (RFP). BMP components plus phosphorus and albumin levels.
  2. Complete blood count (CBC) with differential.
    a. Provides information about the current hematologic and infection status.
    b. Can impact or be impacted by kidney dysfunction.
    c. Hemoglobin/hematocrit (Hgb/Hct) – level of anemia, which is directly affected by production of erythropoietin by the kidneys.
      (1) Systemic dysfunction causing abnormal production (bone marrow suppression) or loss (bleeding, hemolysis) can also affect degree of anemia.
      (2) Evaluating for anemia caused by a nonrenal condition is important to remember, including assessing the components related to production of RBCs (erythropoietin, iron, B12, folate).
    d. White blood count (WBC) – elevation shows an indication of the degree of systemic infection.
    e. Platelet – basic assessment of one component of clotting mechanism. Low levels in patients who are on dialysis need to be assessed for heparin induced thrombocytopenia (HIT) and other possible disorders.
  3. Endocrine.
    a. Thyroid stimulating hormone (TSH) abnormality can cause systemic dysfunction.
      (1) Increased.
        (a) Hypertension.
        (b) Arrythmias.
      (2) Decreased.
        (a) Edema.
        (b) Hyponatremia.
        (c) Hypotension.
    b. Hemoglobin A1C (HbA1C) helps determine the level of diabetic control.
      (1) Important to check if significant proteinuria is present. If HbA1C is normal, evaluate for a nondiabetic cause for the proteinuria. It may indicate a primary

glomerular abnormality (acute or chronic glomerulonephritis) or hematologic cause (multiple myeloma).

    (2) In patients with diabetes who are on dialysis, the HbA1C is significantly underestimated due to the shortened red cell survival in patients with CKD stage 5. A more accurate test for these patients is a glycated albumin (Freedman et al., 2010; Peacock et al, 2008), which provides a measure of glycemic control over approximately the past 2 to 3 weeks (Furusyo et al., 2011).

  c. Parathyroid hormone (PTH) is elevated in secondary hyperparathyroidism.

    (1) Very often seen in CKD stages 3 and above.

    (2) Essential to check in hypocalcemia and hypercalcemia to evaluate if a primary or secondary hyperparathyroidism is present.

  d. Vitamin D 25-hydroxy is the measurement of levels of previtamin D present in the body.

    (1) An essential precursor to the production of active vitamin D by the kidneys.

    (2) Essential to check in hypocalcemia and hypercalcemia to evaluate if low or elevated levels are the cause.

    (3) Often low in patients with CKD; supplementation is required.

4. Arterial blood gas (ABG).

  a. Provides valuable information about the acid-base balance of the patient. When compared to the serum levels, ABG can help determine the degree of kidney vs. respiratory impairment.

  b. Necessary data to obtain before initiating treatment for suspected metabolic acidosis caused by kidney disease and to determine the degree of respiratory compensation.

5. Microbiology is the blood, urine, and samples of other body fluids that are cultured and tested for possible infection.

6. Specialty tests.

  a. Iron studies.

    (1) Ferritin.

      (a) A measurement of the iron stores of the body.

      (b) Is an acute phase reactant, so an elevated level can be seen during acute inflammation or infectious conditions leading to a functional iron deficiency. With this deficiency there is plenty of iron stored up, but it is not available for use by the body.

    (2) Iron/TIBC/transferrin saturation percentage is the measurement of the iron and TIBC levels; can then determine the percentage of iron available for use by the bone marrow to make RBCs.

Transferrin saturation % = Serum iron x 100 / TIBC

  b. Eosinophil.

    (1) An elevated absolute eosinophil count will be seen in acute interstitial nephritis, very often caused by a medication. Used less often due to the low sensitivity and specificity, making the accuracy of the results a concern.

    (2) It is often difficult to determine which medication triggered the allergic reaction.

      (a) Many antibiotics used acutely can be the trigger.

      (b) Some chronic medications, such as proton pump inhibitors (PPIs) and xanthine oxidase inhibitors (allopurinol), can serve as the trigger.

    (3) It is helpful to look at the timeline to determine when the AKI occurred and correlate that to any new medications.

  c. Uric acid.

    (1) Is the end product of purine metabolism.

    (2) Often elevated in CKD since two thirds of uric acid production is excreted by the kidneys (Fischbach, 2000).

    (3) Elevated.

      (a) Decreased GFR.

      (b) Gout.

      (c) Tumor lysis syndrome.

      (d) Metabolic acidosis.

      (e) Liver disease.

      (f) Hypothyroidism.

    (4) Decreased.

      (a) SIADH.

      (b) Multiple myeloma.

      (c) Hodgkin's lymphoma.

  d. Cortisol.

    (1) Measurement of adrenal glucocorticosteroid.

    (2) Most often measured during a hyponatremia workup as low serum cortisol levels can cause a hypersecretion of ADH (Oelkers, 1989).

  e. Osmolarity.

    (1) Evaluation of both urine and serum osmolarities is used to help determine water and electrolyte (especially serum sodium) levels.

    (2) Measuring the osmolar gap is important when possible overdoses are a concern or in severe shock or acidosis.

  f. Renin/aldosterone.

    (1) Often measured to evaluate for severe hypertension or hypokalemic states that can occur due to adrenal or kidney tumors.

    (2) Should be considered if a patient has unexplained hypokalemia, or if there is severe and uncontrolled hypertension.

IV. Chronic kidney disease (CKD) vs. acute kidney injury (AKI).

A. General information.
1. The most important factor in determining if a kidney abnormality is acute or chronic is time.
   a. Obtaining past lab data can provide important clues to how rapid a change occurred.
   b. Past lab data can also provide information that may help influence the course of treatment.
2. Acute kidney injury can be caused by many factors that upset the metabolic equilibrium of the body.
   a. Determining the pathophysiologic triggers is an important step in determining the plan of care for treatment. There is always a reason for an imbalance.
   b. Resolving AKI may take hours, days, weeks, or months depending upon many factors, including:
      (1) Cause of the AKI.
      (2) Length of time the impact has occurred.
      (3) Baseline clinical condition of the patient.
      (4) Effectiveness of treatment of the AKI.
      (5) Many other subtle factors.
3. Sometimes the kidney injury is never fully resolved and becomes chronic in nature.
4. The Kidney Disease Outcomes Quality Initiative states that a patient cannot be considered to have chronic kidney disease until "either kidney damage or GFR < 60 mL/min/1.73 m^2 for ≥ 3 months. Kidney damage is defined as pathologic abnormalities or markers of damage, including abnormalities in blood or urine tests or imaging studies" (NFK, 2002).

B. Kidney Disease Improving Global Outcomes (KDIGO) defines AKI as any of the following (KDIGO-AKI, 2012):
1. An increase in serum creatinine by ≥ 0.3 mg/dL within 48 hours.
2. An increase in serum creatinine to ≥ 1.5 times baseline, which is presumed to have occurred within the prior 7 days.
3. Urine volume < 0.5 mL/kg/hour for 6 hours.

C. AKI can be staged by severity according to the following criteria.
1. Patients can also have an acute injury on top of chronic disease. For instance, if a patient has a baseline creatinine of 2.2 and develops an AKI that further declines the kidney function to a creatinine of 3.8, the patient may or may not improve with treatment.
2. The postacute kidney function may settle out at some value between these two and thus establish a new baseline.
3. See Table 4.2 to see KDIGO's staging of AKI.

Table 4.2
Staging of AKI

STAGE	SERUM CREATININE	URINE OUTPUT
1	1.5–1.9 baseline OR ≥ 0.3 mg/dL (≥ 26.5µmol/l increase	< 0.5mL/kg/h for 6–12 hours
2	2.0–2.9 times baseline	< 0.5 mL/kg/h for ≥ 12 hours
3	3.0 baseline OR Increase in creatinine to ≥ 4.0 mg/dL (≥ 353.6 µmol/l) OR Initiation of renal replacement therapy OR In patients < 18 years, decrease in eGFR to < 135 mL/min per 1.73 m^2	< 0.3 mL/kg/h for ≥ 24 hours OR Anuria for ≥ 12 hours

Used with permission from KDIGO (2012). *Clinical practice guideline for acute kidney injury.* Retrieved from http://kdigo.org/home/guidelines/acute-kidney-injury

V. Acute kidney injury (AKI).

A. AKI is a common clinical condition.
1. It is seen in 5–7% of all hospitalized patients (Drawz et al., 2008).
2. More than 35% of critically ill patients will experience AKI (Palevsky et al., 2008).
3. However, due to the lack of consensus of which measurement criteria to use, the prevalence can be wide ranging from 1–70% (Case, 2013).

B. Patients who develop AKI have mortality rates that range from 40–70%, depending upon severity and the course of treatment (Palevsky et al., 2013).

C. Classification of AKI can often be difficult to quantify.
1. The RIFLE (Risk, Injury, Failure, Loss, End-stage) criteria was developed by the Acute Dialysis Quality Initiative (ADQI) in 2002 to help give some objective measurement of when AKI occurs as well as the degree of severity.
2. These criteria were subsequently modified by the AKI Network (AKIN) to set an absolute increase in creatinine and adjust the time factor when determining if AKI has occurred (Palevsky et al., 2008).
3. See Figure 4.1 for the RIFLE and the AKIN criteria.

D. AKI differentiation. Determining when AKI has occurred is one important factor when evaluating a patient, but diagnosing the etiology of the AKI is just as important. The causes of AKI are commonly categorized into three areas.

1. Prerenal.
   a. Prerenal etiology is any condition causing hypo-perfusion to the kidneys.
   b. The pathophysiology of AKI is any process that can directly decrease the effective kidney blood flow, such as the following (Windus, 2008).
      (1) Intravascular volume depletion or dehydration.
      (2) Kidney vasoconstriction or blockage.
         (a) Sepsis.
         (b) Hypercalcemia.
         (c) Nonsteroidal antiinflammatory (NSAIDs) medications.
         (d) Renal artery stenosis or thrombus.
      (3) Decreased effective circulating volume.
         (a) Decreased cardiac output.
         (b) Cirrhosis.
         (c) Third spacing of fluid from intravascular to extravascular spaces.
      (4) Efferent arteriolar vasodilatation. ACE inhibitors or ARB antihypertensives.
   c. Assessment.
      (1) Measuring blood pressures and determining if any hypotension has occurred.
      (2) Evaluating for other comorbid conditions that would cause poor kidney blood flow.
      (3) Reviewing medication list for any pharmacologic cause.
      (4) Fractionated secretion of sodium, uric acid, and urea. Low values will show that there is poor intravascular volume.
      (5) Physical exam shows signs and symptoms of dehydration, poor skin turgor, dry mucous membranes, and/or orthostatic hypotension.
   d. Treatment.
      (1) Restore effective circulatory volume by infusing a crystalloid solution (intravenous 0.9% normal saline is primary choice in AKI).
      (2) Treat the possible cause.
         (a) Stop offensive medications.
         (b) Restore effective renal blood flow.
         (c) Improve cardiac output and perfusion.
2. Intrinsic.
   a. The etiology can be further broken down into subcategories (Windus, 2008).

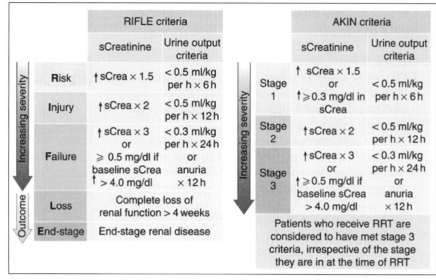

Figure 4.1. Comparison of RIFLE (Risk, Injury, Failure, Loss, and End-stage) and Acute Kidney Injury Network (AKIN) Criteria for the diagnosis of AKI.

Open source paper. Used with permission from Seller-Pérez, G., Herrera-Gutiérrez, M.E., Maynar-Moliner, J., Sánchez-Izquierdo-Riera, J.A., Marinho, A., & Luis do Pico, J. (2013). Estimating kidney function in the critically ill patients. *Critical Care Research and Practice*. doi:10.1155/2013/721810.

   (1) Microvascular.
      (a) Atheroembolic.
      (b) Hypertension nephrosclerosis.
      (c) Scleroderma.
   (2) Glomerulus.
      (a) Glomerulonephritis.
      (b) Lupus nephritis.
      (c) Wegener's granulomatosis.
      (d) Henoch-Schonlein purpura.
      (e) Goodpasture's syndrome.
   (3) Tubule.
      (a) Acute tubular necrosis (ATN) (see Figure 4.2).
      (b) Ischemia.
      (c) Toxins.
      (d) Contrast nephropathy.
      (e) Sepsis.
      (f) Multiple myeloma.
      (g) Rhabdomyolysis (see Figure 4.3).
         i. Local features include muscle pain, tenderness, swelling, bruising, and weakness.
         ii. Systemic features include tea-colored urine, fever, malaise, nausea, emesis, confusion, agitation, delirium, and anuria.
   (4) Interstitium.
      (a) Acute interstitial nephritis (AIN).
      (b) Infiltrative diseases.
         i. Lymphoma.
         ii. Leukemia.

iii. Amyloidosis.
(c) Pyelonephritis.
(5) Hereditary.
(a) Polycystic kidney
disease (PCKD).
(b) Alport's syndrome.
b. Pathophysiology.
(1) Depends upon the etiology
of the disease.
(2) History and assessment are
essential in providing clues
to which subcategory may
be impacted, which can
then narrow the differential
cause.
(3) Acute tubular necrosis is a
general term often used
when there is an unknown
or questionable cause that
has caused AKI.
c. Assessment.
(1) Detailed blood and urine
analysis provides initial
clues and can point to
which area to search more
in-depth.
(2) If no clear cause is identified, and
depending upon the degree of AKI, a
kidney biopsy may be warranted.
(3) Blood.
(a) An elevation in creatinine indicates
AKI.
(b) Many other blood tests specific for
individual disease processes can be
ordered.
(4) Urine.
(a) Obtaining a UA with micro is helpful.
(b) Presence of abnormal sediment, casts,
or cells can point to specific disease
processes. Actually looking at the urine
under the microscope with the
assistance of a trained lab technician is
a good way to learn about urinary
sediment (see Table 4.3).
(5) Biopsy.
(a) A last resort option due to the invasive
nature of a biopsy.
(b) But a biopsy can provide an exact
determination of the cause of AKI,
thereby providing a targeted clinical
treatment regimen.
(c) The risks and benefits of obtaining a
biopsy must be weighed and potential
contradictions considered.
i. Relative contraindications include
active infections and anatomic

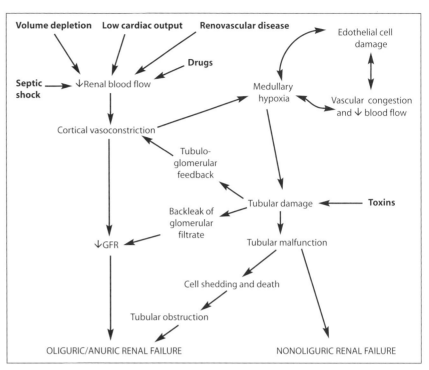

Figure 4.2. Mechanisms of acute tubular necrosis.

Source: Fry, A.C., & Farrington, K. (2006). Management of acute renal failure. *Postgraduate Medicine Journal, 82*, 106-116. Used with permission.

abnormalities that would increase
the biopsy's risk.
ii. Absolute contraindications include
a solitary native kidney,
uncontrolled severe hypertension,
or an uncooperative patient.
(d) A biopsy is inherently risky due to the
potential for bleeding.
i. It cannot be done safely if someone
is prone to bleeding due to intrinsic
or extrinsic causes.
ii. Medications that affect bleeding
(e.g., aspirin, clopidogrel, warfarin)
need to be held 1 to 2 weeks prior to
the biopsy.
[a] The specific time for
withholding the medication is
determined by the clinician
performing the procedure.
[b] Use of desmopressin just prior
to the procedure can help
minimize bleeding.
(e) Postbiopsy hemoglobin and/or
ultrasound is essential to make sure no
significant bleeding has occurred.
d. Treatment.
(1) Varies widely based on the etiology of the
AKI.

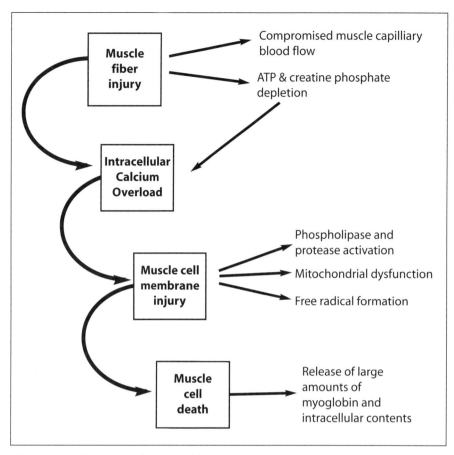

Figure 4.3. Pathogenesis of exertional rhabdomyolysis.

Source: Russell, T.A. (2005). Acute renal failure related to rhabdomyolysis: Pathophysiology, diagnosis, and collaborative management. *Nephrology Nursing Journal, 32,* 409-417. Used with permission.

(2) Once the specific etiology is determined, start following standard treatment guidelines for that disease with close follow-up and serial labs.

(3) Very often, however, the exact cause is not clear and treatment of the clinical situation is necessary, such as providing fluids to maintain euvolemia, antibiotics for possible infection, and hypertensive medication to keep BP under control until more data is available to finalize the cause of the AKI.

(4) Improvement in AKI can take days, weeks, or months if it happens at all, which should be included in the discussion with the patient and family about treatment options.

3. Postrenal.
 a. Etiology is usually a consequence of an obstruction of urinary flow due to a structural or functional change of the urinary tract.
 b. The pathophysiology can be caused by many abnormalities.

(1) The overall presence is approximately 3% of hospitalizations, with both genders being affected equally (Windus, 2008).

(2) Can be unilateral or bilateral depending upon where along the urinary tract the blockage has occurred.
 (a) Benign prostatic hyperplasia (BPH).
 (b) Nephrolithiasis (kidney stones).
 (c) Tumor – benign or malignant.
 (d) Neurogenic bladder.
 (e) Urethral strictures.

 c. Assessment.
 (1) Can occur acutely or establish itself as a chronic condition.
 (2) Establishing a time line of AKI as well as old data for comparison and a detailed history helps to distinguish the acuity of the obstruction.
 (3) Urinalysis can provide clues to the cause as well as the length of time of the obstruction. Bland urine is often seen in uncomplicated obstruction, while a more

Table 4.3

Typical Findings in Prerenal and Intrarenal Acute Renal Failure

	Prerenal	Intrarenal
Volume	Oliguria	Oliguria or nonoliguria
Urinary sediment	Normal (hyaline and granular casts)	RBC casts Cellular debris
Specific gravity	High	Low
Osmolality (mOsm/Kg H_2O)	High	Low (Isosthenuria)
Ratio Osm Urine to Osm Plasma	> 1.5	< 1.2
Urine Na (mEq/L)	Low (< 20)	Increased over prerenal (> 20)
Urine urea (g/24 hrs)	Low (15)	Low (5)
Urine creatinine (g/24 hrs)	Normal (> 1.0)	Low (< 1.0)
Ratio urine creatinine to plasma creatinine	> 15:1	< 10:1

Source: Lancaster, L.E. (1990). Renal response to shock. *Critical Care Nursing Clinics of North America, 2*(2), 221-223. Used with permission.

active urine sediment can be seen in nephrolithiasis (hematuria, crystals) or tumor (neoplastic cells).

(4) Imaging is the key to diagnosing the presence of an obstruction.

  (a) Basic bladder scan can be done by the bedside nurse to evaluate for urinary retention, but does not confirm an obstruction.

  (b) Kidney ultrasound is > 90% sensitive and specific for obstruction.

  (c) CT scan can be used with a stone protocol (noncontrast) to evaluate the presence of kidney stones or to compare and confirm findings from the ultrasound.

  (d) More invasive imaging tests such as a urography, pyelography, or renography can be obtained but are usually done by urology once an obstruction is documented and are used during treatment (i.e., stent or percutaneous nephrostomy placement).

d. Treatment of an obstruction.

  (1) Treatment centers on management of the cause of the obstruction.

  (2) In general, if an obstruction is found, a urologic consult is warranted, both to treat the current acute abnormality and often to follow up afterward as an acute event often leads to a chronic condition.

  (3) Resolving the obstruction by creating some pathway for the urine to flow is the goal, either through a Foley catheter or a more invasive percutaneous nephrostomy.

  (4) If the AKI was primarily caused by the obstruction and is fairly acute, then resolution of the AKI is often fairly rapid (hours to days). If there was some other disease process, with the obstruction being secondary, then the AKI may take longer to resolve, if it does.

  (5) Once a patent urinary tract is obtained, there is often a postobstructive diuresis that occurs; can lead to polyuria and subsequent electrolyte losses.

  (a) Dehydration and a prerenal state can often develop, blunting the resolving AKI, so starting the patient on intravenous fluids is often necessary.

  (b) Replacing approximately two thirds of urinary losses, with close monitoring of intake and output, is essential during the first few days.

  (c) Close monitoring of serum electrolytes during the diuretic phase is needed, with supplementation as needed (Windus, 2008) (see Figure 4.4).

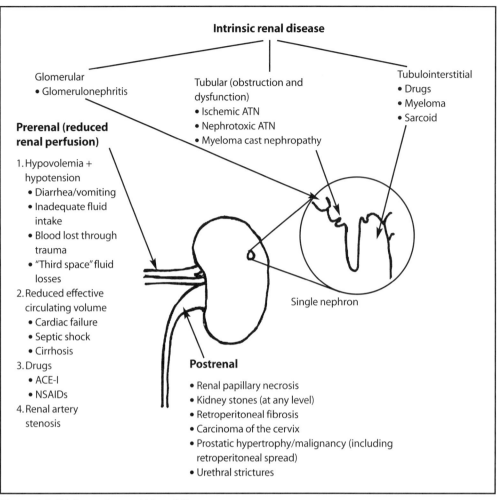

Figure 4.4. Etiology of acute kidney failure.

Source: Fry, A.C., & Farrington, K. (2006). Management of acute renal failure. *Postgraduate Medicine Journal, 82,* 106-116. Used with permission.

VI. Acute kidney replacement therapies.

A. Despite aggressive treatment, a patient's clinical condition will deteriorate to the point that kidney replacement therapy (KRT) must be considered. That point is based upon a variety of clinical factors such as the following.
   1. Hyperkalemia refractory to medical therapy.
   2. Uremic syndrome (encephalopathy or pericarditis).
   3. Metabolic acidosis refractory to medical therapy.
   4. Volume overload refractory to medical therapy.
   5. Overdose of dialysis responsive drugs.

B. Patient and family discussion.
   1. As a patient's clinical condition changes, it is important to keep the patient and family updated. If it looks like KRT will be needed, it is wise to explain this early on as a potential option.
   2. Deciding to proceed with an invasive mode of treatment, such as KRT, is often viewed quite differently, and often negatively, than more noninvasive therapies, such as pharmacologic treatment or hydration.
   3. Discussion with the patient and family should address three possible pathways of therapy.
      a. Aggressive therapy, including use of KRT.
      b. Aggressive therapy, without the use of KRT.
      c. Nonaggressive or more conservative therapy, including possible hospice.
   4. The pros and cons of each pathway should be discussed so that the patient and family can make an informed decision and understand the potential consequences of that decision.
   5. Emphasize that they can change their mind and that an open communication path will be maintained between them and the APRN.
   6. Appropriate documentation and a signed consent for dialysis, as well as consent for placement of appropriate dialysis catheter, should be completed.
   7. Based upon the prehospital kidney function and the patient's clinical condition, the APRN can

often have some sense if the initiation of dialysis will be permanent.
  a. A patient who has had a longstanding progressive decline of CKD who now needs dialysis must be approached differently than a patient who had normal kidney function and now presents with AKI.
  b. For the former, the APRN must look at managing the acute situation as well as keeping in mind that the patient may end up requiring dialysis permanently.
  c. For the latter, the APRN generally focuses on managing the acute situation, with the hope that with aggressive treatment the patient will be able to come off dialysis.
  d. Emphasize that resolution of AKI is always an unknown factor and that even if they do come off dialysis, they are at risk of being left with some CKD.

C. Deciding which modality of KRT to use is based upon a variety of factors.
  1. Hemodynamic stability.
    a. A patient may not be clinically stable enough for intermittent hemodialysis (IHD); a continuous renal replacement therapy (CRRT) may need to be considered.
    b. Acute peritoneal dialysis (APD) is also a possibility as it provides gentler hemodynamic shifts than IHD and is often better tolerated in acute situations.
  2. Clinical history of the patient.
    a. APD may not be an option if the patient has an absolute contraindication to PD (e.g., recent abdominal surgery or a chronic ostomy).
    b. A patient who is hypercoagulable or who has an allergy to heparin or anticoagulant may do better with APD.
  3. Current infection status.
    a. Placement of a tunneled hemodialysis catheter or a PD catheter is contraindicated if there is any question of sepsis or active infection.
    b. Clearance from infectious disease is often requested by the vascular or PD surgeons prior to placement of a catheter.
    c. Use of a nontunneled hemodialysis catheter is preferred when KRT is urgently needed. It is important to limit the catheter's use to the shortest amount of time possible.
  4. The cause of the AKI or need for dialysis. Caring for a patient being treated for an overdose, where dialysis may only be needed for a couple of sessions, will be very different than caring for a patient being treated for uremic encephalopathy, who has underlying CKD, and will require extended dialysis sessions that may be permanent.
  5. The decision of the patient and family based upon

discussion and education of modalities by the APRN and other healthcare providers.

D. Acute and intermittent hemodialysis (IHD).
  1. Upon deciding that the patient needs dialysis and can tolerate IHD, the APRN should obtain a signed consent based upon the hospital's policies.
  2. Initial acute hemodialysis prescription should be based upon the following variables.
    a. Placement of a tunneled vs. nontunneled hemodialysis catheter as inserted by vascular surgery or interventional radiologist.
    b. Length of time.
      (1) Initial treatment times are generally limited to 2 hours unless specific needs are present. For example:
        (a) The need to remove more fluid.
        (b) Certain overdose situations.
      (2) Subsequent dialysis session times are generally titrated up in a step format of 30-minute increments until a final time (in general 3 minutes per kg) is reached.
      (3) Session times can be adjusted based upon the need for fluid removal or degree of azotemia.
      (4) If severe azotemia is present, there is a risk for dialysis disequilibrium.
        (a) Initially, a shorter time on dialysis is used with a lower blood flow and a lower efficiency dialyzer.
        (b) For the first treatment the goal is to limit the reduction of urea to no more than 30%.
        (c) These steps will lessen the solute shift and minimize the neurological risk associated with dialysis disequilibrium. Table 4.4 summarizes the signs and symptoms of DDS.
    c. Dialysis frequency.
      (1) The frequency of dialysis depends upon the patient's clinical condition.
      (2) Usually a patient starting dialysis will dialyze for 3 consecutive days and then transition to the standard 3 times a week.
      (3) Individual factors, such as the need for aggressive fluid or solute removal, demand that these initial orders be patient-specific.
    d. Dialysate prescription.
      (1) Base.
        (a) Usual range 30 to 35mEq/L.
        (b) Use of bicarbonate base is the standard.
        (c) Acetate is not often used as it is associated with hemodynamic instability.
      (2) Sodium (Na^+).
        (a) Usual range from 140 to 145mEq/L Na^+.
        (b) Higher levels may predispose the

Table 4.4

DDS Signs and Symptoms

Mild To Early Disequilibrium
Nausea/vomiting
Blurred vision
Restlessness
Headache
Hypertension
Increased pulse pressure
Muscle cramps
Dizziness not related to BP
Asterixsis

Severe Disequilibrium
Confusion
Disorientation
Muscle twitching/tremors
Seizures
Arrhythmias
Coma (improved within 24 hours)
Death

Courtesy of DCI Acute Program, Omaha, Nebraska.
Used with permission.

patient to increased thirst and interdialytic weight gain.

(c) Lower levels induce intradialytic hypotension, cramps, headaches, nausea, vomiting, and, in acute situations, with severe azotemia dialysis disequilibrium.

(3) Potassium (K^+).

(a) Range from 1 to 4 mEq/L K^+ bath levels.

(b) Lower concentrations (0 to 1 K^+) should be reserved for patients with excessive hyperkalemia with electrocardiovascular compromise and only used for a short and partial treatment (30 to 60 minutes) to minimize potential life-threatening arrhythmias.

(c) When a < 2 K^+ potassium concentration bath is used, it is vital that the patient's EKG be monitored during dialysis and is suggested that a plasma potassium level be checked immediately after the low potassium bath is finished to avoid overcorrection and hypokalemia.

(d) For hyperkalemic patients who already have a vascular access and can be effectively dialyzed within a reasonable time period, it is more effective and less problematic for the patient to receive HD than be given Kayexalate®

or a "high K^+ cocktail" (D50/insulin/bicarb/calcium). If predialysis medical management of hyperkalemia was initiated (i.e., Kayexalate®, D50/insulin/bicarb/calcium), the patient should be monitored for postdialysis hypokalemia as well.

(e) Higher concentrations (4 K^+) may be needed for patients with severe cardiac disease who are at increased risk for developing dysrhythmias. Higher concentrations may also be needed for those patients with hypokalemia related to nonrenal etiologies, such as GI losses.

(f) As acidosis is corrected with hemodialysis, a shift of potassium from extracellular to intracellular lowers the serum potassium.

(g) A potassium rebound will occur in 1 to 2 hours postdialysis. Do not supplement if the patient is hypokalemic during this time.

(4) Calcium (Ca^+).

(a) Range from 2.0 to 3.5 mEq/L Ca^+ bath levels.

(b) Standard calcium concentration for most hemodialysis patients is 2.5 mEq/L.

(c) Higher or lower calcium concentrations should be reserved for acute clinical abnormalities when the patient has shown symptomatic hypercalcemic or hypocalcemic changes.

(d) If higher or lower calcium baths are used, then corrected serum calcium levels should be closely monitored.

(5) Dextrose.

(a) Usually set at 200 mg/dL.

(b) Dextrose is needed to prevent hypoglycemia.

(c) Monitor for signs and symptoms of hypoglycemia during hemodialysis. A decreased GFR, especially in an acute situation such as AKI, makes patients more prone to hypoglycemia if they were on a diabetic management regimen.

(6) Dialysate flow rate.

(a) Range 400 to 800 mL/min.

(b) For acute situations, including initial hemodialysis, a lower dialysate flow rate is used, 400 to 500 mL/min, especially in severe azotemia, to lessen the risk of dialysis disequilibrium.

(c) In subsequent dialysis sessions, the

flow rate can be titrated up to near normal range (600 to 800 mL/min) to provide adequate solute clearance.

(d) For stable clinical patients or those on chronic hemodialysis, a flow rate of twice the blood flow rate, up to 800 mEq/L, is used.

(7) Blood flow rate.

(a) Range 100 to 500 mL/min.

(b) For acute situations, including initial hemodialysis, a lower blood flow rate is used, 100 to 200 mL/min, especially in severe azotemia, to lessen the risk of dialysis disequilibrium.

(c) In subsequent dialysis sessions, the flow rate can be titrated up to near normal range (350 to 500 mL/min) to provide adequate solute clearance.

(d) Maximum flow rates will often be dependent upon the type of vascular access used.

(8) Dialysate solution temperature.

(a) Range 35° to 37°C.

(b) Bath temperature can be reduced to 35.5° to 36°C to help minimize intradialytic hypotension.

(9) Ultrafiltration.

(a) Range from 0 to 5 liters per session.

(b) Amount of fluid to be removed should be assessed predialysis and throughout the treatment with fluid goals adjusted based upon the patient's clinical situation.

(c) Avoid intradialytic hypotension in the following.

i. AKI, as hypotension/hypoperfusion risks blunting the resolution of the AKI.

ii. Newly placed AV fistulas or grafts which risks causing thrombosis.

iii. Acute stroke, as this may risk further cerebral hypoperfusion. A discussion with neurologist or neurosurgeon as to blood pressure limits is often helpful.

E. Acute peritoneal dialysis.

1. Peritoneal dialysis is a nonvascular approach to treating AKI. Reasons for using acute peritoneal dialysis (APD) are listed below (Ponce, 2011; KDIGO-AKI, 2012).

a. Hemodynamically unstable patients.

b. Hemorrhagic conditions contraindicating placement of vascular access for hemodialysis or anticoagulation, such as hypercoagulable conditions.

c. Patients with difficult vascular access placement.

d. KRT in the treatment of AKI in children.

e. Removal of high molecular weight toxins (> 10 kD [kilodaltons]).

f. Patients at risk for increased intracranial pressure.

2. Contraindications of the use of peritoneal dialysis are listed below (Ponce, 2011).

a. Recent abdominal surgery.

b. Pleuroperitoneal communication.

c. Diaphragmatic severe respiratory failure.

d. Life-threatening hyperkalemia not responding to medical therapy.

e. Extreme hypercatabolic state.

f. Severe volume overload in nonventilatory patients.

g. Severe gastroespohageal reflux disease (GERD).

h. Low peritoneal clearance.

i. Active peritonitis or sepsis.

j. Abdominal wall cellulitis.

k. AKI in pregnancy is a relative contraindication depending upon weeks of gestation (Coffman, 2012).

3. Order insertion of peritoneal catheter.

a. A temporary stylet catheter can be inserted if a longer dwelling peritoneal catheter cannot be placed.

b. The temporary catheter should not stay in longer than 3 days.

4. Postop care after insertion of a new PD catheter.

a. Minimize bacterial colonization of the exit site and tunnel.

b. Immobilize catheter to prevent trauma to exit site and traction on catheter.

c. Minimize intraabdominal pressure.

d. Until healed, sterile dressing changes should be performed only by trained staff.

e. Exit site should be kept dry (no showers or baths).

f. Teach patient how to do self-care after healing completed, usually 2 weeks postinsertion.

5. Acute peritoneal dialysis prescription. Order for 24 hours. Review and update daily. Hourly exchanges may be required for the patient with acute kidney injury for the first few days.

a. Choose type of therapy: continuous ambulatory peritoneal dialysis (CAPD – manual exchanges) vs. automated peritoneal dialysis (APD – cycler).

b. Session length.

c. Cycle fill volume.

d. Exchange time.

(1) Inflow.

(2) Dwell.

(3) Drain.

e. Dialysis solution (1.5%, 2.5%, 4.25%).

f. Dialysis solution additives.

(1) Potassium.
(2) Heparin.
(3) Insulin.
(4) Antibiotics.
(5) Lidocaine.
6. Order intake and outtake and daily weights.
7. Review total ultrafiltration daily.
8. Monitor volume status.
9. Monitor and manage uremic symptoms.
10. Monitor clearance daily.
   a. Goal of therapy is blood urea nitrogen levels < 80 mg/dL.
   b. Increase clearance by increasing dwell times or by decreasing exchange times.
11. Monitor for complications of acute PD.
   a. Incomplete drainage and abdominal complications.
   b. Infection (peritonitis, tunnel infection, exit-site infection).
   c. Catheter malfunction.
   d. Hypovolemia and hypervolemia.
   e. Hypotension.
   f. Hyperglycemia.
   g. Hypokalemia.
   h. Hypernatremia.
   i. Hypoalbuminemia.

F. Continuous renal replacement therapy (CRRT).
   1. For use with critically ill patients who are hemodynamically unstable. Advantages are listed below (KDIGO-AKI, 2012).
      a. Slower but steady fluid removal providing more control over hemodynamics and fluid balance.
      b. Improved control over solute concentrations and removal.
      c. Greater flexibility allowing adaption to changes in the patient's clinical condition.
      d. User friendly machines.
   2. Disadvantages of CRRT (KDIGO-AKI, 2012).
      a. The need for immobilization over an extended period of time.
      b. Use of continuous anticoagulation.
      c. Risk of hypothermia.
      d. Often a higher cost, compared to intermittent hemodialysis.
   3. A variety of types of CRRT are available. The decision as to which type to use depends upon the degree of azotemia, volume status, and clinical condition of the patient. Modalities of CRRT are listed below (see Figures 4.5, 4.6, 4.7 and 4.8 for various CRRT possibilities).
      a. Slow continuous ultrafiltration (SCUF).
      b. Continuous venovenous hemofiltration (CVVH).
      c. Continuous venovenous hemodialysis (CVVHD).
      d. Continuous venovenous hemodialfiltration (CVVHDF).
      e. An alternative to CRRT is slow, low efficiency

dialysis (SLED), which allows for many of the benefits of CRRT without the disadvantages (KDIGO-AKI, 2012).
      (1) Allows for "down-time" diagnostic and therapeutic procedures.
      (2) Reduced exposure to anticoagulation.
   4. APRN management of CRRT should include the following.
      a. Perform comprehensive patient assessment.
      b. Order insertion of dialysis catheter.
      c. Educate patient and family regarding the goals of CRRT.
      d. Order the CRRT prescription.
         (1) Type of CRRT modality to be used.
         (2) Type of filter to be used.
         (3) Blood flow rate.
         (4) Dialysate flow rate.
         (5) Replacement fluid rate.
         (6) Patient hourly fluid removal rate goal.
         (7) Anticoagulation.
            (a) Heparin.
            (b) Citrate. If citrate is used, replacement IV calcium must be given to prevent hypocalcemia from developing. Close monitoring of serum calcium is essential.
         (8) Labs are based on the patient's clinical condition, typically every 4 to 12 hours.
            (a) Chemistry panel, including phosphorus, magnesium, and ionized calcium.
            (b) Coagulation profile.
            (c) CBC.
         (9) Specific parameters in which the APRN should be notified (e.g., filter clotting, hemodynamic changes).
         (10) Strict bed rest.
         (11) Strict intake/output documentation.
         (12) Daily weights.
      e. Evaluate patient's status daily and adjust prescription accordingly.
      f. Manage electrolyte replacements and parenteral nutrition orders while patient is on CRRT.
      g. When patient is stable, coordinate transition to IHD if needed.
      h. Prepare patient and family regarding transition to IHD.

G. Vascular access.
   1. Required once the decision is made for hemodialysis/CRRT.
   2. Placement is made by the vascular surgeon or interventional radiology.
   3. Use of fluoroscopy for placement can minimize complications.
   4. The position of the tip of any central catheter should be verified radiologically.

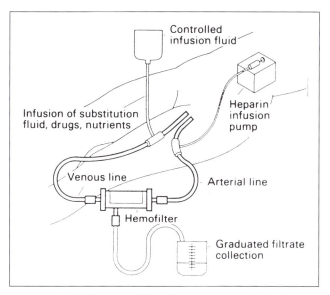

Figure 4.5. CAVH circuit: CAVH using a femoral cannulation.

Reprinted with permission from Millipore Corporation.

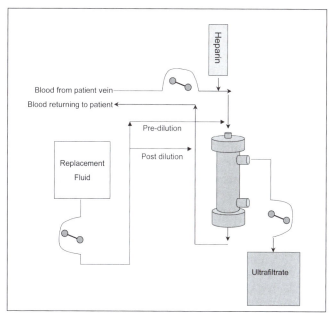

Figure 4.6. CVVH circuit: CVVH circuit with heparin anticoagulation.

Courtesy of Maureen Craig, UC Davis Medical Center, Sacramento, California.

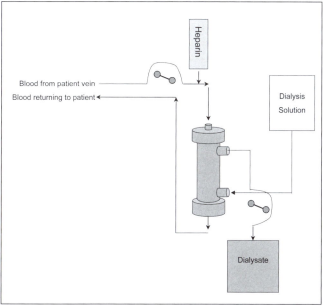

Figure 4.7. CVVHD circuit: CVVHD circuit with heparin anticoagulation.

Courtesy of Maureen Craig, UC Davis Medical Center, Sacramento, California.

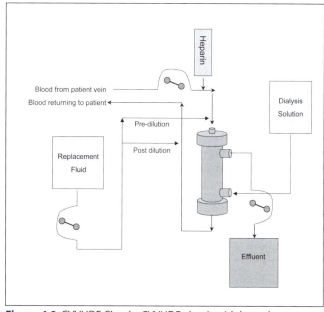

Figure 4.8. CVVHDF Circuit: CVVHDF circuit with heparin anticoagulation.

Courtesy of Maureen Craig, UC Davis Medical Center, Sacramento, California.

5. Insertion sites by order of preference (KDIGO-AKI, 2012).
   a. Right internal jugular vein.
   b. Left internal jugular vein.
   c. Right or left external jugular veins.
   d. Femoral veins.
   e. Subclavian veins should be limited to last resort due to the higher risk of stenosis and potential for pneumothorax.
6. Nontunneled (noncuffed) catheter is preferred for acute hemodialysis/CRRT.
   a. Can be placed quickly.

   b. Should be used instead of a tunneled catheter if patient is currently septic or is at risk of bleeding.
   c. Should not be left in place for longer than 7 days.
      (1) Higher risk of infection than tunneled catheters.
      (2) Track time of insertion.
      (3) Order new catheter insertion as indicated.
   d. Femoral temporary catheters.

(1) Easier insertion technique.

(2) Can be placed if at risk of bleeding or pulmonary compromise.

(3) Order strict bed rest and knee immobilizer to prevent kinking of the catheter.

(4) Associated with increased risk of infection so should be switched to nonfemoral site as soon as possible, preferably within 72 hours.

7. Tunneled (cuffed) catheter.

a. Placed when patient more hemodynamically stable.

b. For patients who will likely be dialysis dependent.

c. Need to be nonseptic for placement; may require infectious disease clearance.

8. Vein preservation.

a. If underlying CKD or severe AKI requiring KRT is present, then vein preservation of upper extremities should be made.

b. Use of "Save the Vein" wristband on nondominant arm.

c. Avoid use of peripherally inserted central catheter (PICC) lines.

d. For unstable patient or those who require extended IV access placement of a tunneled central catheter, a Hohn® (or Broviac®, etc.) may be used instead.

9. Arteriovenous fistulas (AVF) or grafts (AVG).

a. Should be considered once the patient is considered dialysis dependent, hemodynamically stable, and infection free.

b. If CKD stages 4 or 5 persist after the AKI has been resolved or if the patient remains dialysis dependent, a vascular access referral should be made for an AVF/AVG prior to discharge.

VII. Acute care management of chronic kidney disease (CKD).

Often, patients present with an AKI on top of preexisting CKD. In-hospital management of both AKI and CKD should include the following.

A. Performing a comprehensive health history, clinical data review, and physical exam.

B. Establishing euvolemia.

C. Maintaining blood pressure for adequate perfusion.

D. Avoiding nephrotoxic agents.

E. Treating infections.

F. Reviewing medications and dose adjustment if needed based on eGFR.

G. Coordinate and collaborate treatment regimen with other members of the healthcare team.

H. Treating comorbid conditions.

1. Anemia.

a. Evaluate iron stores, B12, and folate.

(1) Supplement if B12 or folate levels are low.

(2) Intravenous (IV) iron is preferred (KDIGO–Anemia, 2012).

(a) If iron saturation ≤ 30% and ferritin ≤ 500 ng/mL.

(b) Avoid IV iron if ferritin > 500 or if active systemic infection.

(c) Monitor for anaphylaxis.

b. Monitor for any gastrointestinal losses.

c. Evaluate for any hematologic cause.

d. Evaluate for signs of inflammation or infection that could be blunting erythrocyte production.

e. Start erythropoiesis-stimulating agent (ESA) therapy if workup indicates chronic kidney disease as cause, other causes have been corrected, and hemoglobin < 10 (KDIGO–Anemia, 2012).

f. Transfuse patient with packed red blood cells (PRBCs) if: (KDIGO–Anemia, 2012)

(1) Rapid correction is needed to stabilize the patient's condition (e.g., acute hemorrhage, unstable myocardial ischemia).

(2) Hemoglobin < 7.0.

(3) ESA therapy is not effective or warranted.

g. Limit blood transfusions in patients who may meet transplantation criteria in the future.

2. Bone and mineral metabolism.

a. Evaluate calcium and phosphorus.

b. Treatment will often be deferred to outpatient management.

c. If calcium levels are abnormal, do the following.

(1) High: evaluate for malignancy, hyperparathyroidism (primary or secondary), or excessive calcium or vitamin D intake.

(2) Low: evaluate for vitamin D deficiency, hypoparathyroidism, or malnutrition.

(3) Check ionized calcium, intact parathyroid hormone (I-PTH), alkaline phosphatase, and Vit D25 Hydrox.

(4) Review and adjust calcium based binders if needed.

(5) Adjust calcium level when low albumin is present.

d. If phosphorus levels are as follows, conduct the following.

(1) High: evaluate need for phosphate binders and dietary restriction.

(2) Low: evaluate for malnutrition, GI losses, or need to adjust phosphate binders.

3. Hypertension.

a. In an acute/in-hospital setting:

(1) Review and adjust hypertension

medications to make sure they are not contributing to any acute clinical abnormality, such as hyperkalemia caused by an ACE inhibitor.
(2) Individualize hypertension targets and medications according to age, co-existent cardiovascular disease, and other comorbidities (KDIGO–HTN, 2012).
(3) Adjust medications keeping these considerations in mind.
  (a) Know the patient's regimen at admission to eliminate the burden of purchasing all new medications.
  (b) Consider what the patient can realistically afford.
  (c) Identify what the patient's insurance will cover.
(4) Choose a medication that benefits two comorbidities; for example:
  (a) ACE inhibitor for hypertension management and anti-proteinuric effect.
  (b) Diuretic for hypertension management and control of congestive heart failure.
b. Encourage and educate lifestyle modifications that promote stable hypertension management.
  (1) Low salt, heart-healthy diet.
  (2) Smoking cessation.
  (3) Medication adherence.
  (4) Encourage weight control management strategies.
c. Monitor for orthostatic or relative hypotension when adjusting medication regimen.
d. Follow hypertension management goals based on current guidelines.
  (1) KDIGO (KDIGO–HTN, 2012).
    (a) ≤ 140 / ≤ 80 for nondiabetic patients.
    (b) ≤ 130 / ≤ 80 for diabetic patients or those with proteinuria > 300 mg/day.
  (2) Joint National Committee (JNC) 8 (James et al., 2013). The JNC 8 hypertension guidelines are not without controversy due in part to the significant treatment change from previous guidelines. Any treatment should be initiated after a careful review of the patient's overall clinical presentation; the effects of the treatment must be monitored carefully.
    (a) General population ≥ 60 years old should initiate pharmacologic therapy to keep SBP ≤ 150 mmHg or DBP ≤ 90.
    (b) General population < 60 years old should initiate pharmacologic therapy to keep SBP < 140 mmHg or DBP < 90 mmHg.
    (c) In CKD or diabetic patients ≥ 18 years, initiate pharmacologic therapy to keep

SBP < 140 mmHg or DBP < 90 mmHg.
    (d) Pharmacologic therapy in the general nonblack population, including those with diabetes, should include a thiazide diuretic, calcium channel blocker, ACE inhibitor, or ARB.
    (e) Pharmacologic therapy in the general black population, including those with diabetes, should include a thiazide diuretic or calcium channel blocker.
    (f) Pharmacologic therapy for patients ≥ 18 years old with CKD should initially begin with (or added on to) an ACE inhibitor or ARB.
e. Monitor for changes in kidney function and potassium after changes made to hypertension regimen, especially ACE or ARB medications.
f. Try to limit making more than one medication change at a time to determine its effect.
g. Target patient to achieve euvolemia.
h. If unable to achieve hypertension goals and malignant hypertension is a possibility, further workup is needed.
  (1) Kidney ultrasound to evaluate for renal artery stenosis.
  (2) Urine toxicology screen.
  (3) Pheochromocytoma workup.
  (4) Check TSH to evaluate for hyperthyroidism.
4. Fluid and electrolyte management.
a. Daily weights, preferably standing scale.
b. Strict intake and output documentation.
c. Low salt diet.
d. Review effects of diuretic regimen daily; adjust as needed.
  (1) Understand the mechanism of action of different classes of diuretics.
    (a) Loop diuretics.
    (b) Thiazide diuretics.
    (c) Potassium sparing diuretics.
    (d) Carbonic anhydrase inhibitor (e.g. acetazolamide).
  (2) Choose a diuretic based upon the clinical presentation and effect desired.
  (3) Within each class different drugs can have different effects, half-lives, and side effects that can result in varying diuretic results and electrolyte levels.
  (4) Target patient to achieve euvolemia.
e. Monitor daily (or more frequently if clinically unstable) kidney function and electrolytes until clinically stable. Supplement enterally or intravenously as needed.
5. Acid-base management.
a. The most common acid-base abnormality in CKD is metabolic acidosis due to the decreased ability of the kidneys to excrete hydrogen ions

along with a corresponding decrease in bicarbonate production resulting in a blunting of the buffering effect by the kidneys.

b. Review chemistry lab data.
   (1) Serum bicarbonate.
   (2) Anion gap (AG) [normal 8 to 12mmol/L]. Serum AG = (sodium + potassium) – (chloride + bicarbonate).
   (3) Cause for an abnormal anion gap acidosis.
      (a) High – GI losses, kidney tubular acidosis.
      (b) Low – mnemonic GOLDMARK (Mehta et al., 2008).
         i. **G**lycols (ethylene).
         ii. **O**xoproline.
         iii. **L**-Lactate.
         iv. **D**-Lactate.
         v. **M**ethanol.
         vi. **A**spirin.
         vii. **R**enal failure.
         viii. **K**etones.

c. Goal is to keep serum bicarbonate concentration in the normal range (23 to 29 mEq/L) (KDIGO-CKD, 2013).
   (1) Oral sodium bicarbonate can be used to maintain this goal.
   (2) Target range will be affected if there are other comorbidities that would affect acid-base balance such as chronic obstructive pulmonary disease (COPD).
   (3) Aggressive diuresis will cause a contraction alkalosis, so adjustment of bicarbonate supplements would be needed.

d. If the patient presents with severe acidosis or is clinically unstable, further clinical workup is needed to clarify the acid-base abnormality and potential cause.
   (1) Arterial blood gas (ABG).
   (2) Lactic acid and lactate dehydrogenase (LDH).

e. Serum bicarbonate and potassium have an inverse effect on each other. Treating one will affect the other. Serum potassium must be normalized or supplemented before aggressive bicarbonate therapy is initiated.

f. If intravenous bicarbonate is being supplemented, daily chemistry panels should be obtained to monitor for changes.

g. If patient is clinically unstable or ventilated and with acid-base abnormalities, daily ABG's should be obtained to monitor for changes.

6. Dyslipidemia.
   a. Check lipid panel if newly identified CKD or if not currently on lipid lowering medication.
   b. Initiate lipid lowering medication therapy based on current KDIGO guidelines (KDIGO–Lipid, 2013).
   c. Hyperlipidemia is often seen in the following.
      (1) Nephrotic range proteinuria.
      (2) Diabetes.
      (3) Hypothyroidism.
      (4) Liver disease and alcoholism.
   d. If clinically indicated, initiate dietary restriction and refer to registered dietician (RD) for low-fat diet education.
   e. Low cholesterol in CKD patients is a sign of malnutrition and a poor prognostic indicator.

7. Malnutrition.
   a. As kidney function declines, the degree of malnutrition increases. Steps in evaluation are listed below.
      (1) Review recent nutritional intake, including calorie counts if needed.
      (2) Measurements often abnormally low with malnutrition include the following.
         (a) Albumin.
         (b) Prealbumin, which can be abnormally low in inflammation or infectious conditions, and is most accurate when monitored serially (Fouque et al., 2011).
         (c) Cholesterol.
         (d) Blood urea nitrogen (BUN).
         (e) Creatinine, if chronically malnourished with low muscle mass.
      (3) Calculate BMI and review weight trends.
   b. If malnutrition is suspected, refer to RD for dietary evaluation and support.
   c. CKD patients without malnutrition should be placed on a protein-restricted diet, 0.8 g/kg/day (KDIGO–CKD, 2013).
   d. Once on dialysis, a patient's protein intake should be increased to 1.0 to 1.2 g/kg/day (NKF, 2002).
   e. With both acute and chronic illnesses, many factors can affect a patient's overall nutritional status. Preventative treatment with RD support is often beneficial.
   f. Treatment and nutritional support.
      (1) Enteral. Primary choice of dietary support. Diet should be tailored to the patient's current clinical condition, including electrolyte levels and volume status.
      (2) Parenteral. Discuss with RD concerning the most appropriate tube-feed formula to use, including rate, regimen and overall caloric needs.
      (3) Total parenteral nutrition (TPN).
         (a) To be used if enteral and parenteral route is not available.
         (b) Obtain baseline chemistries to calculate electrolyte needs. Daily labs should be ordered to review and adjust TPN as needed.
         (c) Discuss with RD concerning calculation of protein and lipid requirements.

(d) Monitor blood glucose levels while on TPN and order short-acting insulin coverage.

(e) Placement of a central venous catheter for TPN use. If unable, then adjust formula to peripheral parenteral nutrition (PPN).

(f) Obtain baseline prealbumin, with serial follow-up to document nutritional trends.

(g) Monitor patient's volume status, with adjustments in diuretics or dialysis U, to keep euvolemic.

(h) Switch to enteral or parenteral route as soon as able.

(4) Intradialytic parenteral nutrition (IDPN).

(a) Used with outpatient IHD in community dialysis centers.

(b) Obtain baseline in-hospital chemistries and discuss continuing with IDPN or converting to TPN and following above pathway.

VIII. Acute care management of patients with kidney failure.

A. Obtain copy of outpatient dialysis regimen.

B. Hemodialysis patients.
1. Review current laboratory and radiologic data.
   a. Adjust in-hospital dialysis regimen accordingly based on electrolytes and volume status.
   b. Order labs to be drawn with dialysis unless clinically indicated otherwise to minimize vein trauma and loss of blood due to multiple blood draws.
   c. Review anticoagulation needs and adjust if needed based on current clinical situation.
2. Continue same dialysis schedule (MWF vs. TTS) as outpatient unless clinically indicated.
3. Measures to minimize intradialytic hypotension while hospitalized.
   a. Ensure patients eat prior to their hemodialysis session and not during hemodialysis session.
   b. Order antihypertensive medications to be held prior to dialysis (as appropriate depending on patient and timing of dialysis).
   c. Minimize hypotension by avoiding excessive ultrafiltration.
   d. Slow the ultrafiltration rate.
   e. Perform isolated ultrafiltration.
   f. Increase the dialysate sodium concentration as appropriate.
   g. Switch from acetate to bicarbonate-buffered dialysate.
   h. Proper positioning of patient during HD session.

i. Reduce the dialysate temperature.
j. Administer Amantine® (Midodrine) predialysis.
k. Correct anemia.
l. Administer supplemental oxygen.
m. Reevaluate dry weight systematically after each hemodialysis session.
4. Evaluate dialysis access.
   a. If signs and symptoms of systemic or access infection.
      (1) Vascular evaluation if access involved.
      (2) Obtain appropriate cultures, preferably before antibiotics are started.
      (3) If sepsis is suspected, obtain infectious disease consult.
      (4) Removal of infected catheter or graft if clinically indicated.
      (5) Antibiotics started, dose adjusted for kidney failure.
   b. If signs and symptoms of abnormal access flow.
      (1) Vascular evaluation.
      (2) Review adjustment of anticoagulation.
      (3) If history of multiple systemic thrombosis, consider hypercoagulation work up.
   c. If admitted with dialysis catheter only.
      (1) Order vascular consult and plan for placement of AVF/AVG as soon as medically stable.
      (2) Educate nursing staff that only dialysis staff members are to change the dialysis catheter dressing and access dialysis catheter.
      (3) Protect the nondominant arm.
         (a) Place "Save the Vein" wristband on arm.
         (b) Hang a sign above bed and note in the EMR indicating: No IV's, phlebotomy, BP's in nondominant arm. No PICC lines or midlines at all.
      (4) Obtain vein mapping of bilateral extremities.
   d. If AVF/AVG, notify nursing staff to remove dressing over access within 24 hours after each dialysis. Notify APRN if any postdialysis bleeding or signs of infection observed.
   e. Have the nursing staff monitor the AVF/AVG for a bruit or thrill every shift; notify the APRN if abnormal or absent.
5. Upon discharge from the hospital, the APRN should update the outpatient dialysis center with any clinically pertinent changes in the patient's condition.
   a. Dry weight.
   b. Potassium or calcium baths.
   c. Access interventions or problems.
   d. Need for antibiotic therapy.
   e. Changes in outpatient medications.
   f. Brief overview of inpatient clinical findings and new problems.

C. Patients on peritoneal dialysis.
1. Review current laboratory and radiologic data.
   a. Adjust in-hospital dialysis regimen accordingly based on electrolytes and volume status.
   b. Review labs as clinically indicated.
2. Continue same PD regimen as outpatient unless clinically indicated otherwise and review and adjust daily as needed.
3. Care of the PD catheter and PD exchanges should be performed by staff trained in PD or the trained patient and family members themselves.
4. Evaluate PD catheter.
   a. Aseptic technique should be used with exit-site care and dressing changes per standard PD guidelines.
   b. Ensure that the catheter is anchored and secured to the abdomen.
5. Surgical procedures may increase the risk for peritonitis.
   a. Consider prophylactic antibiotics prior to certain high-risk procedures.
   b. Drain the peritoneal cavity prior to any procedures involving the abdomen or pelvis.
6. Monitor daily weights.
   a. Standing scale is preferred.
   b. Drain the peritoneal cavity prior to each weight.
7. Bowel program.
   a. Constipation predisposes PD patients to bowel sources of infection and can impair adequate solute and electrolyte transport leading to inadequate dialysis clearance.
   b. Assess patient's bowel patterns daily.
   c. Target patient to achieve euvolemia.
   d. Order cathartics as needed to reduce constipation while hospitalized.
   e. Limit narcotic pain medications.
   f. Encourage ambulation as tolerated.
   g. Treat hypokalemia.
8. Prevent infection.
   a. Meticulous hand hygiene among all visitors, caregivers, and staff.
   b. Remove all unnecessary invasive lines promptly (e.g., IV catheters, Foley catheter).
   c. Administer appropriate vaccinations before discharge (influenza, pneumococcal, hepatitis B).
9. Upon discharge from the hospital, the APRN should update the outpatient PD center with any clinically pertinent changes in the patient's condition.
   a. Weight changes.
   b. Change to dialysis regimen.
   c. PD catheter interventions or problems.
   d. Need for antibiotic therapy.
   e. Changes in outpatient medications.
   f. Brief overview of inpatient clinical findings and new problems.

IX. Infectious disease considerations.

A. Assess for signs and symptoms of infection.
1. Systemic vs. localized (catheter/access).
2. Obtain cultures from appropriate source.
   a. Blood cultures if possible systemic or severe local/access infection.
   b. Peritoneal fluid if possible peritonitis in patients on PD.
   c. Urine culture.
   d. Other nonkidney sources if clinically indicated.

B. Infectious disease evaluation if clinically unstable, recurrent infection, or if multisystem involvement.

C. Antibiotics to be dose-adjusted to eGFR.
1. Obtain cultures if able prior to starting antibiotics.
2. Monitor drug levels for appropriate antibiotics.

D. Hemodialysis considerations.
1. Use of catheters for hemodialysis is the most common risk factor for bacteremia.
2. Obtain blood cultures.
3. *Staphylococcus aureus* is the leading cause of exit-site infections and bacteremia in hemodialysis patients.
4. Order appropriate antibiotic coverage.
5. Infectious diseases consultation (IDC).
6. Remove dialysis catheter, if indicated.
7. If dialysis catheter is removed, coordinate insertion of a new catheter. Criteria is as follows.
   a. Surveillance blood cultures negative.
   b. Afebrile for > 24 hours.

E. Peritoneal dialysis considerations.
1. Peritonitis.
   a. Symptoms include cloudy effluent, abdominal pain, and fever.
   b. Obtain stat cell count and differential.
   c. Obtain gram stain and culture on initial drain.
   d. Obtain abdominal film if bowel source suspected.
   e. Diagnosis of peritonitis is supported by an elevated effluent count of white blood cells (WBC) of more than 100 mm^3, of which at least 50% are polymorphonuclear neutrophils (PMNs).
   f. Initiate empiric therapy covering both gram-positive and gram-negative organisms.
      (1) Empiric therapy should target organisms that are causing peritonitis at your institution and the patient's history of previous organisms.
      (2) Gram-positive may be covered by vancomycin or a cephalosporin. Gram-negative may be covered by a third-generation cephalosporin or aminoglycoside.

g. Narrow antibiotic coverage once sensitivities are obtained. Refer to the International Society for Peritoneal Dialysis (ISPD) Peritonitis Guidelines to guide therapy.

h. Clinical improvement should be seen within 72 hours after therapy is initiated.

i. Patients who fail to improve within 72 hours should be evaluated closely on a day-to-day basis.
   (1) Consider catheter removal if symptoms persist after appropriate antibiotic therapy.
   (2) Continue antibiotics for 1 week after catheter removal.
   (3) Consider a CT to evaluate for abscess formation.
   (4) Consider surgical consult.

j. Duration of treatment is based on organism.
   (1) Gram-positive peritonitis and culture-negative peritonitis should be treated for at least 1 week after a clear dialysate (< 100 leukocytes/mm3) and negative cultures have been obtained (total length of therapy typically 10 to 14 days).
   (2) Uncomplicated peritonitis due to a gram-negative organism should be treated for 21 days.
   (3) Multigram-negative organism peritonitis has high relapsing rates, so catheter removal should be considered. If catheter is not removed, antibiotic therapy should continue for 21 days. CT scan should be considered to evaluate for abscess formation.
   (4) Fungal peritonitis.
      (a) The peritoneum should be lavaged until the returning fluid is clear.
      (b) Antifungal therapy for 4 weeks.
      (c) Removal of PD catheter.

k. Order pain medications.

l. Promote protein intake.

m. If patient unable to continue peritoneal dialysis, transition patient to hemodialysis.

2. Exit-site infection (ESI).
   a. An ESI is defined by the "presence of purulent drainage with or without erythema of the skin at the catheter epidermal interface."
   b. Obtain gram stain and culture of drainage.
   c. *S. aureus* and *P. aeruginosa* are the most common exit-site pathogens.
   d. Initiate empiric antibiotic therapy based on gram stain if condition warrants, or delay therapy until sensitivities available.
   e. Avoid the use of vancomycin in routine treatment of exit-site infections due to the threat of vancomycin-resistant *Enterococcus* (VRE).

f. Oral therapy is as effective as intraperitoneal, with the exception of methicillin-resistant *S. aureus* (MRSA).

g. Order appropriate antibiotic coverage.
   (1) Gram-positive organism: oral penicillinase-resistant penicillin, cephalexin, or sulfamethoxazole trimethoprim. Add rifampin 600 mg if slow to respond or severe case of *S. aureus*. Avoid the use of vancomycin.
   (2) Gram-negative organism: oral fluoroquinolone.
   (3) Continue therapy until exit site appears normal. Minimum length of treatment is 2 weeks.
   (4) Increase exit-site care to twice daily.
   (5) If infection persists after 3 to 4 weeks of appropriate antibiotic therapy, catheter removal should be considered.

3. Tunnel infection.
   a. A tunnel infection is defined by erythema, edema, and/or tenderness over the subcutaneous pathway, and may be characterized by intermittent or chronic, purulent, or bloody drainage, which discharges spontaneously or when pressure is placed on the cuff.
   b. Usually occurs in the presence of an exit-site infection.
   c. Most common organisms are *S. aureus*, *S. epidermidis*, and *P. aeruginosa*.
   d. Diagnosis is made based on ultrasound findings of fluid around the subcutaneous tunnel.
   e. Tunnel infections usually require catheter removal.

X. Pharmacologic considerations (Aronoff et al., 2007).

As kidney function declines, there is a proportional rise in the dysfunction associated with medication use. To effectively manage kidney dysfunction, APRNs must have a basic understanding of the biochemical and physiologic effects of drugs in patients with kidney disease.

A. APRN prescriptive authority.
   1. Regulated by individual state nurse practice laws.
   2. Implemented by each individual state's board of nursing.
   3. Prescriptive formulary for APRNs varies by state and practice role.

B. Bioavailability.
   1. How much of the unchanged drug given reaches the systemic circulation.
   2. Uremia affects gastrointestinal absorption as well

as protein binding, complicating first-pass hepatic metabolism.

C. Distribution.
1. How the drug disperses throughout the body.
2. Water soluble vs. lipid soluble drugs can be greatly impacted by the resultant edema, ascites, and muscle wasting often seen in CKD.
3. Proteinuria with resulting hypoalbuminemia results in more free drugs available for both physiologic activity as well as excretion.

D. Metabolism.
1. The intended metabolic effect of a drug is often substantially affected by CKD.
2. Active or toxic metabolities may not be renally excreted increasing the likelihood of adverse drug reactions.

E. Kidney excretion.
1. Affected by GFR, tubular secretion, and reabsorption.
2. The molecular size and protein binding of the drug impacts excretion rates.

F. Pharmacokinetics.
1. How long the drug is active within the body.
2. Peak and trough levels.

G. Current kidney function and estimated glomerular filtration rate (eGFR).
1. Calculate eGFR based on formula available.
2. MDRD formula is currently used by many laboratories in calculating eGFR.
3. The variability of kidney function in AKI limits the accuracy of formulas to predict eGFR. As kidney function changes, serial calculations must be done.

H. Dosing regimen: load and maintenance.
1. Load: a larger initial drug dose given to produce a therapeutic plasma drug concentration rapidly.
2. Maintenance: subsequent drug doses given to produce a stable systemic effect.

I. KRT dosing: HD, PD, CRRT.
1. Effects often difficult to predict due to multiple variables.
2. Use reference material specific for drug dosing in KRT and/or discuss with a pharmacist.

J. Therapeutic drug monitoring.
1. Measurement of plasma drug concentrations.
2. Provides ability to individualize drug dosing based on a current clinical situation, while maximizing positive drug effects and minimizing negative drug effects.

K. Adverse drug reactions.
1. Remain common in patients with kidney disease due to the unpredictable nature of CKD and multiple variables involved.
2. Can occur rapidly as AKI develops.
3. Unexplained clinical symptoms developing should alert the APRN for a possible adverse drug effect.
4. Monitor for reactions carefully after starting or adjusting a medication.
5. Document reactions in EMR or chart so that future problems can be prevented.

XI. General nephrology care.

A. Cardiac.
1. Malignant hypertension. See section VII.3 for discussion concerning hypertension as it relates to patients with CKD. The information provided below focuses on malignant hypertension in patients without CKD.
    a. Etiology.
       (1) Blood pressure ≥ 180/120 mmHg (Chobanian et al., 2003; Kaplan, 1994).
       (2) Acute life-threatening hypertensive emergencies.
       (3) Often seen in patients with longstanding uncontrolled hypertension or with patients who discontinued their antihypertensive medications.
       (4) Renal artery stenosis, more commonly seen in Caucasian patients.
    b. Pathophysiology.
       (1) Retinal hemorrhages, exudates, or papilledema.
       (2) Hypertensive nephrosclerosis.
          (a) Acute kidney injury.
          (b) Hematuria.
          (c) Proteinuria.
       (3) Hypertensive encephalopathy.
          (a) Change in mental status or confusion.
          (b) Severe headache.
          (c) Nausea and vomiting.
          (d) Seizures and coma.
    c. Assessment.
       (1) Review of prior medications and hypertension trend.
       (2) Assessment of possible illicit medications. Obtain toxicology screen.
       (3) Ocular evaluation to evaluate retinal changes.
       (4) Neurologic assessment, and if severe changes, found then neurology consult with possible CT/MRI scan to exclude ischemic stroke or hemorrhage.
       (5) Renal assessment of current labs and volume status.

d. Treatment (Kaplan, 2006; Vaughan & Delanty, 2000).
   (1) Intravenous antihypertensive medications.
      (a) Nitroprusside®.
      (b) Nicardipine®.
      (c) Labetalol®.
      (d) Fenoldopam®.
   (2) Lower diastolic blood pressure to 100 to 105 mmHg within 2 to 6 hours, not exceeding a 25% drop from the initial reading.
   (3) Once blood pressure is controlled, transition to oral antihypertensive therapy.
   (4) Gradual reduction in diastolic pressure to 85 to 95 mmHg over the next 2 to 3 months.
   (5) Limit aggressive hypotensive therapy as this may cause a relative hypotension, which may lead to a hypoperfusion and possible ischemic events such as AKI, stroke, or myocardial infarction.
   (6) Outpatient follow-up is strongly suggested to continue to monitor and adjust hypertensive therapy.
2. Orthostatic hypotension.
   a. Etiology.
      (1) Autonomic failure (multiple disorders).
         (a) Neurodegenerative disease (i.e., Parkinson's disease).
         (b) Neuropathies (i.e., diabetes, amyloidosis).
      (2) Volume depletion and dehydration.
      (3) Medication side effects.
         (a) Can cause or exacerbate orthostasis from other causes.
         (b) Common medications seen in CKD include antihypertensives (i.e., alpha blockers, calcium channel blockers, diuretics) and selective serotonin re-uptake inhibitors or serotonin-specific re-uptake inhibitor (SSRIs).
      (4) Aging.
      (5) Cardiac dysfunction.
   b. Pathophysiology.
      (1) Decrease in baroreceptor sensitivity.
      (2) Neuropathies of the peripheral nerves that limit response to changes in posture.
      (3) Intravascular volume depletion.
   c. Assessment.
      (1) Significant reduction of blood pressure upon standing (Freeman et al., 2011).
         (a) Systolic drop ≥ 20 mmHg.
         (b) Diastolic drop ≥ 10 mmHg.
      (2) Increase in heart rate, which can be blunted by the use of beta blockers.
      (3) Neurologic symptoms such as dizziness and syncope.
      (4) Review of causal medications.
      (5) Evaluation of volume status.
      (6) Detailed medical history.
      (7) Lab tests: kidney function, anemia, diabetes, thyroid.
      (8) Cardio evaluation: electrocardiogram (ECG) and transthoracic echocardiogram (TTE).
   d. Treatment.
      (1) Removal of offending medications.
      (2) Orthostatic precautions.
         (a) Slow postural changes.
         (b) Use of compression stockings to legs.
         (c) Maintain euvolemia.
         (d) Exercise.
      (3) Pharmacologic.
         (a) Florinef®.
         (b) Midodrine®.
3. Cardiorenal syndrome (CRS) (see Table 4.5).
   a. Etiology.
      (1) The heart and renal systems are closely tied together so that dysfunction with one affects the other.
      (2) All types of CRS (1 to 5) include some level of decreased GFR and corresponding heart failure or cardiac dysfunction (i.e. arrhythmias, reduced cardiac output).
   b. Pathophysiology.
      (1) Varies depending on the cause of both the kidney and cardiac dysfunction.
      (2) All types of CRS (1–5) include the following.
         (a) Neurohumoral adaptations.
            i. Sympathetic nervous system.
            ii. Renin angiotension-aldosterone system.
            iii. Stimulation of vasopressin release.
         (b) Reduced renal perfusion.
         (c) Increased renal venous pressure.
         (d) Right ventricular dilatation and dysfunction.

Table 4.5

Cardiorenal Syndrome

1	Acute heart failure results in AKI.
2	Chronic cardiac dysfunction/heart failure causes progressive CKD.
3	AKI causes acute cardiac dysfunction, heart failure.
4	CKD causes chronic cardiac dysfunction, heart failure, arrhythmias.
5	Acute or chronic systemic disorders cause *both* cardiac and renal dysfunctions.

c. Assessment.
  (1) Decreased GFR.
  (2) Radiologic and clinical exam confirmation of heart failure.
d. Treatment.
  (1) Treat the cause of the decreased GFR and cardiac dysfunction (e.g., stabilize the arrhythmia).
  (2) Diuretics should be used to the degree the BP and kidney function will allow. A decrease in the GFR up to 20% is acceptable during aggressive diuresis. In the long term, the patient will do better with less fluid on even if GFR is a bit lower (Hunt, 2009).
  (3) Low salt diet and limited fluid restriction.
  (4) ACE inhibitors or angiotension receptor blockers (ARBs) once the patient is euvolemic.
  (5) Ultrafiltration.
  (6) Other treatments, such as the uses of intravenous vasodialators and inotropic drugs, may help the heart failure but worsen the GFR. Intensive observation must be provided if these drugs are used.
4. Congestive heart failure (CHF).
  a. Etiology.
    (1) Left-sided heart failure resulting from a structural or functional cardiac dysfunction. Risk factors include the following (He et al., 2001).
      (a) Myocardial infarction.
      (b) Cigarette smoking.
      (c) Hypertension.
      (d) Obesity.
      (e) Diabetes.
      (f) Valvular heart disease.
    (2) Can be an acute, chronic, or acute on chronic illness.
    (3) Systemic fluid overload causes.
      (a) Decreased GFR.
      (b) Excessive volume intake.
      (c) Excessive salt intake.
      (d) Hormonal stimulation, such as antidiuretic hormone release.
    (4) High output arteriovenous fistula (AVF) (Basile et al., 2008; MacRae et al., 2004), although more commonly seen in patients with preexisting cardiac disease (Lazarides et al., 1998).
  b. Pathophysiology.
    (1) Left ventricle impairment results in increased hydrostatic pressure in the capillaries of the lungs causing a shift of fluid from intravascular to interstitial tissue.
    (2) Neurohormonal stimulation, often in a dysfunctional feedback loop, resulting in

increased hypertension, fluid gains, and excessive stress placed back on the heart.
  c. Assessment.
    (1) Chest radiograph (x-ray) showing pulmonary edema. Cardiomegaly is also an indication for chronic heart dysfunction.
    (2) Physical exam.
      (a) Crackles upon lung auscultation.
      (b) Jugular vein distention.
      (c) S3 gallop.
    (3) Electrocardiogram (ECG) to evaluate for any arrhythmias.
    (4) Transthoracic echocardiogram (TTE) to evaluate an abnormal ejection fraction and any valvular abnormalites.
    (5) Laboratory tests.
      (a) B-type natriuretic peptide (BNP) is elevated in CHF. However, BNP levels are often elevated with a decreased GFR and therefore difficult to interpret in patients with kidney disease. A low BNP value helps exclude CHF in patients with kidney disease (McCullough et al., 2003; Mueller et al., 2005; Takami et al., 2004).
      (b) CBC: anemia can predispose a patient to CHF.
      (c) Sodium: hyponatremia is often seen in CHF.
      (d) BUN/creatinine: evaluation of kidney status.
  d. Treatment (Yancy et al., 2013).
    (1) Reduce systemic volume through either diuretics or aggressive ultrafiltration.
    (2) ACE inhibitors or ARB's are started after the patient is euvolemic. Initiating during aggressive diuretic phase can often lead to worsening AKI.
    (3) Dietary salt (and often fluid) restriction.
    (4) Beta blockers are started once diuretics and ACE/ARB have been used and the patient is stable.

B. Fluid and electrolytes.
  1. Hyperkalemia.
    a. Etiology.
      (1) Shift from intracellular to extracellular. 90% of the body's potassium is located intracellular (Fischbach, 2000).
        (a) Cellular trauma causing hemolysis.
          i. Crush injuries.
          ii. Gastrointestinal bleed.
          iii. Rhabdomyolysis.
          iiii. Tumor lysis syndrome.
        (b) Metabolic acidosis.
        (c) Hyperglycemia.

(d) Pseudo-hyperkalemia due to poor venipuncture technique.

(2) Excessive enteral or parenteral intake.

(3) Decreased excretion with decreased GFR.

(4) Hypoaldosteronism.

(5) Pharmacologic causes.

    (a) Nonsteroidal antiinflammatories (NSAIDs).

    (b) ACE inhibitors or ARB's.

    (c) Potassium sparing diuretics.

    (d) Potassium supplements.

    (e) Potassium salt products, such as penicillin V potassium (Pen VK®).

    (f) Beta 2 adrenergic use (Beta 2 beta blockers).

b. Pathophysiology.

(1) Cardiac abnormalities.

    (a) Conduction abnormalities.

    (b) Arrhythmias.

(2) Severe skeletal muscle weakness.

(3) Figure 4.9 depicts the mechanisms of hyperkalemia in acute kidney injury.

c. Assessment.

(1) Serum potassium level.

(2) If pseudohyperkalemia is suspected, then drawing peripheral venipuncture without a tourniquet should be done.

(3) ECG obtained to evaluate for arrhythmias.

(4) Review of medications as cause.

(5) Evaluate degree of kidney dysfunction.

(6) Detailed history looking for precipitating factors and timing of when hyperkalemia occurred.

d. Treatment.

(1) Confirm that the patient is truly hyperkalemic.

(2) Remove offending agent, such as intravenous potassium or ACE/ARB.

(3) An intravenous high-potassium "cocktail" is usually given sequentially as a rapid but temporary way to lower the potassium.

    (a) 10 units regular insulin.

    (b) Dextrose (one ampule D50).

    (c) Sodium bicarbonate (one ampule).

    (d) Calcium gluconate 1 gram.

(4) Kayexalate, orally or rectally.

(5) Diuretics. Not often used during acute/severe hyperkalemia.

(6) Hemodialysis with a low potassium bath.

(7) Monitor serial potassium levels posttreatment. Depending on the cause of hyperkalemia and the treatment given, there can be a rebound effect that produces a rise in serum potassium.

2. Hypokalemia.

a. Etiology.

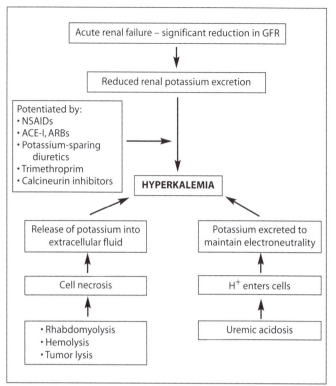

Figure 4.9. Mechanisms of hyperkalemia in acute kidney injury.

Source: Fry, A.C., & Farrington, K. (2006). Management of acute renal failure. *Postgraduate Medicine Journal, 82,* 106-116. Used with permission.

(1) Decreased potassium intake. Usually has to be a severe, prolonged restriction to see an effect on the serum potassium level (Gallen et al., 1998).

(2) Shift from extracellular to intracellular.

    (a) Insulin.

    (b) Increased beta-adrenergic activity.

        i. Stress-induced catecholamine release.

        ii. Albuterol therapy.

        iii. Pseudoephedrine (Sudafed®) use.

    (c) Metabolic alkalosis.

(3) Increased urinary excretion.

    (a) Diuretic use.

    (b) Polyuria.

    (c) Renal tubular acidosis.

    (d) Hypomagnesemia.

    (e) Hyperaldosteronism.

(4) Gastrointestinal losses.

(5) Dialysis losses.

(6) Licorice intake.

b. Pathophysiology.

(1) Severe muscle weakness.

(2) Cardiac arrhythmias (see Figure 4.10).

(3) Gastrointestinal hypomotility.

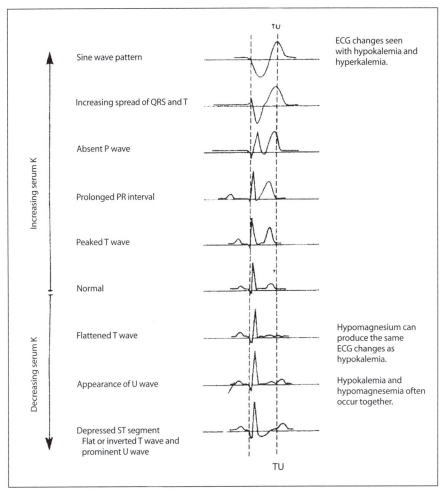

Figure 4.10. ECG changes with hypo/hyperkalemia.

Courtesy of DCI Acute Program, Omaha, Nebraska. Used with permission.

c. Assessment.
   (1) Serum potassium level.
   (2) Urine electrolytes: potassium, creatinine.
   (3) Serum renin and aldosterone levels, and evaluate ratio.
   (4) Calculation of transtubular potassium gradient (TTKG) (Choi & Ziyadeh, 2008).
   TTKG = urine potassium/plasma potassium ÷ urine osmolarity/plasma osmolarity
   Differentiates between renal vs. gastrointestinal losses. Formula only valid when urine osmolarity > 300 and urine sodium > 25.

d. Treatment.

> If the patient presents with metabolic acidosis and hypokalemia, treat the hypokalemia first as long as the acidosis is not severe. Treatment of the acidosis will shift potassium from extracellular to intracellular space thereby lowering the potassium even further. Close monitoring of serum potassium and acid-base balance with an arterial blood gas is often needed.

   (1) Confirm that the patient is truly hypokalemic.
   (2) Supplement potassium intravenously until stable, then may switch to oral supplements.
   (3) Supplement magnesium if indicated.
   (4) Use of potassium sparing diuretics. Note: Draw serum renin/aldosterone before starting or results will be difficult to interpret.
   (5) ECG if severely hypokalemic or medically unstable.
   (6) Treat reversible causes.
   (7) Serial monitoring of serum potassium posttreatment.

3. Hypernatremia.
   a. Etiology.
      (1) Dehydration causing free water depletion.
         (a) Gastrointestinal losses.
         (b) Impaired fluid intake.
         (c) Osmotic diuresis.
         (d) Hypothalmic lesions impairing the thirst stimuli.

(e) Insensible losses from sweat and respiratory deficits.

(2) Diabetes insipidus (DI).

(3) Excessive sodium intake.

   (a) Intravenous hypertonic solution.

   (b) Excessive oral salt intake.

(4) Osmostat reset with mineralocorticoid excess. .

(5) Third spacing shift.

(6) Lithium use can cause a permanent nephrogenic diabetes insipidus state which will persist even after being off of lithium (Grünfeld & Rossier, 2009).

b. Pathophysiology.

(1) Mental status changes due to a cerebral shift of fluid out of the brain.

(2) Generalized weakness and lethargy.

c. Assessment.

(1) High serum sodium.

(2) Patient exam showing volume deficit.

   (a) Poor skin turgor and dry mucous membranes.

   (b) Positive orthostatic hypotension.

   (c) Low jugular vein pressure.

   (d) Oliguria.

(3) Elevated urine and serum osmolarity relative to the etiology. If antidiuretic hormone (ADH) secretion is altered, then the osmolarity can be affected by specific abnormalities.

(4) Low fractionated secretion of sodium (FeNa$^+$).

(5) Elevated BUN/creatinine ratio.

(6) Elevated hematocrit and serum albumin concentration relative to the patient's clinical status.

d. Treatment.

> Estimate of free water deficit (Alshayeb, 2011).
> Water deficit = current TBW x ([serum sodium ÷ 140] - 1)
> Estimate of total body water (TBW)
> Young men/women = 50% to 60%
> Older men/women = 45% to 50%
> If severely hypernatremic subtract 10%

(1) Intravenous hypotonic fluid.

(2) Rate of correction should be no more than a decrease of 10 mEq/L per day to minimize potential neurologic symptoms (Alshayeb et al., 2011).

(3) Encourage oral intake of free water.

(4) Treat reversible cause.

(5) If diabetes insipidus is suspected, then a desmopressin suppression test can be performed to differentiate central vs. nephrogenic DI.

(6) Serial sodium measurements until stable and within normal limits.

4. Hyponatremia.

a. Etiology.

(1) Hypovolemia.

(2) Diuretic induced, which can be seen with loop diuretics, but much more common with thiazides.

(3) Heart failure.

(4) Cirrhosis.

(5) Polydipsia, often seen in patients with psychiatric illnesses.

(6) Low solute dietary intake, such as beer potomania.

(7) Hyperglycemia will cause a pseudohyponatremia due to the osmotic changes induced by the high glucose concentrations (Hillier et al., 1999).

   (a) For glucose levels 100 to 400 mg/dL, the sodium concentration will fall by 1.6 mEq/L for every 100 mg/dL rise above 100.

   (b) For glucose levels > 400 mg/dL, the sodium concentration will fall by 4 mEq/L per 100 mg/dL increase.

(8) Syndrome of inappropriate antidiuretic hormone (SIADH) secretion.

   (a) Hypothyroidism.

   (b) Cortisol deficiency.

   (c) Advanced CKD.

   (d) Central nervous system (CNS) disorders. Pain itself is also a potent cause of ADH release.

   (e) Malignancies, especially those of the lung.

   (f) Many pharmacologic agents can enhance ADH release or effect. Some common drugs seen with patients with kidney disease include the following (Liamis et al., 2008).

     i. Selective serotonin reuptake inhibitors (SSRIs).

     ii. NSAIDs.

     iii. Ciprofloxacin.

     iv. Amiodarone.

   (g) Acute or chronic pulmonary diseases.

   (h) HIV infection.

b. Pathophysiology.

(1) Causes a fall in serum osmolarity that predisposes a patient to cerebral edema.

(2) Symptoms are primarily neurologic and relative to the degree of impairment (Ellis, 1995).

   (a) Nausea and malaise when the sodium falls below 125 to 130 mEq/L.

   (b) Headache, lethargy, seizures, and/or coma when the sodium falls below 115 to 120 mEq/L.

(c) The rate of change is even more important than the severity.

(3) Higher risk of gait impairment and falls, especially in the elderly (Renneboog et al., 2006).

(4) Osmotic demyelination can occur when the sodium is rapidly corrected. This can lead to a potentially severe neurological impairment, which may be irreversible.

c. Assessment.

(1) Thorough assessment looking for the cause, including medications, fluids status, and acute/chronic illnesses.

(2) Neurologic status, current vs. baseline. A change in mental status can necessitate more aggressive treatment of the hyponatremia.

(3) Laboratory tests.

   (a) Osmolarity.

      i. Serum osmolarity is usually low.

      ii. Urine osmolarity is variable depending upon the cause of the hyponatremia.

   (b) Low urine fractionated secretion of sodium.

   (c) Serum uric acid that is often low in SIADH.

   (d) Thyroid stimulating hormone (TSH) can be low.

   (e) Cortisol level will be low if the cause is due to adrenal insufficiency.

   (f) Kidney function.

(4) Orthostatic hypotension will often be positive if hypovolemia is contributory.

(5) If the cause of the hyponatremia is not readily apparent after initial evaluation, further testing can be done which may include the following.

   (a) Transthoracic echocardiogram (TTE) to evaluate heart function, as cardiac dysfunction can precipitate hyponatremia.

   (b) Chest x-ray and/or CT of chest to evaluate for any lung lesions or acute/chronic pulmonary conditions that would predispose the patient to SIADH.

d. Treatment.

(1) Evaluation of current serum sodium, and trends to determine how acute or chronic the hyponatremia is.

(2) Remove any contributing cause and treat underlying disease.

(3) Fluid restriction is to be used in the vast majority of cases, although will depend upon the cause of the hyponatremia.

(4) Treatment will vary greatly depending upon the following variables.

   (a) The cause of the hyponatremia.

   (b) The acuity of the drop in sodium.

   (c) The patient's neurologic status.

   (d) Underlying comorbid diseases.

   (e) Current hemodynamic condition.

(5) Treatment may include the following.

   (a) Saline, hypertonic 3% or isotonic 0.9%.

   (b) Sodium chloride tablets orally.

   (c) Vasopressin receptor antagonists.

   (d) Loop diuretic if the cause is hypervolemic.

   (e) Demeclocycline (off label use) works by diminishing the renal tubules' response to ADH. It can take days to weeks to have an effect and must be monitored carefully as it can have a nephrotoxic effect itself (Forrest, 1978).

(6) Rate of sodium correction in severe hyponatremia (< 120 mEq/L) should be no more than an increase of 4 to 6 mEq/L in 24 hours to lessen the chance of osmotic demyelination syndrome (Sterns et al., 2009; Verbalis et al., 2007).

(7) Follow-up with serial sodium levels is needed.

5. Anasarca.

a. Etiology.

(1) Increased capillary hydraulic pressure.

   (a) Heart failure.

   (b) Kidney disease.

   (c) Drugs such as NSAIDs, vasodilators, and calcium channel blockers.

   (d) Sodium and fluid retention and overload.

   (e) Cirrhosis.

   (f) Pregnancy.

(2) Hypoalbuminemia.

   (a) Nephrotic syndrome.

   (b) Cirrhosis.

   (c) Malnutrition.

(3) Increased capillary permeability.

   (a) Inflammation.

   (b) Sepsis.

   (c) Allergic reactions.

   (d) Diabetes mellitus.

   (e) Burns or trauma.

(4) Lymphatic obstruction.

   (a) Malignancy.

   (b) Hypothyroidism.

   (c) Lymph node dysfunction.

b. Pathophysiology.

(1) Abnormalities in capillary hemodynamics that causes the movement of fluid from intravascular spaces to the interstitium.

(2) Retention of sodium and/or water by the kidneys.

c. Assessment.
   (1) Evaluate for comorbid conditions that could be precipitating edema.
   (2) Physical exam to evaluate degree and distribution of edema.
   (3) Pitting vs. nonpitting edema, with nonpitting often seen with lymphatic obstruction or hypothyroidism.
   (4) Laboratory data.
       (a) Proteinuria evaluation.
       (b) BUN/creatinine.
       (c) Thyroid stimulating hormone (TSH).
       (d) Serum albumin.
       (e) Liver function tests if cirrhosis is suspected.
   (5) Transthoracic echocardiogram (TTE) to evaluate for degree of heart failure.
   (6) Evaluate for possible deep vein thrombosis (DVT) if edema specific to an extremity, especially if unilateral.

d. Treatment.
   (1) Diuretics as blood pressure and kidney status allow the following.
       (a) Oral loop diuretics and evaluate effectiveness.
       (b) Intravenous loop diuretic, bolus.
       (c) Intravenous loop diuretic, bolus then continuous infusion.
       (d) Add thiazide and/or potassium-sparing diuretic as needed.
       (e) Monitor electrolytes and kidney function. Supplement as needed. Balance expected mild to moderate AKI due to aggressive diuresis with need to remove fluid.
       (f) Use of albumin intravenously in conjunction with diuretics has shown limited effectiveness (Chalasani et al., 2001).
   (2) Low salt diet, with fluid restriction if needed.
   (3) Remove any contributing cause and treat underlying disease.
   (4) Daily weights to monitor volume change.
   (5) Ultrafiltration/hemodialysis for severe anasarca edema that is refractory to diuretic regimen.

C. Gout.
   1. Etiology.
      a. Increased urate production can be seen due to many causes.
         (1) Malignancies.
         (2) Obesity.
         (3) Excessive dietary purine ingestion.
         (4) Alcohol ingestion.
         (5) Inherited enzyme defects.
      b. Decreased kidney clearance contributes to secondary hyperuricemia.
      c. Many drugs can induce hyperuricemia, including the following.
         (1) Diuretics, both thiazides and loop.
         (2) Cyclosporine and tacrolimus.
         (3) Low-dose salicylates.
   2. Pathophysiology.
      a. Monosodium urate crystals are a product of purine metabolism.
      b. Hyposecretion of uric acid by the kidneys is the primary cause of hyperuricemia (Richette & Bardin, 2010).
      c. Serum uric acid is an independent risk factor for CKD (Jalal et al., 2013; Weiner et al., 2008).
      d. Uric acid or urate crystal deposits can cause three different types of kidney disease.
         (1) Acute uric acid nephropathy/tumor lysis syndrome.
            (a) Overproduction and excretion of uric acid particularly in patients with lymphoma and leukemia, especially after chemotherapy leading to tumor lysis syndrome.
            (b) Marked serum uric acid levels >15 mg/dL.
            (c) If significant tissue breakdown develops releasing intracellular substances, then expect electrolyte abnormalities, including as follows.
               i. Hyperkalemia.
               ii. Hyperphosphatemia.
               iii. Hypocalcemia.
            (d) Prevention is the best treatment in patients at high risk, but for those patients who do present with these signs and symptoms, treatment should include the following.
               i. Aggressive hydration.
               ii. Allopurinol®.
               iii. Rasburicase®.
               iv. Hemodialysis if anuric and clinically indicated.
         (2) Chronic urate nephropathy (Johnson et al., 1999).
            (a) Gradual deposition of urate crystals in the kidneys.
            (b) Chronic inflammation causes fibrosis and eventual CKD.
            (c) Clinical features are fairly nonspecific with bland urinary sediment and mild proteinuria.
            (d) Treatment is preventative by lowering the serum uric acid level with the following.

i. Low purine diet.
ii. Euvolemic status.
iii. Allopurinol®, Febuxostat®, Colchicine®.
(3) Uric acid nephrolithiasis.
(a) Precipitating factors.
i. A high urine uric acid concentration.
ii. A low urine pH.
iii. Systemic gout.
iv. Dehydration and low urine output.
v. Diabetic mellitus.
vi. Chronic diarrhea, due to predisposition for ii and iv.
(b) Present with acute flank pain.
(c) If stone causes urethral blockage, can cause obstructive AKI.
(d) Treatment.
i. Alkalinization of the urine.
ii. Aggressive hydration.
iii. Medications to lower the serum uric acid level.
(4) High serum uric acid in CKD patients does not necessarily mean the hyperuricemia is the cause for the CKD (Sorensen, 1980). Unless obvious clinical conditions are present, i.e., tumor lysis syndrome, or urate nephrolithiasis, a kidney biopsy is the only way to know that the CKD has been caused by the high uric acid levels.
3. Assessment.
a. Hyperuricemia (high serum uric acid levels).
b. Polarized light microscopy of synovial fluid showing urate crystals.
c. Unilateral joint involvement presenting with inflammation, erythema, and/or pain.
d. Rule out pseudogout (calcium pyrophosphate), septic arthritis, or other arthritic state.
e. If the serum uric acid level is high, obtaining a urine uric acid/creatinine ratio helps to differentiate tumor lysis vs. prerenal. If the ratio is greater than 0.7, then it's likely to be tumor lysis.
4. Treatment.
a. Low purine diet.
b. Hydration initially, then euvolemic status as goal.
c. Colchicine® for acute gout attacks not chronic treatment, and should be dose adjusted for eGFR.
d. Allopurinol® (dose adjusted for eGFR) or Febuxostat® for preventative treatment.
e. Avoid NSAIDs in CKD patients.
f. Short-term steroid therapy for significant gout flares.

D. Diabetic ketoacidosis (DKA).
1. Etiology.
a. Shortage of insulin.
b. Metabolism switches to utilizing fatty acids, with ketones as byproduct.
c. Characterized by a triad of symptoms.
(1) Hyperglycemia.
(2) Metabolic acidosis with an elevated anion gap.
(3) Ketosis.
d. Most common precipitating factors (Kitabchi et al., 2003; Randall et al., 2011).
(1) Infection.
(a) Pneumonia.
(b) Urinary tract infection.
(c) Sepsis.
(2) Inadequate insulin therapy.
(3) Acute major illness.
(a) Myocardial infarction.
(b) Stroke.
(c) Pancreatitis.
(4) Alcohol or drug abuse.
e. Evolves rapidly over hours with rapidly changing symptoms.
(1) Polyuria.
(2) Polydipsia.
(3) Neurologic changes.
(a) Lethargy.
(b) Confusion.
(c) Stupor and coma.
(4) Abdominal pain, nausea, and vomiting.
(5) Hyperventilation.
2. Pathophysiology.
a. Two hormonal abnormalities that contribute to DKA that result in a net insulin deficiency.
(1) Decreased insulin production and/or resistance.
(2) Glucagon excess.
b. Ketoacidosis occurs then from the breakdown of fatty acids resulting in the production of acidic ketone bodies.
c. Hyperglycemia then causes polyuria resulting in a net dehydration and significant electrolyte instability.
d. AKI, if it occurs, results primarily from a prerenal state, but also due to hypotension/hypoperfusion from the net volume loss.
3. Assessment.
a. Stage of severity (Kitabchi et al., 2009).
(1) Mild.
(a) pH 7.25 to 7.30.
(b) Serum bicarbonate 15 to 18 mmol/L.
(c) Patient is alert.
(2) Moderate.
(a) pH 7.00 to 7.25.
(b) Serum bicarbonate 10 to 15 mmol/L.

(c) Mild drowsiness or lethargy.
  (3) Severe.
    (a) pH below 7.00.
    (b) Serum bicarbonate below 10 mmol/L.
    (c) Stupor or coma.
 b. Laboratory data.
  (1) CMP/BMP/RFP.
  (2) Calculation of anion gap.
  (3) Urinalysis.
  (4) Urine and serum ketone level.
  (5) Serum and urine osmolarity.
  (6) Arterial blood gas (if + anion gap or ketones present).
  (7) Electrocardiogram (ECG) if hyperkalemic.
 c. Evaluation of potential precipitating event leading to DKA.
  (1) Infection workup.
  (2) Drug, alcohol, or medication-induced.
  (3) Cardiovascular event.
  (4) GI or pancreatic event.
 d. If no ketones are present, then it is not true DKA but rather a hyperosmolar hyperglycemic state, with similar presentation and treatment.
4. Treatment.
 a. Treat the cause/trigger of DKA.
 b. Aggressive hydration with intravenous fluids, usually with isotonic saline (0.9%) until euvolemic.
 c. Intravenous insulin infusion.
  (1) Titrating to stable blood sugar.
  (2) Addition of intravenous dextrose if needed to keep blood sugars stable.
 d. Continue until serum ketones are negative, then switch to standard diabetic management.
 e. Use of bicarbonate therapy is usually NOT warranted unless pH < 7.0 with an unstable cardiovascular status or in life-threatening hyperkalemia. Acidosis will resolve on its own with aggressive hydration. Bicarbonate use can cause a posttreatment metabolic alkalosis and slow the DKA recovery (Narins & Cohen, 1987; Okuda et al., 1996).
 f. Frequent (often hourly until stable) blood work to monitor rapidly changing glucose and electrolytes. Adjust therapy as needed.
  (1) Expect hypokalemia to result from therapy as there is usually a net potassium deficit within the body that becomes apparent with rehydration and normalizing glucose levels as the potassium gets shifted into the cells.
  (2) Serum phosphorus and magnesium levels are often low and need frequent supplementation.
 g. Once medically stable, readdress appropriate diabetic management and educate about signs of DKA to help the patient avoid future events.

E. Diabetes insipidus (DI).
1. Etiology.
 a. Polyuric presentation of greater than 3 liters per day of urine due to non-DI stimuli such as the following.
  (1) Diuretics.
  (2) Excessive fluid intake such as psychogenic polydipsia.
  (3) Hyperglycemic induced osmotic diuresis.
 b. Neurogenic (central) diabetes insipidus.
  (1) Deficient secretion of antidiuretic hormone (ADH).
  (2) Causes can include the following (Maghnie et al., 2000; Rose & Post, 2001).
    (a) Tumors.
    (b) Infiltrative diseases such as Sarcoidosis.
    (c) Trauma.
    (d) Neurosurgery.
    (e) Idiopathic.
 c. Nephrogenic diabetes insipidus.
  (1) Normal ADH secretion.
  (2) Kidney insensitivity to ADH effects.
  (3) Causes can include the following.
    (a) Lithium toxicity, which may cause permanent nephrogenic DI (Grünfeld & Rossier, 2009).
    (b) Hypercalcemia, when levels are persistently above 11 mg/dL (Rose & Post, 2001).
    (c) Posturethral obstruction (Frøkiaer et al., 1996).
    (d) Polycystic kidney disease.
    (e) Genetic/inherited.
 d. Neurogenic and nephrogenic DI present with similar signs and symptoms. Differentiating between the two is important since the treatment of each is different.
 e. Onset of polyuria.
  (1) If polyuria develops in children, evaluation of a genetic origin, which can cause either neurogenic or nephrogenic DI, should be considered.
  (2) Neurogenic DI is usually more abrupt while nephrogenic DI is more gradual.
  (3) Newly developed nocturia in absence of other causes may indicate the development of DI.
2. Pathophysiology.
 a. Excessive thirst due to the neurohormonal stimulus to maintain euvolemia.
 b. Polyuria due to the excessive fluid intake and/or decreased ADH effect.
 c. Decreased ability to concentrate urinary solutes leading to severely dilute urine.
3. Assessment.
 a. Obtaining a detailed history from the patient or family can help determine the following.

(1) Time of onset of polyuria.
(2) Potential non-DI causes.
(3) Medication effect.
(4) Genetic cause.
(5) Psychiatric cause.
b. Serum and urine osmolarity.
c. Serum sodium.
d. Water restriction test.
e. Giving Desmopressin® (DDAVP), which is an exogenous ADH, can differentiate between neurogenic and nephrogenic cause.
(1) If neurogenic cause, the serum and urine osmolarity will increase, with a corresponding drop in urinary output.
(2) If nephrogenic cause, the serum and urine osmolarity and polyuria will not change.
4. Treatment.
a. Neurogenic DI.
(1) Thiazide diuretics.
(2) Nonsteroidal anti-inflammatory medications, especially indomethacin.
(3) Low salt, low protein diet.
(4) Chronic Desmopressin® administration.
(5) Monitor for fluid retention and hyponatremia with use of Desmopressin®.
b. Nephrogenic DI.
(1) Treat the cause.
(2) Low salt, low protein diet.
(3) Combination of thiazide and potassium sparing diuretics.
(4) Nonsteroidal anti-inflammatory medications, especially indomethacin.
(5) Nonrestrictive fluid intake. Allow patients to drink as much as they want.
(6) Intravenous fluids if the patient is symptomatic, has other causes for fluid loss such as GI losses, or cannot take oral fluids.
(7) Serial monitoring of electrolytes and ability to maintain euvolemia.

F. Hepatorenal syndrome (HRS).
1. Etiology.
a. Associated with patients with underlying liver cirrhosis and usually presents with chronic ascites and volume overload.
b. Signs and symptoms (Ginès et al., 2003; Wadei et al., 2006).
(1) Progressive AKI.
(2) Benign urine with minimal sediment and very low proteinuria.
(3) Low urinary sodium excretion.
(4) Oliguria in later stage HRS.
(5) Asymptomatic hypotension in severe cases.
c. Diagnosis is one of exclusion and clinical criteria; there is no one test that can establish the diagnosis (Wadei et al., 2006).
(1) Hepatic cirrhosis with portal hypertension.

(2) Serum creatinine > 1.5 mg/dL that may be acute or chronic.
(3) Absence of other cause for AKI/CKD.
(4) Benign urine with minimal proteinuria.
(5) Lack of improvement of serum creatinine after intravenous volume expansion.
d. Often is precipitated by some acute insult such as infection or gastrointestinal bleeding.
e. Two types of HRS.
(1) Type 1 HRS.
(a) Rapid AKI.
(b) Oliguric.
(c) Hypotensive.
(d) Poor prognosis compared to type 2 (Arroyo et al., 2002).
(2) Type 2 HRS.
(a) AKI is less severe than type 1.
(b) Resistant to diuretic therapy.
(c) Low urine sodium (<10 mmol/L) (Ginès et al., 1987).
2. Pathophysiology.
a. Level of serum creatinine often does not correlate with degree of HRS due to liver disease, poor diet/protein intake, and often low muscle mass.
b. Arterial vasodilatation in the hepato-mesenteric circulation due to increased nitric oxide production results in kidney hypoperfusion (Martin et al., 1998).
c. Intravascular volume depletion due to shunting of fluid into peritoneal space (ascites) or extremities (anasarca) due to 2b above as well as loss of oncotic pressure from hypoalbuminemia.
3. Assessment.
a. Abnormal hepatic function tests demonstrating underlying cirrhosis.
b. Ensure that the AKI is not precipitated by a nonhepatic cause since the diagnosis of HRS is one of exclusion.
c. Kidney function labs to evaluate AKI trends to establish how rapid and severe the kidney failure is; this will help determine if it is type 1 or type 2 HRS.
d. Fractionated secretion of sodium (FeNa$^+$).
e. Urinalysis with microscopic analysis.
4. Treatment.
a. Gastrointestinal consult and co-management.
b. Intravascular volume expansion.
(1) Albumin is preferred as it helps improve oncotic pressure.
(2) Crystalloid solution can be used but can lead to volume overload as it shifts fluid to the extravascular space.
c. Midodrine to help with hypotension as a systemic vasoconstrictor.
d. Octreotide inhibits endogenous vasodilator release.

e. Low salt diet to prevent further fluid retention.

f. GI evaluation for a transjugular intrahepatic portosystemic shunt (TIPS) procedure, if indicated.

g. Diuretic therapy with loop diuretics is used for symptom control if there is massive systemic anasarca that is impairing the patient's clinical status.

h. Dialysis is indicated only as ancillary support for patients awaiting liver transplant or in patients with acute, potentially reversible liver failure.

i. Referral for liver transplant.

G. Dialysis related amyloidosis (DRA).

1. Etiology.

a. DRA occurs specifically from the accumulation of beta2-microglobuin (B2-M) since B2-M is excreted by the kidneys and is poorly cleared by hemodialysis. A reduction of GFR directly correlates to a rise in B2-M levels (Dember, 2006).

b. Older low flux dialyzers are impermeable to B2-M while newer high flux dialyzers do provide some clearance.

c. Peritoneal dialysis offers less clearance of B2-M than high flux hemodialysis filters and increases the risk of DRA (Evenepoel et al., 2006).

d. DRA causes deposits primarily in the following (Noël et al., 1987; Winchester et al., 2003).
   (1) Bone.
   (2) Articular cartilage.
   (3) Synovium.
   (4) Muscle.
   (5) Tendons and ligaments.

e. The most common symptoms associated with DRA are as follows (Sprague & Moe, 1996).
   (1) Shoulder pain.
   (2) Carpel tunnel syndrome.
   (3) Intervertebral disk pain.

f. DRA risk increases with:
   (1) Age of the patient.
   (2) Length of time on dialysis.
   (3) Lack of residual kidney function.

2. Pathophysiology.

a. Amyloidosis deposits of proteins that have become insoluble into the extracellular space of various organs or tissues causing a disruption of normal function.

b. Various types of proteins can cause amyloidosis with symptoms that vary depending on the location of the protein deposits.

c. Reactive inflammation occurs at the site of B2-M deposits contributing to further dysfunction.

3. Assessment.

a. Physical exam.

(1) Hypertrophy of muscles of scapula, shoulder, rotator cuff, and bicep area due to deposition of amyloid.

(2) Weakness and atrophy of the hand consistent with carpel tunnel syndrome.

b. Increased serum B2-M level can be seen in DRA, but may also be due to other causes (Winchester et al., 2003).

c. Radiography or CT/MRI scans can show hypertrophic lesions in affected areas caused by the amyloid deposits.

d. Tissue biopsy is the "gold standard" but is rarely obtained; the diagnosis is usually made upon a combination of clinical and radiologic findings (Dember & Jaber, 2006).

4. Treatment.

a. No specific medical treatment is available for DRA other than ensuring adequate dialysis, which only slows the progression of the amyloid deposits. The longer the dialysis time, the better the B2-M clearance. Daily home hemodialysis or nocturnal hemodialysis should be encouraged.

b. Maximize residual kidney function for those patients who still have some function left.

c. Kidney transplant.

d. Symptomatic treatment of affected area.

XII. Collaborative management.

A. Working with nursing staff.

1. Resource for nursing staff.

2. Resource for hospital dialysis staff.

3. Education for nursing staff about CKD.

a. Predialysis care.
   (1) Daily weights.
   (2) Predialysis medications.

b. Postdialysis care.
   (1) Check blood pressure before giving BP medications.
   (2) Remove AVF/AVG dressings 24 hours postdialysis.
   (3) Nursing staff should not use or change catheter dressing since dialysis staff will perform the task.
   (4) Call if any bleeding or signs/symptoms of infection from access.

c. Medications.
   (1) No Fleet® enemas.
   (2) No NSAIDs.
   (3) Phosphate binders – when and how to give.
   (4) Check labs before giving medications.
   (5) Diabetic hypoglycemia – do not give orange juice.
   (6) Appropriate pain management medications for CKD patients.

d. Anemia management.
  (1) Erythropoiesis-stimulating agents (ESAs).
  (2) Iron supplements – oral vs. intravenous.
  (3) Blood products.
    (a) Prefer to administer blood on dialysis treatments.
    (b) Limit blood products for patients with CKD/kidney failure who may one day receive a kidney transplant.
e. General nursing care.
  (1) Appropriate kidney diet, with fluid restriction if needed.
  (2) Daily weights.
  (3) Strict intake and output documentation.
  (4) Laboratory data related to the effects of kidney disease.
  (5) Postsurgical kidney follow-up.
    (a) Appropriate IV fluids.
    (b) Postoperative diet: kidney-appropriate.
f. Vascular access.
  (1) Vein preservation – "Save the Vein."
  (2) No PICC lines.
  (3) Evaluating dialysis access every shift.
  (4) Reason to prefer AVF vs. AVG vs. catheter for hemodialysis.
4. Organizational healthcare committees.

B. Interaction with other APRNs, physicians, physician assistants (PA), and other healthcare professionals.
  1. Patient advocate.
  2. Nursing advocate.
  3. Active communication.
  4. Collaboration.
  5. Education about the involvement of the kidneys relative to their area of practice.

C. Coordination with outpatient, dialysis, and community organizations.
  1. Dialysis discharge orders.
  2. Office follow-up.
  3. Community kidney organization(s) referral and support.

D. CKD clinics.
  1. Identify patients who qualify for the CKD clinic and follow up with appropriate referral. Outpatient management and education of clinical comorbid conditions by the APRN and CKD clinic staff can be an effective way to slow the progression of CKD, keep patients out of the hospital, and be cost effective.
    a. CKD stage 3+.
    b. Fluid and electrolytes management.
    c. Anemia management.
    d. Hypertension management.
    e. Vascular access monitoring.
  2. Resource for CKD clinic nurses.
  3. Review of CKD clinic protocols.

References

Alshayeb, H.M., Showkat, A., Babar, F., Mangold, T., & Wall, B.M. (2011). Severe hypernatremia correction rate and mortality in hospitalized patients. *American Journal of the Medical Sciences, 341*(5), 356-360. PMID: 21358313. doi:10.1097/MAJ.0b013e31820a3a90

Aronoff, G.R., Bennett, W.M., Berns, J.S., Brier, M.E., Kasbekar, N., Mueller, B.A., ... Smoyer, W.E. (2007). *Drug prescribing in renal failure: Dosing guidelines for adults and children* (5th ed.). Philadelphia: American College of Physicians.

Arroyo, V., Guevara, M., & Ginès, P. (2002). Hepatorenal syndrome in cirrhosis: Pathogenesis and treatment. *Gastroenterology, 122*(6), 1658-1676. doi:10.1053/gast.2002.33575

Basile, C., Lomonte, C., Vernaglione, L., Casucci, F., Antonelli, M., & Losurdo, N. (2008). The relationship between the flow of arteriovenous fistula and cardiac output in haemodialysis patients. *Nephrology Dialysis Transplantation, 23*(1), 282. PMID: 17942475.

Blowey, D.L. (2005). Nephrotoxicity of over-the-counter analgesics, natural medicines, and illicit drugs. *Adolescent Medicine Clinics, 16*, 31-43. doi:10.1016/j.admecli.2004.10.001

Case, J., Khan, S., Khalid, R., & Khan, A. (2013). Epidemiology of acute kidney injury in the intensive care unit. *Critical Care Research and Practice, 2013*. 1-9. doi: 10.1155/2013/479730.

Chalasani, N., Gorski, J.C., Horlander, J.C., Craven, R., Hoen, H., Maya, J., & Brater, D.C. (2001). Effects of albumin/furosemide mixtures on responses to furosemide in hypoalbuminemic patients. *Journal of the American Society of Nephrology, 12*(5), 1010. PMID: 11316860

Chan, E.J., & Dellsperger, K.C. (2011). Update on cardiorenal syndrome: A clinical conundrum. *Advances in Peritoneal Dialysis, 27*, 82-86.

Choi, M.J., & Ziyadeh, F.N. (2008). The utility of the transtubular potassium gradient in the evaluation of hyperkalemia. *Journal of the American Society of Nephrology, 19*(3), 424-426. doi:10.1681/ASN.2007091017

Centers for Medicare and Medicaid Services (CMS). (2010). *Evaluation and management services guide.* ICN:006764. Baltimore, MD.

Coffman, M.T, Falk, R.J, Molitoris, B.A, Neilson, E.G., & Schrier, R.W. (2012). *Schrier's diseases of the kidney* (9th ed.). Philadelphia: Lippincott.

Dember, L.M., & Jaber, B.L. (2006). Dialysis related amyloidosis: Late finding or hidden epidemic? *Seminars in Dialysis, 19*(2), 105. PMID: 16551286.

Drawz, P.E., Miller, R.T., & Sehgal, A.R. (2008). Predicting hospital-acquired acute kidney injury – a case-controlled study. *Renal Failure, 30*(9), 848-855. doi: 10.1080/08860220802356515

Dugo, M., Gatto, R., Zagatti, R., Gatti, P., & Cascone, C. (2010). Herbal remedies: Nephrotoxicity and drug interactions. *Giornale Italiano di Nefrologia, 27* (Suppl 52), S5-9. Retrieved from http://www.ncbi.nlm.nih.gov/pubmed/21132655

Ellis, S.J. (1995). Severe hyponatraemia: Complications and treatment. *Quarterly Journal of Medicine, 88*(12), 905. PMID: 8593551.

Evenepoel, P., Bammens, B., Verbeke, K., & Vanrenterghem, Y. (2006). Superior dialytic clearance of beta(2)-microglobulin and p-cresol by high-flux hemodialysis as compared to peritoneal dialysis. *Kidney International, 70*(4), 794.

Fischbach, F. (2000). *A manual of laboratory & diagnostic tests* (6th ed.). Philadelphia: Lippincott.

Forrest, J.N., Cox, M., Hong, C., Morrison, G., Bia, M., & Singer, I. (1978). Superiority of demeclocycline over lithium in the treatment of chronic syndrome of inappropriate secretion of antidiuretic hormone. *The New England Journal of Medicine, 298*(4), 173. PMID: 413037

Fouque, D., Pelletier, S., Mafra, D., & Chauveau, P. (2011). Nutrition and chronic kidney disease. *Kidney International, 80*(4), 348-357. PMID: 21562470

Freedman, B.I., Shenoy, R.N., Planer, J.A., Clay, K.D., Shihabi, Z.K., Burkart, J.M., ... Bleyer, A.J. (2010). Comparison of glycated albumin and hemoglobin A1c concentrations in diabetic subjects on peritoneal and hemodialysis. *Peritoneal Dialysis International, 30*(1), 72-79. doi:10.3747/pdi.2008.00243

Freeman, R., Wieling, W., Axelrod, F.B., Benditt, D.G., Benarrach, E., Biaggioni, I., ... van Dijk, J.G.(2011). Consensus statement on the definition of orthostatic hypotension, neurally mediated syncope and the postural tachycardia syndrome. *Clinical Autonomic Research, 21*(2), 69-72. PMID: 21431947

Frøkiaer, J., Marples, D., Knepper, M.A., & Nielsen, S. (1996). Bilateral ureteral obstructiondown regulates expression of vasopressin-sensitive AQP-2 water channel in rat kidney. *American Journal of Physiology, 270*(4), F657. PMID: 8967344

Furusyo, N., Koga, T., Ai, M., Otokozawa, S., Kohzuma, T., Ikezaki, H., ... Hayashi, J. (2011). Utility of glycated albumin for the diagnosis of diabetes mellitus in a Japanese population study: results from the Kyushu and Okinawa Population Study (KOPS). *Diabetologia, 54*(12), 3028-3036. doi:10.1007/s00125-011-2310-6

Gallen, I.W., Rosa, R.M., Esparaz, D.Y., Young, J.B., Robertson, G.L., Batlle, D., ... Landsberg, L. (1998). On the mechanism of the effects of potassium restriction on blood pressure and renal sodium retention. *American Journal of Kidney Disease, 31*(1), 19. PMID: 9428447

Ginès, P., Arroya, V., Quintero, E., Planas, R., Bory, F., Cabrera, J., ... Jiménez, W. (1987). Comparison of paracentesis and diuretics in the treatment of cirrhotics with tense ascites. Results of a randomized study. *Gastroenterology, 93* (2), 234-241. PMID: 3297907

Ginès, P., Guevara, M., Arroyo, V., & Rodés, J. (2003). Hepatorenal syndrome. *The Lancet, 362*(9398), 1819-1827. PMID: 14654322

Grünfeld, J.P., & Rossier, B.C. (2009). Lithium nephrotoxicity revisited. *Nature Reviews Nephrology, 5*(5), 270. PMID: 19384328

He, J., Ogden, L.G., Bazzano, L.A., Vupputuri, S., Loria, C., & Whelton, P.K. (2001). Risk factors for congestive heart failure in US men and women: NHANES I epidemiologic follow-up study. *Archives of Internal Medicine, 161*(7), 996. PMID: 1295963

Hillier, T.A., Abbott, R.D., & Barrett, E.J. (1999). Hyponatremia: evaluating the correction factor for hyperglycemia. *American Journal of Medicine, 106*(4), 399. PMID: 1022524

Hunt, S.A., Abraham, W.T., Chin, M.H., Feldman, A.M., Francis, G.S., Ganiats, T.G., ... Yancy, C.W. (2009). *Circulation, 119*(14), e391. PMID: 19324966

Jalal, D.I., Chonchol, M., Chen, W., & Targher, G. (2013). Uric acid as a target of therapy in CKD. *American Journal of Kidney Diseases, 61*(1), 134-146. Retrieved from http://www.medscape.com/viewarticle/776781

James, P.A., Oparil, S., Carter, B.L., Cushman, W.C., Dennison-Himmelfarb, C., Handler, J., Lackland, D.T., ... Ortiz, E. (2013). 2014 evidence-based guideline for the management of high blood pressure in adults: Report from the panel members appointed to the eighth joint national committee (JNC8). *Journal of the American Medical Association.* doi:10.1001/jama.2013.284427

Johnson, R.J., Kivlighn, S.D., Kim, Y.G., Suga, S., & Fogo, A.B. (1999). Reappraisal of the pathogenesis and consequences of hyperuricemia in hypertension, cardiovascular disease, and renal disease. *American Journal of Kidney Disease, 33*(2), 225. PMID: 10023633

Kaplan, N.M. (1994). Management of hypertensive emergencies. *The Lancet, 344*(8933), 1335. PMID: 7968030

Kaplan, N.M. (2006). *Kaplan's clinical hypertension* (9th ed.). Baltimore: Lippincott, Williams & Wilkins.

KDIGO-AKI: Kidney Disease Improving Global Outcomes Acute Kidney Injury Work Group. (2012). KDIGO clinical practice guideline for acute kidney injury. *Kidney International Supplement, 2,* 1-138.

KDIGO-Anemia: Kidney Disease Improving Global Outcomes Anemia Work Group. (2012). KDIGO clinical practice guideline for anemia. *Kidney International Supplement, 2*(4), 1-138.

KDIGO-HTN: Kidney Disease Improving Global Outcomes Blood Pressure Work Group. (2012). KDIGO clinical practice guideline for the management of blood pressure in chronic kidney disease. *Kidney International Supplement, 2,* 337-414.

KDIGO-CKD: Kidney Disease Improving Global Outcomes CKD Work Group. (2012). KDIGO clinical practice guideline for the evaluation and management of chronic kidney disease. *Kidney International Supplement, 3,* 1-150.

KDIGO-Lipid: Kidney Disease Improving Global Outcomes Lipid Management Work Group. (2013). KDIGO clinical practice guideline for lipid management in chronic kidney disease. *KidneyInternational Supplement, 3*(3), 1-56.

Kitabchi, A.E., Umpierrez, G.E., Murphy, M.B., Barrett, E.J., Kreisberg, R.A., Malone, J.I., Wall, B.M. (2003). Hyperglycemic crises in patients with diabetes mellitus. *Diabetes Care, 26*(Suppl. 1), S109. PMID: 12502633.

Kitabchi, A.E., Umpierrez, G.E., Miles, J.M., & Fisher, J.N. (2009). Hyperglycemia crises in adult patients with diabetes. *Diabetes Care, 32*(7), 1335-1343.

Lazarides, M.K., Staramos, D.N., Panagopoulos, G.N., Tzilalis, V.D., Eleftheriou, G.J., Dayantas, J.N., & Staamos, D.N. (1998). *Journal of the American College of Surgeons, 187*(4), 422-426. PMID: 9783790

Liamis, G., Milionis, H., & Elisaf, M. (2008). A review of drug-induced hyponatremia. *American Journal of Kidney Disease, 52* (1), 144. PMID: 18468754

MacRae, J.M., Pandeya, S., Humen, D.P., Krivitski, N., & Lindsay, R.M. (2004). Arteriovenous fistula-associated high-output cardiac failure: A review of mechanisms. *American Journal of Kidney Disease, 43*(5), e17. PMID: 15112194

Maghnie, M., Cosi, G., Genovese, E., Manca-Bitti, M.L., Cohen, A. Zecca, S., ... Aricò, M. (2000). Central diabetes insipidus in children and young adults. *The New England Journal of Medicine, 343*(14), 998. PMID: 11018166

Martin, P.Y., Ginès, P., & Schrier, R.W. (1998). Nitric oxide as a mediator of hemodynamic abnormalities and sodium and water retention in cirrhosis. *The New England Journal of Medicine, 339*(8), 533. PMID: 9709047

McCullough, P.A., Duc, P., Omland, T., McCord, J., Nowak, R.M., Hollander, J.E. ... Maisel, A.S. (2003). B-type natriuretic peptide and renal function in the diagnosis of heart failure: An analysis from the Breathing Not Properly Multinational Study. *American Journal of Kidney Disease, 41*(3), 571. PMID: 12612980.

Mehta, A.N., Emmett, J.B., & Emmett, M. (2008). GOLDMARK: An anion gap mnemonic for the 21stcentury. *The Lancet, 372*(9642), 892. doi:10.1016/S0140-6736(08)61398-7

Mueller, C. Laule-Kilian, K., Scholer, A. Nusbaumer, C., Zeller, T., Staub, D., & Perruchoud, A.P. (2005). B-type natriuretic peptide for acute dyspnea in patients with kidney disease: insights from a randomized comparison. *Kidney International, 67*(1), 278. PMID: 15610252

Narins, R.G., & Cohen, J.J. (1987). Bicarbonate therapy for organic acidosis: The case for its continued use. *Annals of Internal Medicine, 106*(4), 615. PMID: 3103511

National Kidney Foundation (NKF). 2002. Kidney Disease Outcomes

Quality Initiative (K/DOQI) clinical practice guidelines for chronic kidney disease: Evaluation, classification and stratification. *American Journal of Kidney Disease, 39*(Suppl.1), S1-S266.

Noël, L.H., Zingraff, J., Bardin, T., Atlenza, C., Kuntz, D., & Drüeke, T. (1987). Tissue distribution of dialysis amyloidosis. *Clinical Nephrology, 27*(4), 175. PMID: 3555909.

Oelkers, W. (1989). Hyponatremia and inappropriate secretion of vasopressin (antidiuretic hormone) inpatients with hypopituitarism. *The New England Journal of Medicine, 321*(8), 492. PMID: 2548097.

Okuda, Y., Adrogue, H.J., Field, J.B., Nohara, H., & Yamashita, K. (1996). Counterproductive effects of sodium bicarbonate in diabetic ketoacidosis. *The Journal of Clinical Endocrinology & Metabolism, 81*(1), 314. PMID: 8550770.

Palevsky, P.M., Zhang, J.H., O'Connor, T.Z., Chertow, G.M., Crowley, S.T., Choudhury, D., ... Peduzzi, P. (2008). Intensity of renal support in critically ill patients with acute kidney injury. *The New England Journal of Medicine, 359*(1), 7-20. doi:10.1056/NEJMoa0802639

Palevsky, P.M., Liu, K.D., Brophy, P.D., Chawla, L.S., Parikh, C.R., Thakar, C.V., ... Weisbord, S.D. (2013). KDOQI U.S. Commentary on the 2012 KDIGO clinical practice guideline for acute kidney injury. *American Journal of Kidney Disease, 61*(5), 649-672. doi:10.1053/j.ajkd.2013.02.349

Peacock, T.P., Shihabi, Z.K., Bleyer, A.J., Dolbare, E.L., Byers, J.R., Knovich, M.A., ... Freedman, B.I. (2008). Comparison of glycated albumin and hemoglobin A1c levels in diabetic subjects on hemodialysis. *Kidney International, 73*, 1062-1068. doi:10.1038/ki.2008.25

Perazella, M.A. (2009). Renal vulnerability to drug toxicity. *Clinical Journal of the American Society of Nephrology, 4*, 1275-1283. doi:10.2215/CJN.02050309

Ponce, D., & Balbi, A.L. (2011). Peritoneal dialysis in acute kidney injury: A viable alternative. *Peritoneal Dialysis International, 31*, 387-389. doi:10.3747/pdi.2011.00312

Randall, L., Begovic, J., Hudson, M. Smiley, D., Peng, L, Pitre, N., ... Umpierrez, G. (2011). Recurrent diabetic ketoacidosis in inner-city minority patients: Behavioral, socioeconomic, and psychosocial factors. *Diabetes Care, 34*(9), 1891-1896. PMID: 21775761

Renneboog, B., Musch, W., Vandemergel, X. Manto, M.U., & Decaux, G. (2006). Mild chronichyponatremia is associated with falls, unsteadiness, and attention deficits. *American Journal of Medicine, 119*(1), 71. PMID: 16431193

Richette, P., & Bardin, T. (2010). Gout. *The Lancet, 375*(9711), 318-328. PMID: 19692116

Rose, B.D., & Post, T.W. (2001). *Clinical physiology of acid-base and electrolyte disorder* (5th ed.) NewYork: McGraw-Hill.

Sorensen, L.F. (1980). Gout secondary to chronic renal disease: Studies on urate metabolism. *Annals of the Rheumatic Diseases, 39*(5), 424. PMID: 7436573

Sprague, S.M., & Moe, S.M. (1996). Clinical manifestations and pathogenesis of dialysis-related amyloidosis. *Seminars in Dialysis, 9*(4), 360-368. doi:10.1111/j.1525-139X.1996.tb00699.x

Sterns, R.H., Nigwekar, S.U., & Hix, J.K. (2009). The treatment of hyponatremia. *Seminars in Nephrology, 29*(3), 282. PMID 19523575

Takami, Y., Horio, T., Iwashima, Y., Takiuchi, S., Kamide, K., Yoshihara, F., ... Kawano, Y. (2004). Diagnostic and prognostic value of plasma brain natriuretic peptide in non-dialysis-dependent CRF. *American Journal of Kidney Diseases, 44*(3), 420. PMID: 15332214

Vaughan, C.J., & Delanty, N. (2000). Hypertensive emergencies. *The Lancet, 356*(9227), 411. PMID: 10972386

Verbalis, J.G., Goldsmith, S.R., Greenberg, A., Schrier, R.W., & Sterns, R.H. (2007). Hyponatremia treatment guidelines 2007: Expert panel recommendations. *American Journal of Medicine, 120*(11 Suppl 1), S1-21. PMID: 17981159

Wadei, H.M., Mai, M.L., Ahsan, N., & Gonwa, T.A. (2006). Hepatorenal syndrome: Pathophysiology andmanagement. *Clinical Journal of the American Society of Nephrology, 1*(5), 1066-1079. PMID: 17699328

Weiner, D.E., Tighiouart, H., Elsayed, E.F., Griffith, J.L., Salem, D.N., & Levey, A.S. (2008). Uric acid and incident kidney disease in the community. *Journal of the American Society of Nephrology, 19*(6), 1204-1211. PMID: 18337481

Winchester, J.F., Salsberg, J.A., & Levin, N.W. (2003). Beta-2 microglobulin in ESRD: An in-depth review. *Advances in Renal Replacement Therapy, 10*(4), 279-309. PMID: 14681859

Windus, D. (Ed.). (2008). *The Washington manual: Nephrology subspecialty consult* (2nd ed.). Philadelphia: Lippincott, Williams & Wilkins.

Yancy, C.W., Jessup, M., Bozkurt, B., Butler, J., Casey, D.E., Drazner, M.H., ... Wilkoff, B.L. (2013). 2013 ACCF/AHA guideline for the management of heart failure: Executive summary: A report of the American College of Cardiology Foundation/American Heart Association Task Force on Practice Guidelines. *Circulation, 128*(16), 1810-1852. PMID: 23741057 doi:10.1161/CIR.0b013e31829e8807

Overview of Pediatric Nephrology for the APRN

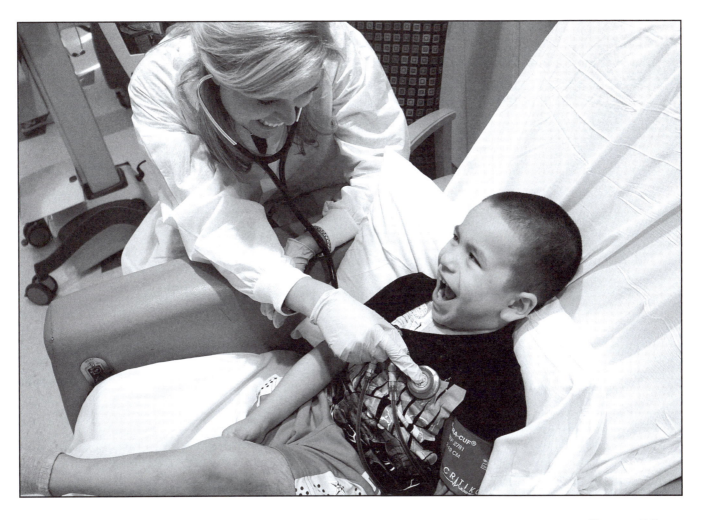

Chapter Editors

Kim Alleman, MS, APRN, FNP-BC, CNN-NP

Katherine Houle, MSN, APRN, CFNP, CNN-NP

Authors

Helen Currier, BSN, RN, CNN, CENP

Jessica J. Geer, MSN, C-PNP, CNN-NP

CHAPTER **5**

Overview of Pediatric Nephrology for the APRN

This offering for **1.9 contact hours** is provided by the American Nephrology Nurses' Association (ANNA).

American Nephrology Nurses' Association is accredited as a provider of continuing nursing education by the American Nurses Credentialing Center Commission on Accreditation.

ANNA is a provider approved by the California Board of Registered Nursing, provider number CEP 00910.

This CNE offering meets the continuing nursing education requirements for certification and recertification by the Nephrology Nursing Certification Commission (NNCC).

To be awarded contact hours for this activity, read this chapter in its entirety. Then complete the CNE evaluation found at **www.annanurse.org/corecne** and submit it; or print it, complete it, and mail it in. Contact hours are not awarded until the evaluation for the activity is complete.

Example of reference for Chapter 5 in APA format. Both authors for entire chapter.

Currier, H., & Geer, J. (2015). Overview of pediatric nephrology for the APRN. In C.S. Counts (Ed.), *Core curriculum for nephrology nursing: Module 6. The APRN's approaches to care in nephrology* (6th ed., pp. 153-200). Pitman, NJ: American Nephrology Nurses' Association.

Interpreted: Chapter authors. (Date). Title of chapter. In ...

Cover photo by Robin Davis, BS, CCLS, Child Life Specialist, Texas Children's Hospital.

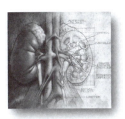

CHAPTER 5

Overview of Pediatric Nephrology for the APRN

Purpose

The purpose of this section is to outline the scope of kidney disease as it relates to neonates and children through 18 years. It differentiates their assessment and treatment from the adult care guidelines and assists in preparing the Advanced Practice Registered Nurse (APRN) who treats children with chronic kidney disease (CKD).

Objectives

Upon completion of this chapter, the learner will be able to:
1. Discuss management and treatment considerations in congenital kidney disorders that affect kidney function.
2. Discuss vascular access challenges in pediatric patients.
3. Discuss the APRN's management and care of the pediatric patient on various types of dialysis.
4. Define pediatric hypertension and discuss management.
5. Discuss management and treatment of chronic kidney disease-mineral bone disease (CKD-MBD) and adynamic bone disease in children.
6. Assess nutrition and growth in the pediatric patient with CKD.
7. Describe the role of the APRN during the transition of the pediatric patient to an adult-care program.

SECTION A
Prenatal and Postnatal Anatomic Development of the Kidneys

I. Stages.

A. The pronephros and mesonephros are primitive kidneys that arise and disappear early in kidney development.

B. The third stage of kidney formation is the metanephros, which becomes the definitive kidney (Avner et al., 2009).
   1. Ureteric bud arises from mesonephric duct near cloaca at 5th week gestation.
   2. Ureteric bud branches repeatedly and at its tip induces differentiation of mesoderm (metanephric blastema) into nephrons of metanephros.
   3. Ureteric bud branches to form collecting system of kidney.
      a. 1st branching forms renal pelvis (8th to 9th week gestation).
      b. 3rd–5th branchings fuse to form major calyces (10th week gestation).
      c. 6th branchings form minor calyces.
      d. 7th–11th branchings form papillary collecting ducts (15th week gestation), and division ceases after the 15th week gestation.
   4. Peripheral growth of ureteric bud without branching induces new nephrons in centrifugal pattern after the 15th week.
   5. Nephronogenesis continues until the 36th week.
   6. Renal vascular system develops from branches of aorta and vena cava and parallels branching pattern of ureteric bud division and nephron induction; vascular system is complete by the 15th week gestation (Avner et al., 2009).
   7. The first urine is found in the bladder between the 9th and 12th week gestation.
   8. Gross structure: fetal lobulation may persist after birth until later in infancy.
   9. The kidneys continue to grow in size after birth until body growth is complete in adolescence. Normal newborn kidneys range in length from 4 to 6 cm, whereas adult kidneys are 8.5 to 13 cm in length.
   10. Failure of formation of ureteric bud results in complete renal agenesis.

11. Failure of ureteric bud to induce metanephros results in the following congenital anomalies.
    a. Agenesis with a malformed or absent ureter.
    b. Renal hypoplasia.
    c. Renal dysplasia.

II. Ascent and rotation.

A. Metanephric kidney formation begins opposite 4th lumbar segment.

B. Kidneys ascend from 1st to 2nd lumbar segment due to rapid growth of the caudal portion of the body.

C. With ascent, kidney rotates 90° and renal pelvis orients medially.

D. Kidney shape results from compression by intraperitoneal viscera during ascent and rotation.

E. Failure to ascend leads to simple or crossed ectopia; fusion then can form horseshoe kidney.

F. Failure to rotate leads to discoid kidney; abnormal rotation leads to unusual direction of renal pelvis and ureter.

III. Lower urinary tract development.

A. Ureteric bud becomes ureter starting at the 6th week of gestation.

B. Initially a membrane (Chwalla's membrane) covers the ureteral opening into the bladder. After the 9th week of gestation, urine formed by the developing kidney creates pressure in the ureter that causes Chwalla's membrane to rupture, creating an opening from the ureter to the bladder.

C. Abnormalities in the formation of ureters lead to the following congenital anomalies.
    1. Failure of membrane rupture results in ureterocele.
    2. Delayed membrane rupture results in physiologic hydronephrosis.
    3. If two ureteric buds develop on one side, two renal units are induced and usually fuse as a duplicated kidney. The upper pole ureter of the duplication often enters the bladder ectopically and is associated with obstruction or ureterocele.

IV. Bladder and urethra.

A. The bladder and urethra arise from the urogenital sinus portion of the cloaca, which is a primitive structure that also gives rise to the rectum. Urogenital sinus forms as anterior division of cloaca at the 4th week of gestation.

B. The ureters separate and enter the bladder at the trigone at the 8th to 9th week of gestation.

C. Endodermal epithelium forms bladder mucosa at 8th to 9th week of gestation.

D. Definitive urethra forms from urogenital sinus at the 9th week of gestation. In males, normal urethral folds are absorbed after prostatic ductules are formed at 12th to 16th week.

E. Bladder is identifiable by fetal ultrasound at 10th to 12th week gestation.

F. Abnormalities in the formation of the bladder and urethra result in congenital anomalies; specifically, failure of absorption of the normal urethral folds in males leads to posterior urethral valves (see "Frequent causes of kidney disease" below).

G. The infant has a coordinated reflex and urinates as often as 15 to 20 times per day.

H. Over time, the bladder capacity gradually increases. The bladder capacity in ounces is equal to the age in years plus 2. This formula applies to children up to 12 to 14 years of age. For example, a 2-year-old child + 2 = 4-ounce bladder capacity.

Section B
Prenatal and Postnatal Developmental Physiology and Pathophysiology Secondary to Abnormal Development of the Kidneys.

I. Prenatal renal physiology.

A. Active urine production begins at 12th to 15th week.

B. Amniotic fluid is nearly all fetal urine after 18th week gestation.

C. Fetal kidneys receive only 2–4% cardiac output in last trimester; newborn kidneys receive 15% cardiac output.

D. Fetal kidneys produce renin, prostaglandins, and kallikreins, which modulate renal vascular tone and blood flow in utero.

E. Sodium reabsorption and urea concentration begin at 12th to 14th week.

F. Loop of Henle is functional for reabsorption at 14th week.

G. Fractional excretion of sodium (FENa) is high in fetus: 12% in fetus, 5% in premature newborn (< 30 weeks), and 3% in full-term newborn.

H. Fetal kidney responds to vasopressin in last trimester, but has limited concentrating ability due to short loops of Henle and poor medullary urea gradient; urine diluting ability is present early in fetal life.

I. Fetal kidneys respond to stress (hypoxemia, asphyxia, volume depletion), but are not needed to maintain electrolyte or volume balance in utero; placenta performs these maintenance functions until birth.

II. Postnatal development of renal blood flow (RBF).

A. Within 24 hours after birth, renal vascular resistance decreases and renal blood flow (RBF) increases to 15% of cardiac output.

B. RBF to outer cortical areas increases at the gestational age when nephrogenesis is completed (36 weeks) and is accompanied by an abrupt increase in GFR.

C. Medullary RBF is increased until the superficial cortical nephrons are fully developed.

III. Postnatal development of glomerular filtration rate (GFR).

A. Nephron formation is complete at birth in full-term infants, but continues after birth in premature infants to gestational age 36 weeks.

B. GFR at 3 to 4 days of age as measured by creatinine clearance is 0.5 to 1.06 mL/min (5 to 8 mL/min/1.73 m^2) in premature infants and as high as 5 mL/min (30 mL/min/1.73 m^2) in full-term infants.

C. Limitation of the newborn kidney: low GFR may limit excretion of substances normally entering the urine by glomerular filtration.

D. GRF normalized to 1.73 m^2 body surface area increases gradually from birth to reach adult values by 3 years.

IV. Plasma creatinine concentration.

Changes of plasma creatinine concentration based on age can be seen in Table 5.1.

V. Changes in body fluid composition.

A. Body fluid composition (% body weight) are listed in Table 5.2 (Avner et al., 2009).

B. TBW normally decreases after birth related to diuresis (1 to 8 mL/kg/hr).

C. Duration (in days) of diuresis depends on:
   1. Degree of excess extracellular fluid (ECF) at birth.
   2. Degree of prematurity: the more premature the infant, the greater the ECF, so postnatal diuresis and weight loss after birth will be greater than in term infants.

Table 5.1

Plasma Creatinine Concentration Based on Age

Age	Plasma creatinine concentration (mg/dL)
Birth	Equal to mother's plasma creatinine
5–7 days (full-term infants)	0.4–0.5
Premature infants	1.0–1.5 (until nephrogenesis is complete)
< 2 years of age	0.4–0.5
2–8 years of age	0.5–0.7

(Avner et al., 2009)

Table 5.2

Changes in Body Fluid Composition

Developmental Age	Total Body Water
Early gestation	90%
1st weeks of 3rd trimester	80%
Term infant	70–75%
Toddler/young child	65–70%
Older child/adolescent	60%
Adult	60% (ECF= 20%, ICF= 40%)

* TBW = total body water; ECF = extracellular fluid; ICF = intracellular fluid

(Avner et al., 2009)

   3. Hemodynamic changes.
      a. Cardiac output to kidneys increases to 15% from 2% to 4%.
      b. Pulmonary circulation opens.

D. Decrease in circulating antidiuretic hormone (ADH) levels after delivery; ADH normally increases during labor.

E. In term infants, the change in ECF volume/body weight during the 1st week follows a parabolic curve.

1. Reaches maximum by day 4.
2. Returns to birth level (40% body weight) at day 6.
3. Plasma volume (PV) decreases first 24 hours, then stays the same.

F. Range of expected values for urine after postnatal diuresis in normal neonate given appropriate fluid intake.
   1. Urine volume = 0.3 to 2.0 mL/kg/hr.
   2. Urine osmolarity = 50 to 800 mOsm/kg water.
   3. Specific gravity = 1.001 to 1.024.

G. The state of hydration in the first month is related to intake (especially in premature infants). ECF increases more in premature infants fed enterally and supplemented parenterally than in those fed enterally only.

VI. Predevelopmental and postdevelopmental pathophysiology: Disorders of body fluid composition in the neonate.

A. Excessive fluid administration.

B. Hydrops fetalis: end stage of severe erythroblastosis fetalis (alloimmune hemolytic anemia).

C. Nonimmune hydrops.
   1. Idiopathic.
   2. Congenital infections (e.g., syphilis, toxoplasmosis, viruses).
   3. Congenital heart disease (e.g., hypoplastic left heart, tricuspid atresia, cardiomyopathy, fibroelastosis).
   4. Noonan syndrome.
   5. Cystic hygroma.
   6. Teratomas (e.g., mediastinal, choriocarcinoma, sacrococcygeal).
   7. Chest masses (e.g., diaphragmatic hernia, sequestered lung).
   8. Chromosome abnormalities (e.g., Trisomy 18, 21, XX/XY).
   9. Brain lesions (e.g., encephalocoele, absent corpus callosum).
   10. Storage disease (e.g., Gaucher's, mucopolysaccharidosis).
   11. Osteogenesis imperfecta.
   12. Bowel obstruction and perforation.
   13. Lymphangiectasis.
   14. Infant of diabetic mother.
   15. Vascular malformations.
   16. Renal vein/vena cava/umbilical vein thrombosis.
   17. Prune belly syndrome (Eagle-Barrett syndrome).
       a. Absent abdominal musculature.
       b. Anomalous development of urinary tract with absent ureteral musculature and hydroureter and hydronephrosis.
       c. Bilateral undescended testicles.

VII. Postnatal development of tubular function.

A. Functional maturation of the nephron is age dependent rather than body weight dependent; increases in tubular length continue to 6 months of age.

B. Enzyme immaturity and decreased tubular transport may result in a variety of medications, ions, and sugars not being reabsorbed or excreted.

C. Reduced ability of the kidney to reabsorb sodium and water produces decreased ability to maximally concentrate urine.

D. Tubules have a decreased response to antidiuretic hormone (ADH).

E. Excretory burden is minimized because the infant is retaining large amounts of electrolytes and nitrogen to meet growth needs.

F. Hydrogen ion excretion is reduced for the first year of life.

G. Infants have a lower renal bicarbonate threshold, thus they lose more bicarbonate.

VIII. Sodium (Na+) reabsorption.

A. At birth, premature infants less than 30 weeks gestational age excrete large amounts of Na+ and develop negative Na+ balance. The fractional excretion of sodium (FENa) falls rapidly by 2 weeks of age and reaches full-term levels (1–3%) by 6 weeks of age, which corresponds to 33 to 36 weeks postconceptual age.

B. Distal tubular Na+ reabsorption is lower in premature than in term infants.

C. Premature (less than 35 weeks) and term infants cannot excrete an acute Na+ load as efficiently as older children.

D. Premature infants are at risk for both hyponatremia and hypernatremia.

IX. Urine diluting and concentrating ability.

A. Newborns can dilute urine effectively to 50 mOsm/kg water, but cannot adequately excrete a water load related to low GFR and lack of tight epithelium in distal tubules; ability to excrete a water load matures within a few weeks after birth.

B. Slight but definite increase in urine concentrating ability occurs during development.

C. Postnatal maturation of ability to maximally concentrate urine occurs at same rate in premature (> 30 weeks) and term infants.

1. 1 week old: 500 to 600 mOsm/kg water.
2. 1 month old: 900 to 1000 mOsm/kg water.
3. 2 year old: 1300 to 1400 mOsm/kg water (same as adult).

D. Factors limiting urine concentrating ability in neonates.
  1. Superficial nephrons have not developed elongated loops of Henle extending into the deeper cortical and outer medullary portions of the kidney.
  2. Greater medullary renal blood flow (RBF) before superficial nephron maturation tends to dissipate the osmotic gradient.
  3. Developing superficial nephrons have decreased Na^+ and Cl^- reabsorption in the thick ascending loop of Henle, which prevents maximal dilution of urine delivered to the distal tubule for water reabsorption.
  4. Distal collecting tubule (DCT) does not have tight epithelial junctions, so back flux of Na^+ to the tubular lumen occurs and a concentrated medullary osmotic gradient cannot be established.
  5. Ability to use urea to enhance the osmotic gradient in medullary interstitium matures over weeks after birth.
  6. DCT has decreased kidney responsiveness to vasopressin in neonatal period.

X. Acid-base balance.

A. Kidney regulates acid-base balance through tubular reabsorption of filtered bicarbonate and synthesis of new bicarbonate secondary to excretion of hydrogen ions as ammonium and titratable acid.

B. Exactly when renal acidification mechanisms become functional is not known, but may be as early as third trimester.

C. Premature infant's kidneys are able to excrete an acid load as well as that of adults, so can dispose of normal infant's daily hydrogen production without becoming acidotic.

D. In premature and term infants, measured renal bicarbonate threshold (defined as plasma bicarbonate concentration at which bicarbonate is no longer completely reabsorbed and excretion in urine begins) appears to be lower than that of adults related to extracellular fluid volume expansion that depresses proximal tubular (PT) bicarbonate reabsorption and to decreased basolateral surface area of the PT at birth compared to a few weeks of age (see "renal tubular acidosis" for more information).

XI. Potassium (K^+) balance.

A. Premature and term infants achieve positive K^+ balance within 10 days of age if orally fed.

B. Urinary K^+ remains high because intake of K^+ in formula is in excess of daily requirements.

C. Hypokalemia most often results from inadequate intake in parenteral nutrition, diuretic therapy, GI losses in vomiting or diarrhea, or alkalotic states in which K^+ moves intracellularly.

D. False hyperkalemia can occur from RBC hemolysis or if the platelet count is high (K^+ extrusion from platelets in the clot).

XII.   Glucose reabsorption.

A. Renal tubular glucose reabsorption is only 92% in premature infant less than 34 weeks, then increases to 99%.

B. Renal glucosuria (glucosuria with normal serum glucose) occurs frequently in very low birth weight (VLBW) infant, probably related to proximal tubular immaturity.

XIII.   Calcium balance.

A. Urinary calcium excretion is increased in premature infants and varies directly with FENa and urine flow rate.

B. Even in premature infants, enough calcium is retained to maintain positive calcium balance and normal bone development.

C. High calcium infant formulas and diuretic therapy, especially with loop diuretics, increase renal calcium excretion and are associated with nephrocalcinosis.

XIV.   Phosphate reabsorption.

A. Phosphate reabsorption is greater in neonates than in adults due to the following.
  1. Higher rate of tubular phosphate reabsorption.
  2. Attenuated phosphaturic response to parathyroid hormone (PTH).
  3. Possible effect of growth hormone to increase reabsorption and decrease urine phosphate excretion.

B. In the premature kidney, the preponderance of deep nephrons with a higher capacity for tubular phosphate reabsorption compared to superficial nephrons may contribute to increased phosphate retention.

C. Hypophosphatemia most often results from inadequate intake in parenteral nutrition.

D. Hyperphosphatemia can occur if phosphate intake is excessive (e.g., cow's milk, goat's milk).

E. See Table 5.3 for age-specific normal ranges of serum phosphorus (KDOQI Guidelines [NKF, 2008]).

XV.   Evaluation of the fetal kidneys.

A. Postnatal evaluation of fetal hydronephrosis.
   1. Kidney ultrasound (RUS) in 1st week of life.
   2. Voiding cystourethrogram (VCUG) to rule out vesicoureteral reflux.
   3. If RUS abnormal and VCUG normal, diuretic radionuclide kidney scan.
   4. Serial serum creatinine measurements (serum creatinine 24 to 48 hours after birth reflects maternal serum creatinine).
   5. Etiology of congenital anomalies with fetal hydronephrosis (Nguyen et al., 2010).
      a. Physiologic: 41% to 88%.
      b. Ureteropelvic junction (UPJ) obstruction: 10% to 30%.
      c. Vesicoureteral reflux: 10% to 20%.
      d. Other anomalies (duplication, posterior urethral valves: 15% to 25%, prune belly

syndrome, megaureter, ureterovesical, junction obstruction).

B. Abdominal masses of renal/adrenal origin found in the newborn.
   1. Developmental anomalies of the kidneys may present as an abdominal mass in the newborn, especially multicystic dysplastic kidney, which is the second most frequent neonatal abdominal mass.
   2. Other important renal/adrenal causes of abdominal masses in the newborn are the following.
      a. Hereditary polycystic kidney disease.
         (1) Autosomal recessive associated with hepatic fibrosis.
         (2) Autosomal dominant associated with cysts of liver and pancreas.
      b. Tumors.
         (1) Mesoblastic nephroma (like Wilms, but mesenchymal origin).
         (2) Neuroblastoma.

SECTION C
Assessment of Kidney Structure and Function in Children

I.   Physical findings in kidney failure.

A. General.
   1. Uremia may affect the state of wakefulness and mood, and the child may be irritable.
   2. Failure to thrive may reflect presence of kidney disease.

B. Vital signs.
   1. Deviations from normal may be the first indication of disease.
   2. Kidney disease is the most common cause of hypertension.
   3. Urinary tract infection should be considered in the child with unexplained fever.

C. Growth: growth retardation, defined as a height below the 5th percentile for age and gender, may result from uremia, metabolic acidosis, or malnutrition associated with kidney failure.

D. Skin.
   1. Pale, sallow skin may be a sign of kidney-induced anemia.
   2. Skin excoriation and infection from scratching may indicate uremia.

Table 5.3

Age-specific Normals for Serum Phosphorus

Age (years)	Serum Phosphorus (mg/dL)
0–5 mo	5.2–8.4
6–12 mo	5.0–7.8
1–5 yr	4.5–6.5
6–12 yr	3.6–5.8
13–20 yr	2.3–4.5

Reprinted from *American Journal of Kidney Diseases, 54* (6), National Kidney Foundation, KDOQI Clinical Practice Guideline for Nutrition in Children with CKD: 2008 Update, S11–S104, with permission from Elsevier.

3. State of hydration can be assessed by examining skin turgor and mucous membranes. Dehydration may be caused by polyuria associated with a child's inability to concentrate urine. Dehydration causes poor skin turgor and dry mucous membranes.
4. Edema reflects fluid and salt retention.
5. Vasculitic rash, such as the malar butterfly rash of lupus, may indicate an underlying systemic disorder involving the kidneys.
6. Hypopigmented lesions on the trunk and extremities and sebaceous adenomas, similar to acne, appearing between ages 4 and 6 on the nose and cheek, are associated with kidney cystic disease.
7. Dysplastic or absent nails can be associated with Nail-Patella syndrome.

E. HEENT.
1. Preauricular pits and/or deafness frequently occur in association with renal anomalies ranging from hypoplasia or dysplasia to complete agenesis.
2. Epiphora (watery eyes), photophobia, and cystine crystals throughout the cornea are associated with cystinosis.
3. Cataracts and glaucoma (e.g., Lowe Syndrome).

F. Cardiovascular.
1. Kidney disease is the most frequent cause of hypertension in children.
2. Hypervolemia associated with kidney failure may result in tachycardia, gallop rhythm, and hypertension.
3. Heart murmur may reflect a high output state related to anemia.
4. Peripheral or periorbital edema may indicate presence of proteinuria (nephrotic syndrome).

G. Pulmonary: dyspnea, coughing, increased respiratory rate, rales, and wheezing may be seen in renal-induced fluid overload.

H. Abdominal.
1. Ascites may be observed in nephrotic syndrome.
2. Liver and spleen enlargement may be evidence of hypervolemia or cystic disease on ultrasound exam.
3. Kidney enlargement may cause abdominal distention.
4. Abdominal masses may be caused by hydronephrosis, neoplasms of the kidney, or polycystic kidney disease.

I. Genitourinary.
1. Undescended testes can be associated with urinary tract anomalies, such as prune belly syndrome.

2. Absence of the vagina in females is associated with congenital renal anomalies.
3. History of crying with urination or foul smelling urine may be signs of urinary tract infection (UTI).
4. Dysuria, urgency, frequency, and hesitancy may or may not be discernible in children.

II. Urinalysis in children.

A. Urine collection.
1. In diapered infants, urine can be collected with a sterile adhesive collection bag, but bagged specimens are easily contaminated with bacteria from stool or the perineal skin. Samples obtained by urinary catheter or suprapubic aspiration are used when greater accuracy is needed.
2. A midstream, clean-catch sample can be obtained with the help of an adult in small children who are toilet trained.

B. Urinalysis findings are similar to adults.
1. Protein may be found transiently in the urine of children, especially febrile children. Persistent proteinuria should be evaluated.
2. Gross hematuria or microscopic hematuria (more than 5 RBCs per high-power field in the sediment of 10 mL of centrifuged urine) on three urinalyses should be evaluated.

III. Blood analysis in children.

A. Some normal ranges are the same as adults. Normal range for serum phosphorus and alkaline phosphatase are higher in children than adults.

B. Plasma creatinine.
1. The neonate's plasma creatinine equals the mother's.
2. At 1 week, the full-term neonate should have a creatinine less than 1 mg/dL, which should continue to decrease to less than 0.5 mg/dL in a few weeks.
3. Premature infants may have a serum creatinine as high as 1.5 mg/dL until postconceptual age (gestational age at birth plus postnatal age) is greater than 36 weeks, when nephrogenesis is complete.
4. Serial serum creatinine values are important. Any increase in the serum creatinine in the neonatal period suggests renal insufficiency.
5. Normal serum creatinine increases with age and body mass.

C. Clearance tests.
1. Creatinine clearance can be used to estimate GFR.
   a. Difficult to collect 24-hour urine in children before toilet training is complete or in those with nocturnal enuresis.

b. Normalized GFR can be estimated using the Schwartz formula (see Table 5.4).

$$eGFR \ (mL/min/1.73 \ m^2) = (k \times ht)/serum \ creatinine$$

2. Inulin, iothalmate, or diethylene triamine pentaacetic acid (DTPA) clearance can be obtained if a more accurate measurement of GFR is needed.
3. Stages of chronic kidney disease are listed in Table 5.5.

D. Imaging studies used to evaluate the cause of kidney failure in adults are used similarly in children. Kidney and bladder ultrasound should be performed in young children with the first urinary tract infection (UTI). If abnormal, obtain voiding cystourethrogram (VCUG) or radionuclide cystography (RNC) (Roberts, 2011).

Table 5.4

Constant Variables for Schwartz Equation

K (preterm infant)	0.33
K (term infant)	0.45
K (child & adolescent female)	0.55
K (adolescent male)	0.70
Ht	Height or length in centimeters
Serum creatinine	mg/dL

Table 5.5

Stages of Chronic Kidney Disease

Stage of Chronic Kidney Disease	Glomerular Filtration Rate (GFR)
Stage 1	> 90 mL/min
Stage 2	60–89 mL/min
Stage 3	30–59 mL/min
Stage 4	15–29 mL/min
Stage 5	< 15 mL/min

(Avner et al., 2009)

Section D

Pediatric End-Stage Renal Disease: Current Statistics from the 2014 USRDS Annual Report

I. **Prevalence:** Children aged 0 to 19 years being treated for ESRD in 2012 constituted 1.2% of the total ESRD population (7,522 of 636,905 ESRD patients).

II. **Incidence:** 1,161 incident patients between 2011 and 2012.

A. Incidence greater for boys than girls; boys have more congenital anomalies of the urinary tract that may lead to ESRD.

B. Treatment modality for incident ESRD patients in 2012 (2014 USRDS Annual Report).
1. Hemodialysis: 45% of children 0 to 19 years.
2. Peritoneal Dialysis: 31% of children 0 to 19 years.
3. Transplantation: 24% of children 0 to 19 years.

III. **All-cause mortality rate:** Patients 0 to 19 years was 35 per 1000 patient years.

A. Infection-related mortality decreased by 37.5%

B. Cardiovascular mortality was 11 per 1,000 patient years.

IV. **Primary disease incidence in pediatric ESRD patients, ages 0 to 19 years, is shown in Figure 5.1** (2014 USRDS Annual Report).

Section E

Frequent Causes of Kidney Disease in Children

I. **Renal agenesis, dysplasia, and hypoplasia.**

A. Renal agenesis (Avner et al., 2009).
1. Lack of formation of the kidney, usually unilateral and not inherited.
2. When bilateral, is associated with Potter's facies and pulmonary hypoplasia (Potter's syndrome).

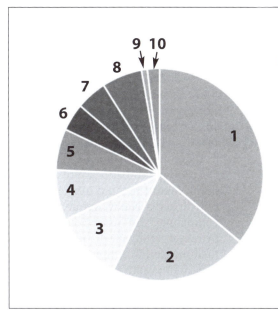

Distribution of reported incident ESRD pediatric patients by primary diagnosis (2008-2012 data)

1. Cystic Hereditary/congenital diseases 35.9%
2. Glomerulinephritis (GN) 21.5%
3. Secondary GN/Vasculitis 10.6%
4. Etiology uncertain 7.7%
5. Miscellaneous 6.3%
6. Hypertension/Large vessel disease 4.2%
7. Interstitial Nephritis/puelonephritis 4.7%
8. Missing 6.3%
9. Diabetes Melllitus 0.9%
10. Neoplasms/tumors 1.9%

Figure 5.1 Distribution of reported incident ESRD pediatric patients by primary diagnosis (2008-2012 data) (USRDS Report, 2014)

B. Renal dysplasia.
  1. Altered differentiation of metanephric tissue with persistence of primitive structures and fibromuscular tissue with or without foci of primitive cartilage.
  2. Primitive glomeruli and tubules in varying numbers.
  3. Cysts frequent. When large cysts are present, the condition is referred to as cystic dysplasia.

C. Multicystic dysplastic kidney (MCDK).
  1. Dysplastic kidney with multiple large cysts, no functioning renal tissue, and an absent or rudimentary ureter.
  2. Usually unilateral and not inherited; congenital condition not to be confused with polycystic kidney.
  3. Incidence for unilateral MCDK: 1 in 4000 live births (Hains et al., 2009).
  4. The most frequent cause of palpable abdominal mass in a newborn.
  5. Suspected by antenatal ultrasonography, but must be distinguished from hydronephrosis.
  6. High incidence of obstruction or vesicoureteral reflux in the contralateral kidney.

D. Kidney hypoplasia.
  1. Abnormally small, nondysplastic kidney with less than the normal number of calyces and nephrons. Distinguish from aplasia, in which the kidney is rudimentary.
  2. Unilateral or bilateral.
  3. Oligomeganephronee: a rare bilateral form with only a few nephrons per kidney that are markedly hypertrophied.

  4. Segmental hypoplasia (Ask-Upmark kidney): only a segment of the kidney is hypoplastic. Associated hypertension is the rule.

E. Evaluation and diagnosis.
  1. Kidney ultrasound.
  2. Consider voiding cystourethrogram (VCUG).
  3. Functional studies [e.g., dimercaptosuccinic acid study (DMSA)] to confirm diagnosis.

F. Treatment.
  1. Control blood pressure.
  2. Monitor serum creatinine and BUN.
  3. Urinalysis to monitor proteinuria.

II. Congenital obstructive uropathy.

A. Posterior urethral valves.
  1. Abnormal mucosal folds that function as a valve to obstruct urine flow.
  2. Suspected prenatally when dilated bladder is observed in association with obstructive uropathy.
  3. Most common childhood cause of obstructive uropathy leading to kidney failure.

B. Prune belly syndrome (Eagle-Barrett syndrome).
  1. Absent abdominal musculature, undescended testicles, and absent ureteral musculature.
  2. Poor peristalsis, hydroureter and hydronephrosis, and varying degrees of kidney dysplasia.

C. Other.
  1. Uteropelvic junction obstruction (UPJ).
  2. Ureterovesical junction obstruction (UVJ).

D. Evaluation and diagnosis.
1. Often detected in utero with prenatal ultrasound.
2. VCUG or endoscopy.

E. Treatment.
1. Serial ultrasound-directed vesiocentesis, vesicoamniotic shunting, fetal cystosopy, and valve ablation are prenatal techniques being done to improve prognosis for PUV.
2. Monitor for urinary tract infections (UTIs).

III. Urinary tract infection (UTI).

A. Before toilet training, is associated with a high incidence of congenital anomalies of kidney development, such as posterior urethral valves, other forms of obstructive uropathy, or vesicoureteral reflux (Roberts, 2011).
1. May be the first indication of underlying kidney anomalies.
2. American Academy of Pediatrics recommends screening with a kidney ultrasound. If the kidney ultrasound is abnormal, obtain voiding cystourethrogram (VCUG) (Roberts, 2011).
3. May occur in uncircumcised boys in the first 6 months of life without underlying congenital kidney anomalies.

B. After toilet training, occurs more frequently in girls than in boys.
1. Screening with kidney ultrasound with first UTI in boys.
2. Screening may be deferred until the second or third UTI in girls, if uncomplicated.

C. Occurs with increased frequency in sexually active adolescent girls.

D. Evaluation and diagnosis. Urinalysis with urine culture.
1. Suprapubic aspiration specimen: > 1,000 colony forming units/mL.
2. Catheter specimen: > 10,000 colony forming units/mL.
3. Clean-catch or midstream specimen: 100,000 colony-forming units/mL or greater.

E. Treatment.
1. Antibiotic therapy is determined by culture sensitivities.
2. Common antibiotics used to treat UTIs in children are amoxicillin/clavulanate (Augmentin®), cefixime (Suprax®), trimethoprim/ sulfamethoxazole (Bactrim®, Septra®).

IV. Enuresis.

A. Defined as uncontrollable leakage of urine (intermittent or continuous) occurring after continence should have been achieved (Chase et al., 2010).
1. Primary nocturnal enuresis-nocturnal wetting in a child who has never been dry on consecutive nights for longer than 6 months (Graham & Levy, 2009).
   a. Evaluation and diagnosis: complete history (including number of events per week/per night, nighttime fluid intake, polyuria, polydipsia, urgency, frequency, dysuria, bowel complaints, and history of sleep disorders); urinalysis (rule out diabetes insipidus, diabetes mellitus, and infection).
   b. Treatment: motivational therapy (sticker chart), wetness alarms, limiting fluid in the evening, and vasopressin analog (for rapid and short-term improvement).
2. Daytime incontinence.
   a. Evaluation: complete history and physical exam (including genitourinary abnormalities, back or sacral abnormalities, and the rectum), urinalysis and urine culture, postvoid residual, and uro-flow test.
   b. Treatment: behavioral therapy (double voiding, timed voiding schedule) (Graham & Levy, 2009).

V. Acquired glomerulonephritis and vasculitis.

A. Acute postinfectious glomerulonephritis.
1. Usually follows group A beta-hemolytic streptococcal throat or skin infection and generally resolves on its own.
2. Varies from asymptomatic hematuria to acute nephritic syndrome (red to brown urine, edema, hypertension, and acute kidney injury).
3. Evaluation and diagnosis.
   a. Urinalysis: hematuria, proteinuria, and often pyruia.
   b. Complement testing: low C3 and often low C4 (return to normal 4 to 8 weeks after presentation).
   c. Serology: streptococcal antibodies (e.g., ASO).
4. Treatment.
   a. Supportive therapy (e.g., loop diuretics for volume overload and hypertension).
   b. May require dialysis, if the loss of kidney function is severe.

B. IgA nephropathy.
1. Often presents in childhood with episodes of gross hematuria associated with febrile illnesses and may progress to kidney failure over time (Wyatt & Julian, 2013).

2. Evaluation and diagnosis.
   a. Urinalysis (hematuria, proteinuria).
   b. Serum creatinine.
   c. Kidney biopsy.
3. Treatment.
   a. Angiotensin-converting enzyme (ACE) inhibitor or angiotensin II receptor blocker (ARB) (reduces protein excretion and preserves kidney function).
   b. Glucocorticoids.
   c. High-dose omega-3 fatty acids.
   d. Intensive immunosuppression if rapid decline in kidney function (e.g., mycophenolate mofetil, cyclophosphamide).

C. Rapidly progressive glomerulonephritis.
1. May be idiopathic or associated with Anti-neutrophil cytoplasmic antibody (ANCA) vasculitis or other diseases.
2. Wegener's granulomatosis: inflammation involving the respiratory tract and necrotizing vasculitis affecting small to medium-sized vessels, usually presents as symptoms related to the upper and lower respiratory tract.
3. Goodpasture syndrome occurs rarely in childhood; it may present with hemoptysis and, less often, pulmonary hemorrhage.
4. Evaluation and diagnosis.
   a. Serologic investigations include complement levels, myeloperoxidase (MPO), or proteinase-3 (PR3), ANCA levels, anti-glomerular basement membrane (GBM) IgG antibodies.
   b. Kidney biopsy.
5. Treatment includes immunosuppressant medications.

D. Henoch-Schönlein purpura.
1. A systemic vasculitis with IgA deposits in the walls of the small vessels.
2. Presents with a characteristic purpuric rash of the lower extremities, abdominal pain (cramping), and arthritis or arthralgias.
3. Symptoms of nephritis, such as hematuria and proteinuria or edema, usually present after the initial symptoms (Trnka, 2013).
4. Evaluation and diagnosis.
   a. Clinical examination and findings.
   b. Urinalysis (red or white cells, cellular casts, and proteinuria).
   c. If unusual presentation, kidney biopsy (e.g., no rash, or those with significant kidney disease).
5. Treatment.
   a. Supportive care by maintaining good hydration, pain control, and monitoring for complications.
   b. The disease is self-limiting and rarely leads to

kidney failure. May require treatment with steroids if symptoms severe (Trnka, 2013).

E. Systemic lupus erythematosus.
1. Occurs more often in girls than boys.
2. Lupus nephritis is more common in childhood lupus, occurring in up to 80% of affected children and adolescents.
3. Most common initial symptoms are fever, malaise, malar rash, and arthritis.
4. Evaluation and diagnosis.
   a. Systemic Lupus International Collaborating Clinics (SLICC) group classification criteria (four or more of the criteria).
   b. Positive antinuclear antibodies (ANAs) or anti-double-stranded DNA antibodies in conjunction with biopsy-proven lupus nephritis.
5. The International Society of Nephrology/Renal Pathology Society (ISN/RPS) classification of lupus nephritis (2003) can be found in Table 5.6.
6. Treatment.
   a. Medications can include hydroxychloroquine (Plaquenil®), glucocorticoids, other immuno-suppressant medications.
   b. Regular ophthalmic evaluations.

F. Hemolytic uremic syndrome (HUS).
1. Characterized by microangiopathic hemolytic anemia, thrombocytopenia, and uremia (Barbour et al., 2012).
2. Typically occurs after a prodromal episode of bloody diarrhea (Shiga-toxin associated) due to a variety of organisms, including enteropathogenic *E. coli* (especially from ingestion of undercooked contaminated beef), Shigella, and perhaps some viruses.
3. May also occur with severe pneumonia due to *Streptococcus pneumoniae*.
4. Pathologic lesion: fibrin thrombi and necrosis in the microvasculature of many organs, including kidney, gut, pancreas, heart, adrenal, retina, and brain.
5. Evaluation and diagnosis.
   a. Screening for Shiga toxin-producing bacterial strains (stool cultures).
   b. Complete blood count: hemolytic anemia (Hgb < 8 g/dL and a peripheral blood smear with schistocytes), thrombocytopenia (platelet count < 140,000/mm^3).
   c. Urinalysis: hematuria, proteinuria.
   d. Assess ADAMTS 13 function (differentiate HUS from thrombotic thrombocytopenic purpura (TTP).
6. Treatment is supportive: red blood cell/platelet transfusions, appropriate fluid and electrolyte

Table 5.6

Abbreviated International Society of Nephrology/Renal Pathology Society (ISN/RPS) Classification of Lupus Nephritis (2003)

Class I	Minimal mesangial lupus nephritis
Class II	Mesangial proliferative lupus nephritis
Class III	Focal lupus nephritis [a]
Class IV	Diffuse segmental (IV-S) or global (IV-G) lupus nephritis [b]
Class V	Membranous lupus nephritis [c]
Class VI	Advanced sclerosing lupus nephritis

[a] Indicate the proportion of glomeruli with active and with sclerotic lesions.
[b] Indicate the proportion of glomeruli with fibrinoid necrosis and cellular crescents.
[c] Class V may occur in combination with class III or IV in which case both will be diagnosed.
Indicate and grade (mild, moderate, severe) tubular atrophy, interstitial inflammation and fibrosis, severity of arteriosclerosis or other vascular lesions.

Republished with permission of *Journal of the American Society of Nephrology*, from [The classification of glomerulonephritis in systemic lupus erythematosus revisited, Weening et al. 15, 2, 2004]; permission conveyed through Copyright Clearance Center, Inc.

management, and initiation of dialysis in patients with symptomatic uremia, severe fluid overload, or electrolyte abnormalities.

G. Atypical HUS (aHUS).
   1. Disease of complement alternative pathway dysregulation, not caused by an external agent.
   2. A diarrheal prodrome is less common. May be familial (either autosomal dominant or recessive) (Barbour et al., 2012).
   3. Evaluation and diagnosis.
      a. Complete blood count: hemolytic anemia (Hgb < 8 g/dL and a peripheral blood smear with schistocytes), thrombocytopenia (platelet count < 140,000/mm³).
      b. Complement testing (C3, C4).
      c. Screening for mutations and antibodies to complement proteins.
      d. Urinalysis: hematuria, proteinuria.
      e. Liver enzymes.
      f. Ophthalmic exam: retinal thrombotic microangiopathy.
   4. Treatment.
      a. Plasma exchange or infusion.
      b. Eculizumab, a humanized monoclonal antibody inhibiting C5 activation, was recently approved by the FDA for first-line treatment of aHUS.
      c. Supportive therapy includes red blood cell/platelet transfusions, initiation of dialysis.
      d. Often rapidly progresses to kidney failure.

VI. Nephrotic syndrome (NS).

A. May be a primary kidney disease or secondary to other systemic diseases, nephrotoxins, or allergic reactions.

B. Clinical presentation: proteinuria with hypoproteinemia, hyperlipidemia, and edema.

C. Causes of primary NS differ in children as compared with adults.
   1. Minimal change disease (MCD): most frequent cause of NS in childhood, accounting for 80% to 90% in children less than 10 years of age. MCD is usually responsive to steroid therapy but has a relapsing and remitting course in most patients.
   2. Focal segmental glomerulosclerosis (FSGS): accounts for about 10% of NS in children and adolescents. About 50% of these patients progress to kidney failure within 5 to 10 years of onset of NS. FSGS recurs frequently (25%) in the transplanted kidney.
   3. Membranoproliferative glomerulonephritis (MPGN): presents with either NS, proteinuria or hematuria with proteinuria, usually in children more than 6 years of age. Without treatment, patients progress slowly to kidney failure over about 10 years.
   4. Membranous glomerulonephritis (MGN): occurs rarely in children, although it is the most frequent cause of NS in adults. MGN may be idiopathic or associated with lupus, hepatitis B infection, or neoplasm like lymphoma.

5. Congenital NS: occurs within the first year of life and may be caused by the Finnish-type mesangial sclerosis, Denys-Drash syndrome (genital abnormalities) (Koziell & Grundy, 1999), congenital infections (e.g., CMV, rubella, hepatitis B, syphilis, malaria), toxins (e.g., mercury, drugs), and other hereditary kidney diseases. Many progress to ESRD during infancy or early childhood. MCD and FSGS rarely occur in the first year of life.

D. Evaluation and diagnosis.
   1. Urinalysis (albumin concentration).
   2. Serum evaluation: electrolytes, creatinine, blood urea nitrogen, cholesterol, albumin, and C3.
   3. Urinary protein excretion greater than 50 mg/kg/day.
   4. Kidney biopsy may be needed.

E. Treatment.
   1. Corticosteroids.
   2. Calcineurin inhibitor or mycophenolate mofetil if steroid resistant.
   3. Patient and parent education to prevent readmission.

VII. Hereditary kidney diseases.

A. Hereditary nephritis (Alport's syndrome).
   1. X-linked dominant (85%): associated with sensorineural hearing loss and lens abnormalities of the eyes in many kindreds. Males are much more likely to have severe disease and nearly always develop kidney failure (Avner et al., 2009).
   2. Autosomal recessive (15%): deafness and kidney failure in all affected individuals before 30 years of age.
   3. Autosomal dominant (< 1%): kidney failure and deafness develop early in life; some patients have thrombocytopenia and others platelet abnormalities.
   4. Affects individuals regardless of geographic or ethnic background.
   5. Presentation: usually hematuria, sometimes episodic macroscopic hematuria; onset of proteinuria considered a poor prognostic sign.
   6. Evaluation and diagnosis.
      a. Thorough clinical examination and family history.
      b. If necessary, kidney biopsy (Avner et al., 2009).
   7. Treatment.
      a. Annual monitoring for microalbuminuria and proteinuria.
      b. Angiotensin blockade with an ACE inhibitor or an angiotensin receptor blocker (ARB).
      c. Regular follow-up with audiology and ophthalmology.
      d. Kidney transplantation.
      e. Genetic counseling.

B. Benign familial hematuria (BFH).
   1. Autosomal dominant, benign condition that does not lead to CKD or kidney failure.
   2. Presentation: persistent or intermittent microscopic hematuria or macroscopic hematuria associated with a febrile illness. Proteinuria is absent. Kidney function is normal.
   3. Evaluation and diagnosis.
      a. Thorough family history.
      b. Exclusion of other causes of hematuria.
      c. Long-term follow-up over years without other symptoms of kidney disease.
      d. Kidney biopsy (characteristic thinning of the glomerular basement membranes) may be useful in situations where the diagnosis is uncertain.
   4. Treatment involves education and supportive therapy.

C. Familial juvenile nephronophthisis (JNPH).
   1. Presents with polyuria and polydipsia, decreased urinary concentrating ability, secondary enuresis, anemia, weakness, and/or growth failure, usually in the first decade of life (Hildebrandt et al., 2009).
   2. Autosomal recessive.
   3. Often have nonrenal-associated anomalies, including skeletal and ophthalmologic abnormalities, cerebellar ataxia, mental retardation, and hepatic fibrosis.
   4. Progresses to kidney failure before adulthood.
   5. Evaluation and diagnosis.
      a. Ultrasound: normal or slightly decreased in size kidneys for age with increased echogenicity.
      b. Kidney biopsy: chronic tubulointerstitial changes with thickening of tubular basement membranes.
      c. Urinalysis: no hematuria or proteinuria.
      d. Genetic testing.
   6. Treatment.
      a. Correction of water and electrolyte imbalances.
      b. Progress to kidney failure. Kidney transplantation is the preferred therapy due to low recurrence rate of primary disease.

D. Primary hyperoxaluria (oxalosis)(PH).
   1. Caused by inborn errors of metabolism of glyoxylate and oxalate. Autosomal recessive disorder due to deficiencies of hepatic enzymes important in the metabolic disposition of glyoxylate.
   2. Characterized by an excessive production of oxalate, a metabolic end-product.
   3. Types of primary hyperoxaluria.
      a. Most frequent type primary hyperoxaluria type 1 (PH1).
         (1) Deficiency or absence of the hepatic enzyme alanine-glyoxylate

aminotransferase (AGT), which leads to excess production and urinary excretion of oxalate.

    (2) Mutation in the AGXT gene that encodes the enzyme AGT accounts for 80% of primary hyperoxaluria.

    (3) Nephrocalcinosis and recurrent calcium oxalate nephrolithiasis result from excessive urinary oxalate excretion and may lead to CKD and kidney failure.

    (4) Calcium oxalate may accumulate in extra renal sites, such as skin, bone, or retina, especially in the presence of CKD (Cochat & Rumsby, 2013).

  b. Primary Hyperoxaluria Type 2.

    (1) Deficiency of glyoxylate reductase/hydroxypyruvate reductase (GRHPR) a cytosolic enzyme.

    (2) Accounts for 15% of PH.

  c. Primary Hyperoxaluria Type 3.

    (1) Linked to the gene DHDPSL, encoding a mitochondrial enzyme; metabolic reactions remain unclear.

    (2) Accounts for ~ 5% of PH.

  d. There is evidence to speculate others will be identified.

4. Onset and severity vary with the severity of the gene mutation.

  a. The median age at onset is 5.5 years.

  b. Patients who present in the first few months of life often have rapid progression to kidney failure.

5. Evaluation and diagnosis.

  a. Clinical diagnosis: recurrent calcium stones, oxalate crystals in the urine sediment.

  b. Metabolic screening: increased urinary oxalate excretion.

  c. Genetic testing.

  d. Liver biopsy: absent or reduced AGT activity.

6. Treatment.

  a. Directed toward reducing stone formation with liberal fluid intake and high intakes of citrate or phosphate.

  b. Pyridoxine, a cofactor for AGT activity, may increase glyoxlate metabolism and decrease oxalate production and stone formation in some patients.

  c. Conventional dialysis is unsuitable for those who reach CKD stage 5 because it cannot clear enough oxalate to prevent continued increase in the body's burden of oxalate.

  d. Short, daily hemodialysis sessions (6 days per week), nocturnal dialysis, or combination of hemodialysis and nocturnal peritoneal dialysis are needed to keep plasma oxalate levels below 20 to 45 mmol/L.

  e. Monitor for caregiver burnout and decreased quality of life due to high burden and rigor of treatment.

  f. Routine follow-up with ophthalmology (crystal deposits in the retina) and orthopedics (deposition in bone and high risk of fracture) (Cochat & Rumsby, 2013).

  g. Combined liver-kidney transplantation is the only way to replace both the defective organ (liver) and the damaged organ (kidney) in PH1 and to reduce the body burden of oxalate.

    (1) Care must be taken to protect the new kidney while the body burden of oxalate is being mobilized and excreted after transplantation (Cochat & Rumsby, 2013). The patient often requires dialysis immediately posttransplant.

    (2) High fluid requirements posttransplant (> 3 L/day).

E. Nephropathy of diabetes mellitus.

1. Infrequent in children as compared to adults because the nephropathy of diabetes usually does not occur until 10 to 20 years after onset of the disease.

2. Evaluation and diagnosis.

  a. Kidney biopsy.

  b. Urinary protein excretion.

3. Treatment.

  a. Adequate blood sugar control to delay progression of chronic kidney disease.

  b. Angiotensin-converting enzyme (ACE) inhibitors.

  c. Early referral to nephrology practitioner for routine follow-up.

F. Sickle cell nephropathy.

1. Hematuria is frequent, and chronic damage to the medulla during sickle cell crises may result in an inability to concentrate the urine in many (Pham et al., 2000).

2. Only about 5% of patients develop CKD, which is usually preceded by the onset of proteinuria (Avner et al., 2009).

3. Evaluation and diagnosis.

  a. Urinalysis with microscopy and quantitation of total proteinuria.

  b. Kidney ultrasound.

  c. Hepatitis C and human immunodeficiency virus (HIV) testing (increased risk due to transfusion-associated infections).

  d. Kidney biopsy may be necessary if rapidly progressive kidney failure.

4. Treatment.

  a. Screen all patients with sickle cell disease regularly for kidney disease and hypertension (serum creatinine, dipstick urinalysis for blood, urine albumin to creatinine ratio, blood

pressure screening at every visit).
    b. Hematuria: hydration using alkaline fluids, with diuretics (increase urine flow rate).
    c. Angiotensin-converting enzyme (ACE) inhibitors or angiotensin II receptor blockers (ARBs) to lower protein excretion and manage hypertension.

G. Nail-patella syndrome.
  1. A rare autosomal dominant disorder whose cardinal features are dysplastic nails, hypoplastic or absent patellae, dysplasia of the elbows, and kidney disease.
  2. Proteinuria may reach nephrotic range and lead to NS.
  3. CKD is infrequent and usually does not develop before adolescence or young adulthood.
  4. If CKD is present, there is a 10% risk of progression to kidney failure (Avner et al., 2009).
  5. Evaluation and diagnosis.
    a. Urinalysis: proteinuria, hematuria.
    b. Blood pressure monitoring.
    c. Decreased urine concentrating ability.
  6. Treatment – there is no specific treatment.

H. Maple sugar urine disease.
  1. Affected newborns typically develop ketonuria within 48 hours of birth.
    a. Present with irritability, poor feeding, vomiting, lethargy, and dystonia.
    b. By 4 days of age, neurologic abnormalities include apnea, seizures, lethargy, and irritability.
  2. Evaluation and diagnosis.
    a. Plasma amino acid concentrations.
    b. Urine organic acid-elevated levels of branched-chain ketoacids, lactate, and pyruvate.
  3. Treatment.
    a. Rapid lowering of tissue and plasma concentrations of leucine by inhibition of protein catabolism.
    b. Rarely, hemodialysis or peritoneal dialysis may be needed to remove branched-chain amino acids and ketoacids.

I. Renal tubular acidosis (RTA).
  1. Characterized by hyperchloremic, non-anion gap metabolic acidosis.
    a. Caused by abnormalities in the renal tubular regulation of bicarbonate concentration.
    b. Classified as proximal or distal depending on which segment of the renal tubule is affected.
  2. The GFR is normal or only mildly decreased.
  3. Distal RTA (type I).
    a. Characterized by persistently alkaline urine in the presence of all degrees of acidosis due to impaired ability of the distal tubule to maintain

a pH gradient and excrete H^+ as ammonium and titratable acids.
    b. Most often in childhood, the disorder is hereditary (autosomal dominant).
      (1) May also be secondary to other disorders like medullary sponge kidney, lupus nephritis, or obstructive uropathy.
      (2) Can also be related to drugs, such as amphotericin B or lithium.
    c. Severe hypokalemia is frequent and requires potassium supplementation as part of the treatment.
    d. Hypercalciuria is present and leads to nephrocalcinosis or nephrolithiasis, if the RTA is untreated for a prolonged period of time.
  4. Proximal RTA (type 2).
    a. Characterized by alkaline urine in the presence of mild to moderate degrees of acidosis, but acid urine in the presence of severe acidosis.
    b. Caused by impaired reabsorption of bicarbonate in the proximal tubule, where 85% of the filtered bicarbonate is normally reabsorbed.
    c. During severe acidosis, the amount of filtered bicarbonate that escapes the diseased proximal tubule is low enough to be completely reabsorbed by the normal distal tubule, so the urine is acidic.
    d. During less severe acidosis, more filtered bicarbonate is delivered to the tubule, exceeding the capacity for reabsorption by the diseased proximal tubule and the normal distal tubule and leading to urinary bicarbonate wasting, so the urine is alkaline.
    e. Often associated with abnormal proximal tubular reabsorption of other substances, including sodium, potassium, phosphorus, amino acids, glucose, and low molecular weight proteins (see Fanconi syndrome below).
    f. Hypokalemia is frequent and requires potassium supplementation as part of the treatment.
  5. Combined distal-proximal RTA (type 3).
    a. Distal RTA with a transient form of proximal RTA.
    b. Can be associated with osteopetrosis (bone disease that makes bones abnormally dense and prone to breakage).
  6. Hyperkalemic distal RTA (type 4).
    a. Characterized by hyperkalemia and the presence of alkaline urine during mild to moderate degrees of acidosis. Urine is acidic when acidosis is severe.
    b. Caused by abnormalities of K^+ and H^+ excretion in the distal tubule secondary to hypoaldosteronism or to end-organ resistance or immature response to aldosterone

(pseudohypoaldosteronism). Infants may outgrow the disorder as the renal tubule matures.
   c. Hyperkalemia may return to normal with treatment of the acidosis; potassium supplements should never be given as part of treatment.
7. Evaluation and diagnosis.
   a. Suspect RTA in an infant or child with failure to thrive and unexplained metabolic acidosis.
   b. Urine pH and urine ammonium excretion.
8. Treatment.
   a. Frequent therapy for all forms of RTA is alkali therapy such as bicarbonate, citrate, or acetate.
   b. The sodium and/or potassium salts of these substances are used as dictated by the need to provide or to avoid potassium supplementation.

J. Fanconi syndrome (FS) (pan-proximal tubular dysfunction).
1. Characterized classically by excessive urinary losses of amino acids, glucose, bicarbonate, and phosphate, but also by losses of calcium, magnesium, uric acid and other organic acids, low molecular weight (tubular) proteins, sodium, potassium, and water.
2. Urinary losses of salts and minerals result in metabolic acidosis, dehydration, hypokalemia, hypophosphatemia, rickets, and growth retardation in children.
3. Frequent causes in childhood.
   a. Cystinosis: rare lysosomal storage disease in which intracellular cystine accumulation is associated with FS, chronic kidney failure, growth failure, corneal opacities, photophobia, and hypothyroidism.
   b. Lowe syndrome is an X-linked recessive disorder that characteristically occurs in males, who present in early infancy with dense congenital cataracts and glaucoma; renal tubular dysfunction, mental retardation, muscular hypotonia, and areflexia appear later in the first year of life.
   c. Idiopathic and there is no identifiable associated disease.
   d. Drug and toxin induced: including aminoglycosides, valproic acid, cis-platinum, ifosfomide, toluene (glue sniffing), and heavy metal poisoning (e.g., lead, mercury, cadimium).
4. Evaluation and diagnosis.
   a. Good history and physical exam (polyuria, polydipsia, genu vulgum, bone pain).
   b. Serum evaluation (hypokalemia, hypophosphatemia).
   c. Urinalysis (glucosuria, proteinuria).

d. Kidney biopsy (chronic tubulointerstitial fibrosis).
5. Treatment.
   a. Fluid and electrolyte management.
   b. Early intervention with fluid management for vomiting, diarrhea, or if being kept NPO for surgery.
   c. Manage and treat growth failure with growth hormone.

K. Nephrogenic diabetes insipidus (NDI).
1. Characterized by resistance of the renal tubule to antidiuretic hormone (ADH), which results in inability to concentrate the urine, polyuria, and compensatory polydipsia (Avner et al., 2009).
2. May be hereditary (X-linked or autosomal recessive) or acquired, secondary to renal medullary tissue injury from diseases like sickle cell disease or interstitial nephritis or to drugs such as lithium, demeclocycline, or cis-platinum.
3. Clinical features include recurrent bouts of dehydration and unexplained fevers, growth failure, and developmental delay.
4. Evaluation and diagnosis.
   a. Obtain plasma sodium and urine osmolality.
   b. Measure urine output.
5. Treatment.
   a. Therapy usually includes maintaining access to large amounts of fluid and diet with a low renal solute load and may require thiazide diuretics or prostaglandin inhibitors (Avner et al., 2009).

L. Bartter syndrome.
1. Characterized by hypokalemia, hypochloremic metabolic alkalosis, and normal BP with elevated plasma renin and aldosterone levels.
2. Magnesium depletion and hypercalciuria are also frequent (Rodriguez-Soriano, 1999).
3. Caused primarily by an abnormality of reabsorption of chloride in the ascending loop of Henle, leading to increased urinary excretion of Cl^- and Na^+.
4. In the presence of hyperaldosteronism, urinary excretion of K^+ and H^+ is also increased.
5. Inherited as an autosomal recessive trait.
6. Evaluation and diagnosis.
   a. Careful history and physical examination.
   b. Measurement of urine chloride and calcium concentration.
   c. Urine diuretic screen.
7. Treatment.
   a. Prostaglandin inhibitors (e.g., indomethocin).
   b. Potassium supplementation as needed to restore normal potassium balance.
   c. Magnesium supplements to correct magnesium depletion, if present (Kleta et al., 2000).

M. Polycystic kidney disease.
1. Autosomal recessive.
   a. Rare disorder, occurring in 1:10,000 to 1:40,000 live births, that usually presents in the neonatal period with markedly enlarged kidneys due to fusiform dilation of the collecting tubules into cysts (Dell, 2011).
   b. Always associated with congenital hepatic fibrosis.
   c. Leads to kidney failure in the first few years of life, and portal hypertension and liver failure later in the first or second decades of life.
2. Autosomal dominant.
   a. Frequent disorder, occurring in 1:1000 individuals (Dell, 2011).
   b. Usually presents in adulthood, but may be identified as early as in utero by fetal ultrasound or in the newborn period.
   c. Cysts in the kidney involve all portions of the nephron, including the glomerulus.
   d. Associated with cysts in other organs, including liver, pancreas, spleen and ovary, and associated with berry aneurysms of the brain.
   e. Clinical features include enlarged kidneys, hypertension, abdominal pain, and urinary tract infection.
   f. Usually progresses to kidney failure in the 4th or 5th decade of life, but kidney failure may be seen as early as the teenage years.
3. Evaluation and diagnosis.
   a. Kidney and liver ultrasound.
   b. If ultrasound results are inconclusive, obtain magnetic resonance imaging (MRI) or computed tomography (CT) scan.
4. Treatment.
   a. Manage hypertension to prevent progression of chronic kidney disease.
   b. Aggressively treat hyperlipidemia with statins.
   c. Nephrectomy is considered for pain that is constant and requires narcotic medications or is associated with reduced quality of life.
   d. Genetic counseling.

N. Other inherited diseases sometimes associated with cystic kidneys.
1. Jeune syndrome (asphyxiating thoracic dystrophy) includes progressive respiratory insufficiency, cystic kidney disease, hepatic insufficiency, and retinal abnormalities.
2. Bardet-Biedl syndrome includes obesity, hypogenitalism in men, mental retardation, retinal dystrophy, hypertension, and kidney malformations with progressive CKD.
3. Tuberous sclerosis develops variety of benign tumors in multiple organs; angiomyolipomas most frequent kidney manifestation.
4. Ehlers-Danlos syndrome is a group of relatively

rare genetic disorders of the connective tissue sometimes associated with cystic kidneys.
5. Von Hippel-Lindau disease is an autosomal dominant syndrome with a variety of benign and malignant tumors. Approximately two thirds of patients develop multiple kidney cysts and kidney cell carcinomas.
6. Joubert syndrome is an autosomal recessive neurologic disorder where cystic kidney dysplasia is seen in approximately one fourth of the cases.

SECTION F
Hypertension in Children

I. Hypertension is often associated with chronic kidney disease in infants and children.

II. Uncontrolled hypertension can accelerate the decline of kidney function in all ages, including children.

III. Mechanisms of hypertension.

A. Plasma volume expansion.

B. Increased renin production.

IV. Major cause of hypertension in children is kidney disease.

A. Causes of hypertension in infants include:
1. Prerenal: renal artery stenosis, renal vein thrombosis, aortic thrombosis, and coarctation of the aorta.
2. Intrarenal: acute renal failure, renal parenchymal anomalies, obstructive uropathy, and renal ischemic events.
3. Pathologic causes: pain, fluid overload, increased intracranial pressure, bronchopulmonary dysplasia, hypercalcemia, and neuroblastoma.

B. Causes of hypertension in children and adolescents include the following:
1. Essential hypertension: rates increasing due to the obesity epidemic in children in the United States. Hypertension present in approximately 30% of overweight children (Sorof & Daniels, 2002).
2. Renal: includes glomerulonephritis, HUS, reflux nephropathy, obstructive uropathy, polycystic kidney disease, and other causes of kidney failure in children.
3. Renovascular disease: includes kidney artery stenosis (fibromuscular dysplasia or associated with neurofibromatosis or William's syndrome),

extrinsic compression from tumors or trauma/hematoma, inflammatory stenosis (Kawasaki, Takayasu, or other arteritis), and vasculitis (lupus, HSP, ANCA vasculitis).

4. Congenital cardiac abnormalities: includes coarctation of the aorta.

5. Endocrine: includes adrenogenital syndrome (17, alpha-hydroxylase or 11, beta-hydroxylase deficiency), hyperaldosteronism, Cushing's syndrome, metabolic syndrome, hyperthyroidism, vitamin D intoxication, neuroblastoma, and pheochromocytoma.

6. Metabolic: includes hypercalcemia, porphyria, and diabetes with kidney involvement.

7. Drug related: includes therapy with exogenous corticosteroids, hormone replacement therapy, birth control pills, theophylline, albuterol, and pseudoephedrine.

8. Other: includes increased intracranial pressure, anxiety, and pain.

V. Assessment of hypertension (*The Fourth Report on the Diagnosis, Evaluation, and Treatment of High Blood Pressure in Children and Adolescents*, 2005).

A. All children 3 years of age or older should have their BP checked during every health visit. BP should be measured with an appropriate sized cuff and compared to the standardized BP table for age, gender, and height of the child (see Tables 5.7 and 5.8).

B. Check BP if < 3 years of age if systemic illness associated with hypertension, known kidney disease, prematurity or other neonatal complications, congenital heart disease, organ transplant, or recurrent UTI, proteinuria, or hematuria (The Fourth Report on the Diagnosis, Evaluation, and Treatment of High Blood Pressure in Children and Adolescents, 2005).

C. Prehypertension is defined as systolic or diastolic between the 90th and 95th percentile for age, sex, and height or > 120/80 mmHg (whichever is lower).

D. Stage I hypertension is defined as systolic or diastolic between the 95th and 99th percentile plus 5 mmHg for age, sex, and height.

E. Stage II hypertension is considered systolic or diastolic greater than the 99th percentile plus 5 mmHg for age, sex and height.

F. Elevated blood pressures must be confirmed on 3 or more occasions. Auscultation is the preferred method for checking the blood pressure. If checked with an automatic machine and the blood pressure is > 90th percentile, repeat with auscultation.

G. Initial evaluation of hypertension in children should include the following.

1. Lab: complete blood count, urinalysis, BUN, creatinine, electrolytes, and lipid panel.

2. Kidney ultrasound to evaluate kidneys and kidney artery blood flow.

3. Echocardiogram to evaluate for left ventricular hypertrophy.

4. Fundoscopic exam to assess for narrowing or arteriovenous nicking.

VI. Treatment of hypertension.

A. In children with CKD, diabetes, or end-organ failure, the goal of therapy is to reduce BP to less than the 90th percentile for age, gender, and height and to prevent long-term effects of hypertension.

B. In children with primary hypertension and no end-organ damage, the goal of therapy is to reduce the BP to less than the 95th percentile for age, gender, and height.

C. Begin with lifestyle modifications.

1. Sodium restriction, exercise, and prevention or treatment of obesity.

2. Initiate lifestyle modifications in children with systolic or diastolic greater than the 90th percentile.

3. Use as complement to drug therapy in children with systolic or diastolic greater than the 95th percentile or when BP is > 90th percentile but presence of end-organ damage, diabetes, or a secondary cause of hypertension.

D. Drug therapy.

1. Should maximize reduction in blood pressure and minimize side effects.

2. Choice of appropriate drug depends on cause of hypertension and existence of comorbid conditions.

   a. As in the adult population, the hemodynamic stability is blocked with beta blockers in the presence of stress by reducing the capacity to augment the heart rate for compensation. Beta blockers are a poor choice for patients with asthma or diabetes.

   b. Angiotensin-converting enzyme (ACE) inhibitor or angiotensin II receptor blocker (ARB) recommended in children with diabetes or proteinuria.

3. Classes of antihypertensive drugs used in children (Blowey, 2012).

   a. If normal kidney function and normal kidney ultrasound, first-line therapy:

      (1) ACE inhibitors (e.g., captopril, enalapril, lisinopril)/ARB (losartan).

Table 5.7

Blood Pressure Levels for Boys by Age and Height Percentile

Age (Year)	BP Percentile ↓	Systolic BP (mmHg) ← Percentile of Height →							Diastolic BP (mmHg) ← Percentile of Height →						
		5th	10th	25th	50th	75th	90th	95th	5th	10th	25th	50th	75th	90th	95th
1	50th	80	81	83	85	87	88	89	34	35	36	37	38	39	39
	90th	94	95	97	99	100	102	103	49	50	51	52	53	53	54
	95th	98	99	101	103	104	106	106	54	54	55	56	57	58	58
	99th	105	106	108	110	112	113	114	61	62	63	64	65	66	66
2	50th	84	85	87	88	90	92	92	39	40	41	42	43	44	44
	90th	97	99	100	102	104	105	106	54	55	56	57	58	58	59
	95th	101	102	104	106	108	109	110	59	59	60	61	62	63	63
	99th	109	110	111	113	115	117	117	66	67	68	69	70	71	71
3	50th	86	87	89	91	93	94	95	44	44	45	46	47	48	48
	90th	100	101	103	105	107	108	109	59	59	60	61	62	63	63
	95th	104	105	107	109	110	112	113	63	63	64	65	66	67	67
	99th	111	112	114	116	118	119	120	71	71	72	73	74	75	75
4	50th	88	89	91	93	95	96	97	47	48	49	50	51	51	52
	90th	102	103	105	107	109	110	111	62	63	64	65	66	66	67
	95th	106	107	109	111	112	114	115	66	67	68	69	70	71	71
	99th	113	114	116	118	120	121	122	74	75	76	77	78	78	79
5	50th	90	91	93	95	96	98	98	50	51	52	53	54	55	55
	90th	104	105	106	108	110	111	112	65	66	67	68	69	69	70
	95th	108	109	110	112	114	115	116	69	70	71	72	73	74	74
	99th	115	116	118	120	121	123	123	77	78	79	80	81	81	82
6	50th	91	92	94	96	98	99	100	53	53	54	55	56	57	57
	90th	105	106	108	110	111	113	113	68	68	69	70	71	72	72
	95th	109	110	112	114	115	117	117	72	72	73	74	75	76	76
	99th	116	117	119	121	123	124	125	80	80	81	82	83	84	84
7	50th	92	94	95	97	99	100	101	55	55	56	57	58	59	59
	90th	106	107	109	111	113	114	115	70	70	71	72	73	74	74
	95th	110	111	113	115	117	118	119	74	74	75	76	77	78	78
	99th	117	118	120	122	124	125	126	82	82	83	84	85	86	86
8	50th	94	95	97	99	100	102	102	56	57	58	59	60	60	61
	90th	107	109	110	112	114	115	116	71	72	72	73	74	75	76
	95th	111	112	114	116	118	119	120	75	76	77	78	79	79	80
	99th	119	120	122	123	125	127	127	83	84	85	86	87	87	88
9	50th	95	96	98	100	102	103	104	57	58	59	60	61	61	62
	90th	109	110	112	114	115	117	118	72	73	74	75	76	76	77
	95th	113	114	116	118	119	121	121	76	77	78	79	80	81	81
	99th	120	121	123	125	127	128	129	84	85	86	87	88	88	89
10	50th	97	98	100	102	103	105	106	58	59	60	61	61	62	63
	90th	111	112	114	115	117	119	119	73	73	74	75	76	77	78
	95th	115	116	117	119	121	122	123	77	78	79	80	81	81	82
	99th	122	123	125	127	128	130	130	85	86	86	88	88	89	90

The Fourth Report on the Diagnosis, Evaluation, and Treatment of High Blood Pressure in Children and Adolescents

Continues on next page

Table 5.7 (continued)

Blood Pressure Levels for Boys by Age and Height Percentile

Age (Year)	BP Percentile ↓	Systolic BP (mmHg) ← Percentile of Height →							Diastolic BP (mmHg) ← Percentile of Height →						
		5th	10th	25th	50th	75th	90th	95th	5th	10th	25th	50th	75th	90th	95th
11	50th	99	100	102	104	105	107	107	59	59	60	61	62	63	63
	90th	113	114	115	117	119	120	121	74	74	75	76	77	78	78
	95th	117	118	119	121	123	124	125	78	78	79	80	81	82	82
	99th	124	125	127	129	130	132	132	86	86	87	88	89	90	90
12	50th	101	102	104	106	108	109	110	59	60	61	62	63	63	64
	90th	115	116	118	120	121	123	123	74	75	75	76	77	78	79
	95th	119	120	122	123	125	127	127	78	79	80	81	82	82	83
	99th	126	127	129	131	133	134	135	86	87	88	89	90	90	91
13	50th	104	105	106	108	110	111	112	60	60	61	62	63	64	64
	90th	117	118	120	122	124	125	126	75	75	76	77	78	79	79
	95th	121	122	124	126	128	129	130	79	79	80	81	82	83	83
	99th	128	130	131	133	135	136	137	87	87	88	89	90	91	91
14	50th	106	107	109	111	113	114	115	60	61	62	63	64	65	65
	90th	120	121	123	125	126	128	128	75	76	77	78	79	79	80
	95th	124	125	127	128	130	132	132	80	80	81	82	83	84	84
	99th	131	132	134	136	138	139	140	87	88	89	90	91	92	92
15	50th	109	110	112	113	115	117	117	61	62	63	64	65	66	66
	90th	122	124	125	127	129	130	131	76	77	78	79	80	80	81
	95th	126	127	129	131	133	134	135	81	81	82	83	84	85	85
	99th	134	135	136	138	140	142	142	88	89	90	91	92	93	93
16	50th	111	112	114	116	118	119	120	63	63	64	65	66	67	67
	90th	125	126	128	130	131	133	134	78	78	79	80	81	82	82
	95th	129	130	132	134	135	137	137	82	83	83	84	85	86	87
	99th	136	137	139	141	143	144	145	90	90	91	92	93	94	94
17	50th	114	115	116	118	120	121	122	65	66	66	67	68	69	70
	90th	127	128	130	132	134	135	136	80	80	81	82	83	84	84
	95th	131	132	134	136	138	139	140	84	85	86	87	87	88	89
	99th	139	140	141	143	145	146	147	92	93	93	94	95	96	97

BP, blood pressure

* The 90th percentile is 1.28 SD, 95th percentile is 1.645 SD, and the 99th percentile is 2.326 SD over the mean. For research purposes, the standard deviations in appendix table B–1 allow one to compute BP Z-scores and percentiles for boys with height percentiles given in table 3 (i.e., the 5th, 10th, 25th, 50th, 75th, 90th, and 95th percentiles). These height percentiles must be converted to height Z-scores given by (5% = -1.645; 10% = -1.28; 25% = -0.68; 50% = 0; 75% = 0.68; 90% = 1.28; 95% = 1.645) and then computed according to the methodology in steps 2–4 described in appendix B. For children with height percentiles other than these, follow steps 1–4 as described in appendix B.

Source: National High Blood Pressure Education Program Working Group on High Blood Pressure in Children and Adolescents. (2004). The fourth report on the diagnosis, evaluation, and treatment of high blood pressure in children and adolescents. *Pediatrics, 114*(2), 555-576. Used with permission.

Table 5.8

Blood Pressure Levels for Girls by Age and Height Percentile

Age (Year)	BP Percentile ↓	Systolic BP (mmHg) ← Percentile of Height →							Diastolic BP (mmHg) ← Percentile of Height →						
		5th	10th	25th	50th	75th	90th	95th	5th	10th	25th	50th	75th	90th	95th
1	50th	83	84	85	86	88	89	90	38	39	39	40	41	41	42
	90th	97	97	98	100	101	102	103	52	53	53	54	55	55	56
	95th	100	101	102	104	105	106	107	56	57	57	58	59	59	60
	99th	108	108	109	111	112	113	114	64	64	65	65	66	67	67
2	50th	85	85	87	88	89	91	91	43	44	44	45	46	46	47
	90th	98	99	100	101	103	104	105	57	58	58	59	60	61	61
	95th	102	103	104	105	107	108	109	61	62	62	63	64	65	65
	99th	109	110	111	112	114	115	116	69	69	70	70	71	72	72
3	50th	86	87	88	89	91	92	93	47	48	48	49	50	50	51
	90th	100	100	102	103	104	106	106	61	62	62	63	64	64	65
	95th	104	104	105	107	108	109	110	65	66	66	67	68	68	69
	99th	111	111	113	114	115	116	117	73	73	74	74	75	76	76
4	50th	88	88	90	91	92	94	94	50	50	51	52	52	53	54
	90th	101	102	103	104	106	107	108	64	64	65	66	67	67	68
	95th	105	106	107	108	110	111	112	68	68	69	70	71	71	72
	99th	112	113	114	115	117	118	119	76	76	76	77	78	79	79
5	50th	89	90	91	93	94	95	96	52	53	53	54	55	55	56
	90th	103	103	105	106	107	109	109	66	67	67	68	69	69	70
	95th	107	107	108	110	111	112	113	70	71	71	72	73	73	74
	99th	114	114	116	117	118	120	120	78	78	79	79	80	81	81
6	50th	91	92	93	94	96	97	98	54	54	55	56	56	57	58
	90th	104	105	106	108	109	110	111	68	68	69	70	70	71	72
	95th	108	109	110	111	113	114	115	72	72	73	74	74	75	76
	99th	115	116	117	119	120	121	122	80	80	80	81	82	83	83
7	50th	93	93	95	96	97	99	99	55	56	56	57	58	58	59
	90th	106	107	108	109	111	112	113	69	70	70	71	72	72	73
	95th	110	111	112	113	115	116	116	73	74	74	75	76	76	77
	99th	117	118	119	120	122	123	124	81	81	82	82	83	84	84
8	50th	95	95	96	98	99	100	101	57	57	57	58	59	60	60
	90th	108	109	110	111	113	114	114	71	71	71	72	73	74	74
	95th	112	112	114	115	116	118	118	75	75	75	76	77	78	78
	99th	119	120	121	122	123	125	125	82	82	83	83	84	85	86
9	50th	96	97	98	100	101	102	103	58	58	58	59	60	61	61
	90th	110	110	112	113	114	116	116	72	72	72	73	74	75	75
	95th	114	114	115	117	118	119	120	76	76	76	77	78	79	79
	99th	121	121	123	124	125	127	127	83	83	84	84	85	86	87
10	50th	98	99	100	102	103	104	105	59	59	59	60	61	62	62
	90th	112	112	114	115	116	118	118	73	73	73	74	75	76	76
	95th	116	116	117	119	120	121	122	77	77	77	78	79	80	80
	99th	123	123	125	126	127	129	129	84	84	85	86	86	87	88

2   The Fourth Report on the Diagnosis, Evaluation, and Treatment of High Blood Pressure in Children and Adolescents

Continues on next page

Table 5.8 (continued)

Blood Pressure Levels for Girls by Age and Height Percentile

Age (Year)	BP Percentile ↓	Systolic BP (mmHg) ← Percentile of Height →							Diastolic BP (mmHg) ← Percentile of Height →						
		5th	10th	25th	50th	75th	90th	95th	5th	10th	25th	50th	75th	90th	95th
11	50th	100	101	102	103	105	106	107	60	60	60	61	62	63	63
	90th	114	114	116	117	118	119	120	74	74	74	75	76	77	77
	95th	118	118	119	121	122	123	124	78	78	78	79	80	81	81
	99th	125	125	126	128	129	130	131	85	85	86	87	87	88	89
12	50th	102	103	104	105	107	108	109	61	61	61	62	63	64	64
	90th	116	116	117	119	120	121	122	75	75	75	76	77	78	78
	95th	119	120	121	123	124	125	126	79	79	79	80	81	82	82
	99th	127	127	128	130	131	132	133	86	86	87	88	88	89	90
13	50th	104	105	106	107	109	110	110	62	62	62	63	64	65	65
	90th	117	118	119	121	122	123	124	76	76	76	77	78	79	79
	95th	121	122	123	124	126	127	128	80	80	80	81	82	83	83
	99th	128	129	130	132	133	134	135	87	87	88	89	89	90	91
14	50th	106	106	107	109	110	111	112	63	63	63	64	65	66	66
	90th	119	120	121	122	124	125	125	77	77	77	78	79	80	80
	95th	123	123	125	126	127	129	129	81	81	81	82	83	84	84
	99th	130	131	132	133	135	136	136	88	88	89	90	90	91	92
15	50th	107	108	109	110	111	113	113	64	64	64	65	66	67	67
	90th	120	121	122	123	125	126	127	78	78	78	79	80	81	81
	95th	124	125	126	127	129	130	131	82	82	82	83	84	85	85
	99th	131	132	133	134	136	137	138	89	89	90	91	91	92	93
16	50th	108	108	110	111	112	114	114	64	64	65	66	66	67	68
	90th	121	122	123	124	126	127	128	78	78	79	80	81	81	82
	95th	125	126	127	128	130	131	132	82	82	83	84	85	85	86
	99th	132	133	134	135	137	138	139	90	90	90	91	92	93	93
17	50th	108	109	110	111	113	114	115	64	65	65	66	67	67	68
	90th	122	122	123	125	126	127	128	78	79	79	80	81	81	82
	95th	125	126	127	129	130	131	132	82	83	83	84	85	85	86
	99th	133	133	134	136	137	138	139	90	90	91	91	92	93	93

BP, blood pressure

* The 90th percentile is 1.28 SD, 95th percentile is 1.645 SD, and the 99th percentile is 2.326 SD over the mean. For research purposes, the standard deviations in appendix table B–1 allow one to compute BP Z-scores and percentiles for girls with height percentiles given in table 4 (i.e., the 5th, 10th, 25th, 50th, 75th, 90th, and 95th percentiles). These height percentiles must be converted to height Z-scores given by (5% = -1.645; 10% = -1.28; 25% = -0.68; 50% = 0; 75% = 0.68; 90% = 1.28; 95% = 1.645) and then computed according to the methodology in steps 2–4 described in appendix B. For children with height percentiles other than these, follow steps 1–4 as described in appendix B.

Source: National High Blood Pressure Education Program Working Group on High Blood Pressure in Children and Adolescents. (2004). The fourth report on the diagnosis, evaluation, and treatment of high blood pressure in children and adolescents. *Pediatrics, 114*(2), 555-576. Used with permission.

(2) Calcium channel blockers (e.g., nifedipine, verapamil, amlodipine).
b. Other available antihypertensive drugs used in children
  (1) Diuretics (e.g., furosemide, hydrochlorothiazide).
  (2) Central alpha-2 agonists (e.g., clonidine, alpha-methyldopa) and beta blockers (e.g., propranolol, atenolol).
  (3) Smooth muscle vasodilators (e.g., hydralazine, minoxidil, diazoxide, nitroprusside).
  (4) Alpha-beta blockers (e.g., labetalol).

E. Hypertension with proteinuria.
  1. In children and adolescents, proteinuria must be defined as fixed proteinuria. Must first rule out postural proteinuria through the use of split 24-hour urines or first morning spot protein to creatinine ratios.
  2. In early stages of CKD, proteinuria should be treated aggressively to try to attain normal protein to creatinine ratios (<0.2) with angiotensin-converting enzyme inhibitors (ACEI) or angiotensin II receptor blockers (ARBs) (Stevens & Levin, 2013).
  3. In the later stages of CKD (3/4/5), the treatment of proteinuria may be more difficult due to decreasing function and hyperkalemia.

VIII. Manual urinalysis microscopic exam. The microscopic examination of urine sediment includes the study of formed elements (e.g., WBCs, RBCs, casts, and crystals) (Berry, 1980).

A. WBC: considered abnormal if > 10 white cells/mm^3 in a midstream urine sample. Neutrophils are seen in UTIs, contaminated samples, proliferative glomerulonephritis, and interstitial nephritis.

B. RBC: abnormal if > 5 red cells/mm^3 in uncentrifuged urine. Microscopy can distinguish anatomically normal RBCs (the lower urinary tract) or dysmorphic RBCs (glomerular origin).

C. Casts: produced by cellular debris in the renal tubule.
  1. Hyaline casts: present in proteinuric states.
  2. RBC casts: glomerular bleeding.
  3. WBC casts: renal inflammation due to pyelonephritis or immunologically mediated disease.
  4. Epithelial casts: may be seen during recovery from acute tubular necrosis.

D. Crystals: cystine, uric acid, or dyhydroxadenine.

Table 5.9

Foods High in Potassium

1. Standard infant formula
2. Tomatoes and tomato products
3. Potatoes (white and sweet)
4. Oranges, orange juice, and bananas
5. Salt substitutes
6. Milk, all types
7. Raisins and prunes (dried fruit)

SECTION G
Treatment of Secondary Issues Related to Chronic Kidney Disease

I. Electrolyte imbalances.

A. Metabolic acidosis.
  1. Can occur as early as CKD stage 1, depending on the underlying disease process.
  2. Maintaining bicarbonate level > 22 mEq/L will optimize growth.
  3. Aggressive management of acidosis can also prevent secondary hyperkalemia.

B. Hyperkalemia.
  1. Can also occur as early as CKD stage 1 depending on the underlying disease process.
  2. Maintaining the potassium level can be challenging.
    a. First line treatment is through dietary potassium restriction. Foods high in potassium are listed in Table 5.9.
    b. Treatment of acidosis with supplemental bicarbonate may be necessary.
    c. Limiting or discontinuing ACEI/ARBs may be necessary.
    d. When moderate to severe hyperkalemia persists despite strict adherence to dietary restrictions, a potassium binder may be needed.

II. Growth and development.

A. Close monitoring of all children with CKD through serial height and weight measurements is imperative to recognize and combat early growth delays.

1. Pay close attention to and intervene aggressively with flat growth curves and those who fall off their own personal growth curves.
2. Variations in height velocity most closely reflect renal causes for growth delays.

B. The greatest velocity of height growth occurs in children up to 3 years of age and only until bones are fused around the mid-teens.

C. Calculation of predicted height should be done early in CKD.
   1. Boys: [Paternal height (cm) + (maternal height (cm) + 5)]/2.
   2. Girls: [Paternal height (cm) + (maternal height (cm) – 5)/2.

D. Evaluate growth velocity at least yearly.

E. If GFR < 70 mL/min/1.73 m^2 and growth velocity is < –2SD/year growth hormone should be considered.

F. See the Nutrition Section at end of chapter.

III. Anemia management in CKD.

A. Early in CKD stage 2, usually once the GFR drops below 70 mL/min/1.73 m^2, the production of erythropoietin decreases and continues to drop with decreasing kidney function.

B. Anemia is equally devastating in children as in adults. Decreased energy levels from anemia can lead to deterioration in the ability to:
   1. Exercise.
   2. Participate in the normal activities of childhood.
   3. Learn.

C. Correcting anemia in children with CKD based on K-DOQI Clinical Practice Guidelines for Anemia Management (NKF, 2007).
   1. Iron management.
      a. Determine degree of iron deficiency: must have enough available iron to produce red blood cell (KDOQI Anemia Guidelines [NKF, 2007]).
         (1) Quarterly serum levels of iron, iron binding capacity, and ferritin (more frequently if medication changes are made).
         (2) Calculated transferrin saturation goal is > 20%. Transferrin saturation and serum levels required to maintain erythropoiesis in pediatric patients are lower than in adults.
         (3) Ferritin goal is between 100–800 ng/mL.
         (4) Ferritin levels > 800 ng/mL constitute iron overload.

      b. Treat iron deficiency.
         (1) Patients who are not iron overloaded: oral iron supplements (elemental iron 3 to 6 mg/kg/day).
         (2) For pediatric patients who are unable to maintain adequate iron stores with oral supplements alone: IV iron, with dose based on the patient's weight.
         (3) The exact dosing, frequency, and appropriate monitoring of IV iron therapy will depend on the iron preparation chosen. Anaphylactoid reactions appear to occur more frequently with iron dextran, and labile or free iron reactions are more frequent with nondextran forms of iron.
   2. Erythropoiesis-stimulating agents (ESAs) treatment.
      a. Therapy benefits.
         (1) Minimizes need for blood transfusions.
         (2) Improved tolerance for exercise and oxygen consumption.
         (3) Leads to regression of ventricular hypertrophy.
         (4) Improved cognitive function.
      b. Administering ESAs.
         (1) Initiate therapy when the hemoglobin is less than the 5th percentile of the normal, adjusted for age and sex (NKF, 2007).
         (2) Darbepoetin alfa (Aranesp®).
            (a) Initial dose: 0.45 mcg/kg/dose once weekly.
            (b) Allow at least 4 weeks of therapy to see full effect before increasing the dose.
         (3) Epoetin alfa (Epogen®).
            (a) Starting dose 50 U/kg subcutaneous three times per week.
            (b) Can be given IV during hemodialysis.
      c. Monitoring therapy with ESAs (KDOQI Anemia Guidelines [NKF, 2007]).
         (1) Monthly CBCs or more frequently after a dose change.
         (2) Maintenance within the target Hgb range: adjustment of ESA dose and detection and correction of etiologies that hinder response, such as low iron stores or high parathyroid hormone (PTH) levels.
         (3) Recommendations for target Hgb levels in children treated with ESAs are the same as for adults.
         (4) Evaluating hyporesponsiveness to epoetin therapy.
            (a) Iron deficiency is frequent in children with CKD and requires treatment with as much or more supplemental iron than in adults. A typical adult male receives only 5% of his daily iron needs from his diet, compared with 30% for a

1-year old infant. Iron deficiency can be exacerbated by blood loss with hemodialysis. Pediatric patients have a comparatively small blood volume, so the obligatory 8 mL/m² of blood lost per treatment in the extracorporeal system can worsen anemia faster than in an adult (Warady et al., 2004).

   (b) Correct secondary hyperparathyroidism.

   (c) Detect and stop blood loss.

   (d) Treat underlying infectious, inflammatory, or malignant processes.

   (e) Diagnose complicating underlying hematologic diseases, such as sickle cell disease or thalassemia.

   (f) Diagnose and treat other vitamin deficiencies, such as folate or B12.

   (g) Detect and treat causes of hemolysis.

  d. Minimizing the trauma of repeated injections.

   (1) Play activities are most useful for children to work through the potential fear and trauma of medical experiences. Types of therapeutic play activities include:

   (a) Handling the medication vial, syringe, and alcohol wipes, especially for young children.

   (b) Using syringes without needles for water play, painting, and decorating sugar cookies (dispensing frosting).

   (c) Free medical play allowing for safe exploration of equipment and supplies without specific guidance (rather than adult-directed).

   (d) Personalizing fabric dolls with fabric markers or paints which can then be used to let the child practice giving injections.

   (e) Sample injection play techniques.

   (f) Create reward stickers for mastering the experience.

   (g) Have the child count to 10 during an injection.

   (h) Have the child exhale to blow the pain away.

   (i) Circle the injection site and draw a smiley face

   (j) Have the child make a drawing of what he or she is feeling.

   (k) Have the child focus on or hold a favorite toy during the injection.

   (2) Patient and family education and support should include the importance of anemia management, not just how to give injections.

   (a) Should include the recognition that repeated injections can become a focus of stress and negotiation between parent or caregiver and child and can reduce the ability to continue with therapy, especially at home.

   (b) Tips for overcoming barriers to patient and family adherence include administering the medication at the same time each day; warming the product to room temperature before administering it; having the patient self-inject, if developmentally age-appropriate; having the parent demonstrate the technique of administration in front of the child; and avoiding the use of terms such as shot, stick, pinch, or bee sting in favor of a descriptive phrase such as medicine under the skin. Similarly, words such as *hurt* or *discomfort* should be used instead of words with a more negative connotation, such as pain. Most importantly, be honest.

   (c) Learning objectives for the patient and family.

   i. State the current ESA dose.

   ii. Demonstrate the ability to give the ESA injection.

   iii. Explain the necessity and method for site rotation.

 3. Blood transfusions of packed red blood cells (PRBC).

  a. Consider when Hgb less than 7 gm/dL (Hct less than 21%), patient is actively bleeding, patient has suffered acute blood loss as in a clotted hemodialysis system, or patient is symptomatic from anemia.

  b. Volume of PRBC transfusion is determined according to the patient's size and desired Hgb: start at 10 to 15 mL/kg body weight given over several hours during dialysis.

IV. Renal osteodystrophy/metabolic bone disease.

A. Basic principles.

 1. A prominent clinical finding in pediatric patients with CKD, especially growing children.

 2. Caused by abnormalities in calcium-phosphorus homeostasis and bone metabolism as well as chronic acidosis associated with CKD.

 3. Signs and symptoms may result as early as stage 3, CKD, when the GFR < 50% of normal.

 4. Should be treated early to prevent severe bony deformities in the growing child.

B. Signs and symptoms of renal osteodystrophy in children. These bone abnormalities can be seen frequently in untreated children with CKD of long duration.

1. Bone deformities.
    a. Swelling and enlargement of wrists, ankles, knees, and medial end of clavicles due to metaphyseal widening at the growth plates of long bones.
    b. Bowing of long bones (bowed legs or knocked knees) in weight-bearing children.
    c. Rachitic rosary (widening of the costochondral junctions) of the ribs.
    d. Ulnar deviation of the hands from epiphyseal fractures.
    e. Slipped femoral capital epiphysis (SCFE).
    f. Fibrous tissue accumulation within and adjacent to the epiphyseal growth plate cartilage in association with secondary hyperparathyroidism.
    g. Adynamic bone disease.
2. Skeletal pain.
    a. May develop gradually over many months.
    b. May be aggravated by weight-bearing, changes in posture, or physical inactivity.
    c. Frequently involves lower back, hips, and legs in weight-bearing children.
3. Radiographic findings.
    a. Normal, if renal osteodystrophy is early or mild.
    b. Widening of and/or fraying of the long bones at the growth plates (epiphyses).
    c. Bowing deformities of the femur, tibia, or fibula.
    d. Subperiosteal erosions from secondary hyperparathyroidism.
    e. Patchy osteosclerosis in the spine, skull, or long bones.

C. Proximal myopathy: associated with hypocalcemia.

D. Extraosseous soft tissue calcification.

E. Impaired height growth.

F. Biochemical features.
    1. Hypocalcemia and hyperphosphatemia from CKD.
    2. Hypophosphatemia is possible if tubular as well as glomerular disease is present, such as in congenital forms of obstructive uropathy.
    3. Uncorrected acidosis: bone becomes a buffer for extra acid in the system.
    4. Secondary hyperparathyroidism.
    5. Elevated serum alkaline phophatase: bone is the source of the highest serum fraction of alkaline phosphatase in normal children and may be used as a marker of the severity of renal osteodystrophy in children. However, serum alkaline phosphatase also increases acutely with therapy before it decreases to normal with bone healing.
    6. Normal or decreased blood levels of 1,25-dihydroxycholecalciferol: depends on whether the diseased kidney can still produce partial or adequate amounts.

G. Monitoring and treatment of osteodystrophy.
    1. The goal is to normalize growth and prevent development of bone deformities.
    2. Monitoring (KDOQI Nutrition Guidelines, 2008).
        a. Monthly monitoring of calcium, phosphorous, alkaline phosphatase, and bicarbonate level.
        b. At least quarterly monitoring of intact PTH.
        c. Annual radiographs for bone age and signs of renal osteodystrophy in children treated with growth hormone and patients at CKD stage 5.
    3. Control serum phosphorous with diet and phosphate binders.
    4. Avoid aluminum-containing phosphate binders in infants and children.
    5. Correct hypocalcemia and avoid hypercalcemia.
        a. Maintain calcium in high normal range for availability for bone formation and to suppress parathyroid hormone production.
        b. Use calcium supplements and vitamin D analogs (e.g., calcitriol (1,25-dihydroxycholecalciferol) as needed.
        c. Prescribe higher or lower hemodialysis or peritoneal dialysate calcium concentration as needed.
    6. Normalize parathyroid hormone.
        a. Maintain levels between 200 and 300 pg/mL (KDOQI Nutrition Guidelines, 2008).
        b. Usually requires treatment with vitamin D analogs (calcitriol). Hypercalcemia may occur with higher doses of calcitriol, especially when used concomitantly with calcium-containing phosphate binders.
        c. Oversuppression of PTH: may retard normal bone growth and contribute to adynamic bone disease.
    7. Maintain normal vitamin D status.
        a. May be maintained with calcitriol.
        b. Treatment with calcitriol is commonly needed in the anephric patient.
        c. Supplement with Ergocalciferol (see Table 5.10).

H. Adynamic bone disease.
    1. May occur frequently in children with renal osteodystrophy; it accounts for 15% to 20% of histologic bone lesions in some studies of children (Salusky & Goodman, 2001).
    2. Caused by factors that directly or indirectly lower osteoblastic activity that results in subnormal rate of bone formation, including:
        a. Decreased PTH secretion.
        b. Calcitriol therapy.
        c. Calcium containing medications.
        d. High dialysate calcium concentration.
        e. Aluminum toxicity (infrequent now because of

avoidance of aluminum-containing phosphate binders in pediatric patients).
3. Signs and symptoms.
   a. Higher incidence of hypercalcemia.
   b. Normal or low serum intact PTH; alkaline phosphatase levels are usually low.
   c. Increased incidence of soft tissue calcification.
   d. Pathologic bone fractures.
4. Treatment.
   a. Currently uncertainty about effectiveness of any treatment.
   b. Consider withholding calcitriol therapy and calcium-containing medications until the serum PTH increases to desired levels.

I. Osteomalacia induced by glucocorticoids.
   1. Characterized by loss of bone and increased risk of fractures as a result of increased osteoclast-mediated bone resorption and decreased osteoblast-mediated bone formation. The severity is dependent on the dose and duration of glucocorticoid therapy (Grossman et al., 2010).
   2. It is a complication of glucocorticoids widely used for treatment of glomerulonephritis and kidney transplantation in children and adolescents.
   3. Very high rates of osteoblast-mediated bone formation are required to maintain adequate bone mineralization in the growing child.
   4. High rates of osteoclast-mediated bone resorption may prevent adolescents from reaching peak bone mass.
   5. Prevention and treatment.
      a. Use lowest possible effective dose of glucocorticoid (Grossman et al., 2010).
      b. Consider calcium and/or calcitriol therapy as needed.

SECTION H

Kidney Replacement Therapies in Children

I. Indications for dialysis.

A. Absolute indications for children same as for adults: hyperkalemia and hypervolemia that are not responsive to conservative treatment.

B. Hyperammonemia is a medical emergency caused by inborn errors of metabolism, usually urea cycle defects.

Table 5.10

Recommended Supplementation for Vitamin D Deficiency and Insufficiency in Children with CKD

Serum 25 (OH)D (ng/mL)	Definition	Ergocalciferol (Vitamin D2) or Cholecalciferol (Vitamin D3) Dosing	Duration (months)
< 5	Severe vitamin D deficiency	8,000 IU/day orally or enterally x 4 weeks or (50,000 IU/week x 4 wks) then 4,000 IU/day x 4 wks or (50,000 IU 2x/month for 2 months) x 2 months	3
5–15	Mild vitamin D deficiency	4,000 IU daily orally or enterally x 12 weeks or 50,000 units every other week x 12 weeks	3
16–30	Vitamin D insufficiency	50,000 IU every 4 weeks or 2,000 IU daily	3

Reprinted from *American Journal of Kidney Diseases, 54*(6), National Kidney Foundation, KDOQI Clinical Practice Guideline for Nutrition in Children with CKD: 2008 Update, S11–S104, with permission from Elsevier.

1. It usually presents in the neonatal period if due to inborn errors of metabolism.
2. The patient may need to be treated with hemodialysis initially to rapidly reduce the blood ammonia level with the option of tandem continuous renal replacement therapies (CRRT) to help prevent rebound of the blood ammonia level.
3. Careful monitoring for hypokalemia and hypophosphatemia is necessary during hemodialysis in children who do not have kidney failure. May need to adjust dialysis solution (see section on Hemodialysis for Children below).

C. Poisoning or intentional overdose with a dialyzable drug, such as theophylline, ethylene glycol, or valproic acid. Careful monitoring for hypokalemia and hypophosphatemia is necessary during hemodialysis in children who do not have kidney failure. (See III. Hemodialysis for Children below.)

D. Relative indications for adults and children.
   1. Congestive heart failure (CHF), fluid overload.
   2. Severe hypertension.
   3. Severe acidosis.
   4. Severe hypernatremia.
   5. Uremic pericarditis.
   6. Uremic encephalopathy.
   7. Severe hypocalcemia.
   8. Severe hyperphosphatemia.

E. Additional relative indications in pediatric patients.
1. Poor growth and development.
2. Fluid restriction that prevents adequate nutritional intake.

F. Subjective indications.
1. Anorexia, fatigue, drowsiness, and general weakness.
2. School absenteeism or deteriorating school performance.

G. Biochemical criteria.
1. Same as adults.
2. Serum creatinine will be lower in smaller children with CKD stage 5. Infants may have serum creatinine as low as 4 to 5 mg/dL with CKD stage 5.

II. Factors to consider when choosing a treatment modality.

A. Effectiveness in controlling problems related to CKD stage 5.

B. Appropriateness for child's potential for vascular or peritoneal access.

C. Ability for family (other-care) or patient to do self-care.

D. Appropriateness in the presence of other medical comorbidities.

E. Appropriateness for developmental progress of the child.

F. Consistent with child's body image.

G. Least disruptive of lifestyle and social interaction with family and peers.

H. Treatment options.
1. Hemodialysis.
2. Peritoneal dialysis.
3. Transplantation.
4. Continuous renal replacement therapies (CRRT).
   a. Continuous venovenous hemofiltration with or without dialysis (CVVH, CVVHD).
   b. Slow continuous ultrafiltration (SCUF).
5. Comfort care only when the above treatments are not acceptable; maintain maximum comfort while not attempting to prolong life.

III. Hemodialysis for children.

A. Vascular access.
1. Acute hemodialysis catheters in children.
   a. Should be smaller than the caliber of the veins into which they are to be placed to prevent obstruction of venous return distal to the catheter.

b. Subclavian vein catheter placement should be avoided to prevent subclavian vein stenosis which may compromise the future potential for permanent access in the upper extremities, either arteriovenous (AV) fistula or graft.
2. Chronic hemodialysis access (Warady et al., 2004).
   a. Whenever possible preserve sites for future access by protecting veins from routine venipuncture by hospital personnel.
   b. The arteriovenous fistula (AVF).
      (1) Can be placed in most children who weigh more than 20 kg.
      (2) Can be placed in children as small as 10 kg by a skilled surgeon using microvascular techniques.
      (3) Vessel mapping (duplex ultrasound of the bilateral upper extremities) should be performed to assess patency and suitability of the arteries and veins for creation of the AVF.
      (4) Maturation of the newly created AVF should be assessed by the most experienced or "expert" nurse at 4 to 6 weeks. If the AV fistula requires transposition, it may require more time to develop.
   c. Arteriovenous graft (AVG).
      (1) An AVG is the next best option if an AVF is not possible.
      (2) In the upper extremity, should be placed in the nondominant arm whenever possible.
      (3) Can be placed in a loop configuration in the lower extremity (thigh), even in a small child weighing greater than 10 kg, to offer a larger surface area for cannulation.
      (4) Will need at least 2 to 4 weeks for maturation.
   d. Semipermanent cuffed catheter.
      (1) May be the only option for some children, including:
         (a) Infants weighing less than 10 kg.
         (b) Children and adolescents with failure of an AVF and/or AVG.
      (2) May be needed as a bridge to permanent access.
   e. Pain management options for AVF or AVG needle insertion (see Principles of Atraumatic Care below).
      (1) Crying may be a response to fear of needle insertion as well as to needle insertion itself.
      (2) The key to success is to offer a variety of pain management options, soothe anxieties, and reinforce desired behaviors.
   f. The APRN's role in managing vascular access complications.
      (1) HD catheter malfunction.
         (a) Order a thrombolytic agent (TPA).

(b) Consider a chest x-ray to verify placement of catheter if no improvement after TPA.

(c) Coordinate replacement of catheter if unable to achieve prescribed blood flows.

(2) HD catheter infection.

(a) Obtain blood cultures from both venous and arterial ports.

(b) Treat the patient prophylactically with gram positive and negative coverage until blood culture results available.

(3) AVF stenosis/thrombosis. Intraaccess blood flow measurements over time are the best surveillance methods for assessing the AV fistula and detecting dysfunction.

B. The hemodialysis prescription.

1. Choice of dialyzer (Warady et al., 2004).

a. The dialyzer's surface area should approximate the child's surface area.

b. The blood volume should be small enough to provide safe extracorporeal volume.

c. The ultrafiltration coefficient should be adequate to remove the desired amount of fluid at the prescribed blood flow.

d. The clearance should allow adequate dialysis at the prescribed blood flow rate.

2. Bloodline options in neonatal-size and pediatric-size provide substantial reductions in blood volume as compared to adult bloodlines.

3. Safe extracorporeal volume (ECV).

a. ECV = dialyzer volume + bloodline volume/estimated blood volume (EBV).

b. ECV should be less than 10% of the child's EBV if possible.

(1) EBV = target weight in kg x 70 mL (80 mL if the patient is less than 6 months old).

(2) If the ECV must be 10% to 12.5% of EBV, prime dialyzer with a volume expander such as 5% albumin in saline.

(3) If the ECV must be 12.5% to 15%, it may be safest to prime the dialyzer with reconstituted whole blood.

(4) If the ECV must be greater than 15%, the dialyzer must be primed with reconstituted whole blood.

(5) If the system is primed with whole blood, the system's contents are not returned at the end of the dialysis treatment.

4. The blood flow rate (QB) is determined by what the access will allow and the desired Kt/V. A QB of 200 to 350 mL/min/1.73 m^2 is usually optimal.

5. The dialysate composition should be based on the metabolic needs of the child, just as for the adult.

C. Adequacy of treatment (Warady et al., 2004).

1. Assessment includes targets plus presence of uremic symptoms.

a. NKF-KDOQI (2006) recommends a prescribed KT/V > 1.3 and delivered KT/V > 1.2 (Clinical Practice Guidelines for Hemodialysis Adequacy Update [NKF, 2006]).

b. The urea kinetic modeling (UKM).

(1) Kt/V from formal UKM is desirable for children.

(2) Double pool kinetics are more accurate because of the child's total body water relative to high clearances.

(3) Urea rebound in most children is independent of size.

(4) The methods for calculating double pool Kt/V and PCR are based on predialysis, 30 seconds, and 15-minute postdialysis BUN samples have been validated for pediatric patients and are acceptable alternatives to formal UKM (Clinical Practice Guidelines for Hemodialysis Adequacy Update [NKF, 2006]).

c. The assessment of clinical condition includes presence of uremic symptoms, nutritional state, growth, development, school performance, and functional status.

2. Special considerations for Kt/V and PCR in children.

a. Needed for growing children because of their dynamic metabolic activity.

b. Should be reassessed at least monthly because of constantly changing growth and metabolic requirements.

D. Reuse of dialyzers for chronic hemodialysis. There is little information available for children.

E. The dialysate delivery system should be volumetrically controlled for safety of fluid removal, especially in small children.

F. The dialysis procedure.

1. Predialysis: assessment.

a. Based on the size and developmental stage of the child.

b. In the acute setting, must also include the severity of illness.

2. Treatment plan.

a. Ultrafiltration (UF). The actual body weight should be reassessed often in children due to growth and frequency of changes in dietary intake, adherence to fluid restrictions, or vomiting and diarrhea.

b. Anticoagulation is based on the target weight.

(1) Heparin prime: 25 to 50 units/kg.

(2) Continuous heparin infusion rate: 10 to 25 units/kg to target the activated clotting time (ACT) to 1.5 times the normal.

(3) Neonates are at increased risk of intracranial hemorrhage and need tight heparinization.

3. Intradialysis. Frequency of vital signs.
   a. Based on size, developmental age, and the individual child's needs.
   b. Vital signs include blood pressure, heart rate, and respiratory rate.
   c. Noninvasive monitors designed to automatically measure BP, mean arterial BP, and heart rate are versatile and effective for neonates and children.
   d. Continuous arterial BP monitoring may be the best choice for acute hemodialysis treatments in unstable patients.
   e. Resist the urge to substitute frequent vital signs for close patient observation just because the patient is a child. Frequent repetition of BP measurements (e.g., every 15 minutes) may lead to patient agitation and result in unreliable values.
      (1) Agitation, vomiting, yawning, and color changes may precede vital sign changes.
      (2) Small children rarely verbalize their symptoms, so observation of behavior is essential.
4. Continuous EKG and pulse oximetry monitoring is desirable for children weighing less than 20 kg.
5. Continuous monitoring with a reliable bed scale may be useful in children weighing less than 10 kg.
6. Blood volume monitoring.
   a. Critical in patients < 35 kg.
   b. Reduces dialysis symptoms and episodes of hypotension.
   c. Helps refine target weight more effectively during a dialysis treatment.
7. Diversionary activities.
   a. Useful for maximizing the child's cooperation with therapy, especially in the chronic setting.
   b. Must be age appropriate.
   c. Include educational as well as entertainment activities.
8. Postdialysis assessment.
   a. Based on the size and developmental stage of the child.
   b. In the acute setting, must also include the severity of illness.
   c. Should include a plan for communication with the family regarding the events of the treatment.

G. Acute complications are similar to adults with the following exceptions.
   1. Hypotension.
      a. Treatment.
         (1) Trendelenburg position and minimization of UF rate.

(2) Normal saline bolus starting at 5 mL/kg.
(3) Assess for hypoalbuminemia in the malnourished or persistently nephrotic child and consider an albumin bolus to acutely raise the oncotic pressure.
   b. Prevention.
      (1) Accurate estimation of actual body weight and careful assessment of intradialytic changes in vascular volume.
      (2) Blood volume monitoring (see above).
      (3) Consideration should be given to increasing treatments to four or more times per week in small children with excessive fluid gains, especially from dietary intake required to provide adequate nutrition.
2. Potential problems related to treatment of hyperammonemia with hemodialysis or CRRT in patients with normal kidney function.
   a. Hypokalemia which can be prevented by adding potassium to the dialysate bath.
   b. Hypophosphatemia which may be severe due to the removal of phosphorus. Serum phosphorus should be monitored frequently during the treatment, and phosphorus supplements should be given as needed by intravenous bolus or addition of extra phosphorus to total parenteral nutrition fluids.

IV. Peritoneal dialysis in children.

A. Indications for peritoneal dialysis (PD).
   1. PD is the dialysis treatment of choice for infants and small children.
   2. The characteristics of the peritoneal cavity.
      a. The peritoneal membrane in children is very large in relation to body surface area.
      b. In males, the peritoneal membrane lines the abdominal cavity covering the abdominal viscera.
      c. In females, the ovaries and fallopian tubes open into the peritoneal cavity.

B. Access placement. Based on the International Society of Peritoneal Dialysis Guidelines, it is suggested to use a double-cuff PD catheter with a downward or lateral subcutaneous tunnel configuration that is placed by a surgeon or nephrologist experienced in PD catheter placement (Warady et al., 2012).

C. Special considerations for the use of peritoneal dialysis in the treatment of acute kidney injury (AKI) and acute kidney failure (AKF) in children.
   1. Manual exchanges in infants when exchange volume is small (less than 50 mL).
      a. Needed when cycler tubing dead-space is high percentage of exchange volume to prevent recirculation.

b. Can be used with commercially available closed tubing sets with buretrol for measuring volume in 1mL increments.

c. Requires external heat source for dialysate to avoid patient hypothermia. Dry heat can be applied to the dialysate bag and/or coiled portion of the delivery tubing to warm the dialysate to 37°C.

2. Automatic PD cyclers.
a. Can deliver a minimum dialysate volume of 50 mL with 10 mL increments.
b. Caution: some cyclers that automatically cycle based upon slowness of the drain rate may not be effective because the drain rate for an exchange volume of less than 700 mL may be so slow that refilling begins before drainage is complete. Patient overfill occurs.

D. Special considerations for the use of peritoneal dialysis in the treatment of CKD stage 5 in children: continuous cycling peritoneal dialysis (CCPD).
1. Preferred to reduce the risk of peritonitis when 4 or more exchanges/day must be performed for adequacy and desired UF.
2. Less demanding and can help prevent caregiver burn-out.
3. Therapy of choice for children with highly permeable peritoneal membranes.
4. Can be done simultaneously with enteral tube feedings to remove the fluid as it is given to prevent fluid overload and still provide desired nutrition.
5. May allow for uninterrupted daily school attendance.

E. The PD prescription.
1. Recommendations for adequacy values currently do not differ from adults; however, little information is available for children.
2. Estimating total body water (V) and body surface area (BSA).
a. V should be estimated by the Mellits-Cheek method in children using actual body weight.
b. BSA can be estimated from a body surface area nomogram (available in The Harriett Lane Handbook) or the method of Dubois.
3. Urine collections for assessing residual kidney function.
a. This is more difficult in infants in diapers, toddlers being toilet trained, and children with enuresis or percutaneous ureterostomies, nephrostomies, or vesicostomies.
b. It is recommended that the collection be done on the same day as the complete dialysate collection.
4. The initial dialysis prescription.
a. The recommended target exchange volume is

1100 mL/m² (KDOQI Practice Guidelines for Peritoneal Dialysis Adequacy [NKF, 2000]).
b. Verify that the delivered dose equals the prescribed dose.
c. Individualize for the patient's growth and nutritional needs which may require frequent changes after the initial prescription.

F. Training.
1. Must be performed by an experienced PD nurse with pediatric training, using a formalized teaching program that has clear objectives and criteria and also incorporates adult-learning principles for care partners.
2. Retraining should be provided to all caregivers periodically.
3. Evaluation of the PD technique should be conducted after development of a peritonitis episode (Warady et al., 2012).

G. Family support.
1. Attention should be given to:
a. The potential for disruptions in family life.
b. The potential for inattention to healthy siblings.
c. The increased caregiver burden associated with providing pediatric care.
2. Caring for the parental caregiver.
a. The effects of caregiving on health and wellbeing can include:
(1) Sleep deprivation.
(2) Poor eating habits.
(3) Failure to exercise.
(4) Postponement of or failure to make medical appointments for their child.
b. Reduce personal stress through the early recognition of warning signs, such as irritability, sleep problems, and forgetfulness.
c. May include respite care offered in-center or in the home depending on institutional or financial resources.
d. Advise the parental caregiver to prepare questions ahead of time and bring someone else along to an appointment with the physician/APRN/PA.
3. School attendance, growth, and developmental progress should be measured serially in pediatric patients on PD.

H. Complications of PD.
1. An umbilical, ventral, or inguinal hernia may occur more often in children.
2. Chylous ascites is rare in infants and children, but must be considered in setting of cloudy peritoneal effluent (Cheung & Khwaja, 2008).
a. Characteristic "milky" appearance of the drained peritoneal fluid due to high concentration of triglycerides (> 110 mg/dL) originating from

lymph within the abdominal cavity.
b. Potential causes:
(1) Damage or obstruction of the lymphatic system during insertion of the PD catheter.
(2) Abdominal malignancy.
(3) Liver cirrhosis.
(4) Infection.
c. Symptoms include abdominal distension, dyspnea, postprandial pain, and nausea.
d. Treatment consists of a low fat diet with supplemental medium-chain triglyercides (MCTs) to reduce lymph flow and allow spontaneous healing of the lymph leak.
3. PD catheter tunnel and exit-site infections.
a. More frequent in diapered infants and children with draining nephrostomies, ureterostomies, or vesicostomies, and in children who pull at their catheter or traumatize the exit site.
b. Oral antibiotics for uncomplicated PD catheter exit-site infections should be initiated depending on culture and sensitivities for a minimum of 2 weeks and for at least 7 days after complete resolution of the infection. If *S. aureus* or *P. aeruginosa*, treatment for 3 weeks is recommended (Warady et al., 2012).
4. Peritonitis.
a. The rate of occurrence is 1 per 18.8 catheter months (NAPRTCS, 2011).
b. Rates higher in pediatric vs. adult patients.
c. Special sources of system contamination in pediatric patients include biting the catheter, undoing the tubing connections for play, pulling on the catheter, and picking at the catheter exit site. These accidents may happen even with the most vigilant care partner's attention.
d. To confirm the diagnosis of peritonitis in the presence of cloudy effluent, obtain cell count, differential count, and culture of the effluent. Empiric diagnosis can be made if the effluent white blood cell (WBC) count is > 100/mm^3, and at least 50% of the WBCs are polymorpho-nuclear leukocytes (Warady et al., 2012).

V. Kidney transplantation in children.

A. Preferred mode of treatment for most children with CKD stage 5.

B. Related statistics (North American Pediatric Renal Transplant Cooperative Study [NAPRTCS] 2010 Report).
1. There were approximately 500 pediatric (ages 0 to 19 years) kidney transplants performed annually from 1987 to 2010.
2. Living related donors accounted for about 42% of all pediatric kidney transplants.
3. The majority of children were greater than 5 years of age when transplanted. However, successful transplantation can be achieved in specialized centers even in the first year of life.
4. 24% of pediatric patients receive preemptive transplants compared with approximately 1% of adult patients.
a. Frequent in children because of an active promotion of transplant by pediatric nephrology programs through educating possible living donor candidates.
b. And, patients are simultaneously listed for deceased donor transplant.

C. Preparation for transplant.
1. Correct or prevent any complications of CKD stage 5 that might affect the kidney transplant procedure.
a. Control or improve renal osteodystrophy.
b. Avoid transfusions to prevent the development of cytotoxic anti-HLA antibodies.
(1) Transfusions are the second most frequent cause of sensitization.
(2) ESAs can be used to treat anemia. (See section on Anemia Management.)
2. Evaluate and correct any lower urinary tract abnormalities before transplant, such as posterior urethral valves, ureterovesical or uretopelvic junction obstruction, bladder abnormalities, or vesicoureteral reflux.
3. Poor bladder function can cause damage to the newly transplanted kidney. Corrective interventions may include double voiding, intiating self-catheterization, bladder augmentation, or Mitranoff procedure (Ohler & Cupples, 2008).
4. Perform native nephrectomy before transplant for specific indications only.
a. Polycystic kidney disease owing to space issues.
b. Severe or poorly controlled hypertension despite medical therapy.
c. Congenital nephrotic syndrome.
d. Drash syndrome because the native kidneys are at high risk for development of Wilm's tumor.
5. Inspect the urinary tract, skin, teeth, and sinuses carefully for infections and treat as needed.
6. Children should be fully immunized prior to transplantation. Live virus immunizations, such as varicella or measles, should be administered at least 2 months before transplant.
7. Common blood tests for transplantation evaluation (Ohler & Cupples, 2008).
a. Blood grouping (ABO typing) and human lymphocyte antigen typing (HLA typing).
b. Panel of reactive antibodies (PRA).
c. Chemistry panel and complete blood count.
d. Urinalysis and urine culture.

e. Lipid panel.

f. Viral screening (Cytomegalovirus (CMV), Epstein-Barr virus (EBV), hepatitis profile, tuberculosis skin test, measles, mumps, rubella, varicella zoster titers, and HIV).

D. Contraindications for transplant in children.
1. HIV infection (varies depending on individual transplant center).
2. Uncontrolled malignancy; generally, a malignancy should be in remission for 2 years with patient off chemotherapy.
3. Elevated levels of anti-GBM antibodies.
4. Multiorgan failure.
5. Presence of cytotoxic antilymphocyte antibodies against the donor.

E. Delay transplant until the following condition or disease is no longer active.
1. Infection.
2. Hemolytic uremic syndrome.
3. Active liver disease.

F. Diseases with high rate of recurrence: focal segmental glomerulosclerosis (FSGS), systemic lupus erythematosus (SLE), and membranoproliferative glomerulonephritis (MPGN).

G. Complications of kidney transplant.
1. Delayed graft function.
   a. Refers to oliguria and decreased GFR or the requirement of dialysis posttransplant.
   b. Associated with decreased graft survival.
   c. Major causes in children.
      (1) Acute tubular necrosis (ATN) (Ohler & Cupples, 2008).
      (2) Results from damage to the proximal tubular membranes.
      (3) Present with oliguria prior to becoming anuric.
      (4) Long, cold ischemic times considered risk factor for developing ATN.
   d. Management includes avoiding nephrotoxic medications, conservative fluid management, monitoring serum potassium levels, and often, dialysis therapy.
2. Thrombosis of the renal artery, vein, or graft.
   a. More frequent complication in pediatric transplantation as compared with adult transplantation.
   b. More likely when a small donor kidney with small vessels is anastomosed to the small vessels of a small child.
   c. More likely when a large donor kidney is placed in the iliac fossa of a small child.
      (1) Swelling of the kidney or fluid collections

in that small space can compromise vascular flow.
      (2) This complication can be prevented by intraperitoneal location of the donor kidney.
3. Urinary tract obstruction or ureteral/bladder leak.
4. Hyperacute rejection.
   a. Results of preformed antibodies from antidonor antibodies and complement.
   b. Onset occurs immediately after reperfusion of the transplant or can occur days after the transplant.
   c. Signs and symptoms include:
      (1) Sudden loss of urine output.
      (2) Fever.
      (3) Systemic toxicity.
      (4) Pain in the area of graft placement.
   d. Ischemia, acidosis, and/or hypoxia occur in the transplanted tissue.
   e. Treatment requires a transplant nephrectomy.
5. Acute rejection.
   a. Onset occurs in days to weeks.
   b. Signs and symptoms include:
      (1) Hypertension.
      (2) Low grade fever.
      (3) Increase in creatinine.
      (4) Decreased urine output.
      (5) Pain over the graft.
   c. Diagnosis: kidney biopsy.
   d. Treatment.
      (1) Acute cellular rejection is treated with high dose corticosteroids.
      (2) Vascular rejection is treated with antibody therapy (choice depends on treatment center protocol).
6. Chronic allograft failure.
   a. The most frequent cause of graft loss in children as well as adults.
   b. Onset occurs in months to years.
   c. Signs and symptoms include a slow rise in serum creatinine, often with proteinuria and hypertension.
7. Failed graft.
   a. Occurs in approximately 10% of kidney transplants in children in the immediate posttransplant period.
   b. Leading cause of sensitization, which may limit future transplantation.
8. Hypertension.
   a. Occurs frequently after kidney transplantation in children, especially as a side effect of steroid and cyclosporine immunosuppressive therapy (Danovitch, 2010).
   b. May also be caused by acute or chronic rejection.
   c. May be the cause of significant morbidity in

children, including encephalopathy and neurologic sequelae.

d. Can have a detrimental effect on graft survival.

e. Treated aggressively with antihypertensive medications.

9. Hyperlipidemia.

a. Occurs frequently in children as a result of steroid and cyclosporine therapy.

b. Treat with dietary measures as appropriate.

10. Infections.

a. Pneumonia and urinary tract infections (UTI) are the most frequent infections that occur after kidney transplantation (Danovitch, 2010).

b. Opportunistic infections.

(1) Includes the same organisms as for adults, including bacterial, CMV, and EBV.

(2) *Pneumocystis carinii* pneumonia (PCP) occurs, especially when multiple immunosuppressive drugs, including prednisone, cyclosporine, MMF, and monoclonal or polyclonal antibodies, are used together.

(a) The highest risk is in the first few months after transplant.

(b) The risk can be reduced with antimicrobial prophylaxis (e.g., Bactrim®, pentamidine).

c. Varicella infection.

(1) The infection may be severe and lead to encephalitis, pneumonitis, hepatic dysfunction, and even death.

(2) Prevention.

(a) Immunization with live varicella vaccine before transplantation is recommended for all children without pretransplant varicella antibodies.

(b) Varicella-zoster immune globulin (VZIG) should be administered within 72 hours of exposure to children with no varicella immunity.

11. Recurrence of primary disease.

a. Similar to the adult experience for the following diseases: membranoproliferative glomerulonephritis, IgA nephropathy, lupus nephritis, membranous GN, and atypical HUS (Danovitch, 2010).

b. Focal glomerusclerosis recurs more frequently when the disease begins after the age of 6 or when the disease progresses rapidly to CKD stage 5.

c. Wilm's tumor has a negligible risk of recurrence or metastasis if the kidney transplant is performed two years after cancer therapy is completed.

d. In primary hyperoxaluria, graft failure is frequently related to oxalate deposits in the transplanted kidney. The best approach is combined kidney-liver transplant to interrupt production of excessive oxalate.

12. Malignancy.

a. There is an increased risk of malignancy in kidney transplant recipients because of chronic immunosuppressive therapy.

b. Lymphoma is the most frequent posttransplant neoplastic disorder in children.

c. Posttransplant lymphoproliferative disease (PTLD) occurs in approximately 1% of pediatric kidney transplants (Danovitch, 2010).

H. Immunosuppression therapy.

1. Corticosteroids.

a. The use of corticosteroids is decreasing due to toxicity (Danovitch, 2010).

b. The initial dose is high and then tapered to a lower maintenance dose. Smaller children often require a higher initial dosage per kilogram of body weight.

c. Acute rejection is treated with oral prednisone or IV methylprednisolone pulses.

d. Side effects are similar to those experienced by adults, except steroids also retard growth and pubertal development, and they may cause hyperactive behavior in the young child.

e. Growth impairment associated with steroid therapy in children.

(1) Is caused in part by steroid inhibition of bone formation.

(2) Improvement may be seen by changing to alternate day corticosteroid therapy; graft function is not affected.

(3) Growth hormone (GH) administration to stable kidney transplant patients.

(a) Results in increased growth velocity.

(b) GH has been associated with acute rejection or worsening of chronic rejection.

(c) To minimize the effects of GH on the immune system, it should not be started until at least 1 year posttransplant and should be discontinued if rejection episodes occur.

2. Azathioprine use is similar to that in adults. The dosage depends on whether azathioprine is used in dual or triple therapy and whether the bone marrow is suppressed.

3. Mycophenolate mofetil (CellCept®).

a. Now widely used instead of azathioprine in the pediatric transplant population.

b. Bone marrow suppression is less likely.

c. Gastrointestinal side effects in children may limit dosage.

4. Calcineurin inhibitors.

a. Cyclosporine.

(1) Has contributed to increased graft survival in children.

(2) May be absorbed or metabolized differently in children.

    (a) Absorption is decreased in young children.

    (b) Metabolism is increased in small children.

(3) It is started at a high dose with subsequent dose adjustments based on drug levels.

b. Tacrolimus (FK506).

    (1) Its mode of action is similar to cyclosporine.

    (2) This drug is used instead of cyclosporine in dual or triple therapy.

    (3) Leads to similar survival rates as with cyclosporine therapy.

5. Polyclonal antibodies, such as anti-thymocyte globulin (ATG), are used in children to reverse and treat acute rejection and for induction therapy.

6. OKT3, monoclonal antibody.

a. This drug is used to reverse and treat acute rejection episodes and for initial transplant induction therapy.

b. A first dose reaction is observed in more than two thirds of patients, including children. To avoid allergic reactions, the patient should receive IV methylprednisolone, diphen-hydramine hydrocholoride (Benadryl®), and acetaminophen (Danovitch, 2010).

7. Newer monoclonal antibodies.

a. Used with success for induction therapy in pediatric patients.

b. Examples:

    (1) Daclizumab (Zenapax®).

    (2) Basiliximab (Simulect®).

8. Other newer drugs (e.g., rapamycin) are used in limited fashion in pediatric patients. Little information was available at the time of writing this chapter.

9. Adherence to drug therapy.

a. May be a problem regardless of the interval since transplant. Nonadherence for even a short time can lead to significant rejection.

b. Adolescents are at a greater risk for poor adherence because of normal adolescent developmental issues.

SECTION I
Acute Kidney Injury in Children

I. Pediatric Risk, Injury, Failure, Loss, End-stage renal disease (pRIFLE) Criteria (Akcan-Arikan et al., 2007) (see Table 5.11).

A. Risk (of kidney dysfunction): Estimated creatinine clearance (eCL) decreases by 25% and urine output < 0.5 mL/kg/hr for 8 hours.

B. Injury (to the kidney): eCL decreases by 50% and urine output < 0.5 mL/kg/hr for 16 hours.

C. Failure (of kidney function): eCL decreases by 75% or eCL < 35 mL/min/1.73 m^2 and urine output < 0.5 mL/kg/hr for 24 hours or anuric for 12 hours.

D. Loss (of kidney function): persistent failure > 4 weeks.

E. End-Stage (kidney disease): persistent failure > 3 months.

II. Indications for continuous renal replacement therapy (CRRT) in children (Avner et al, 2009).

A. Severe fluid overload in patients with cardiovascular instability.

Table 5.11

Pediatric-modified RIFLE (pRIFLE) Criteria

	Estimated CCl	Urine output
Risk	eCCl decrease by 25%	< 0.5 mL/kg/h for 8 h
Injury	eCCl decrease by 50%	< 0.5 mL/kg/h for 16 h
Failure	eCCl decrease by 75% or eCCl < 35 mL/min/1.73 m^2	< 0.3 mL/kg/h for 24 h or anuric for 12 h
Loss	Persistent failure > 4 weeks	
End stage	End-stage renal disease (persistent failure > 3 months)	

eCCl, esitmated creatinine clearance; pRIFLE, pediatric risk, injury, failure, loss and end-stage renal disease

Reprinted with permission from Macmillan Publishers Ltd: [*Kidney International*] (Arikan et al.) copyright 2007).

B. Metabolic imbalance, hyperammonemia, or fluid overload in patients with liver failure, inborn errors of metabolism, or after bone marrow transplant.

III. Continuous hemofiltration.

A. Has been used since the mid-1980s in pediatric patients, either as CVVH with venous access or CAVH with arterial and venous access.

B. Has been used in infants and children requiring extracorporeal membrane oxygenation (ECMO) due to severe cardiovascular or respiratory failure. These patients often have coexisting kidney failure (14% of neonatal ECMO patients; 31% of pediatric ECMO patients), which is associated with a poorer outcome.
1. Requires the hemofilter be placed where there is a pressure differential in the ECMO circuit (e.g., between ECMO circuit preoxygenator port and the circuit bladder).
2. Should only be performed at tertiary or quaternary healthcare facilities with neonatal or pediatric ECMO expertise.
3. Can be used in parallel with a left ventricular assist device (LVAD). Technical difficulty may be experienced in balancing the higher pressure of the LVAD circuit and the lower pressure of the CRRT circuit.

IV. Pediatric challenges.

A. Small size of the patient and the severity of illness.

B. Significant clinical hurdles.
1. Establishing vascular access, especially in the small child.
2. Choosing catheters short in length with a large internal diameter, but not so large as to impede blood flow from a limb or cause superior vena cava syndrome.
3. Operating within the restrictions of a small blood volume.
4. Preventing patient heat loss in the large extracorporeal circuit.
5. Operating with relatively low baseline blood pressure.

C. The small size of the pediatric hemofilters prohibits the rate of replacement fluids in volumes used in adults. The replacement fluid rate should not be in excess of that tolerated by the hemofilter ultrafiltration coefficient and should be appropriate for the patient's body size.

D. Large size of the ECV (priming volume), especially with automated CRRT.

1. Should be less than 10% EBV for safety, as with hemodialysis.
2. If volume exceeds 10–12.5% of patient's EBV, prime the circuit with a volume expander such as 5% albumin in saline or reconstituted whole blood (required for ECV greater than or equal to 15% EBV).
3. There must be separate and accurate pumps and scales for each component of CRRT (i.e., UF, replacement fluid, dialysate).
4. A range of blood flows with a minimum of 20 mL/min.
5. Thermoregulation (warming the extracorporeal circuit).
6. Maximum safety features.

E. Minimum ECV (priming volume) with low resistance.
1. Exchangeable components.
2. Biocompatibility.

F. Microcoagulation measurement to minimize blood sampling.

SECTION J
Nutrition and Growth in Children with Kidney Disorders

I. Chronic kidney disease (CKD) and kidney failure are associated with malnutrition and decreased growth.

A. In children with CKD/kidney failure, sodium wasting in the urine, uncorrected acidosis and renal osteodystrophy, poor calorie intake, and alterations in the growth hormone-insulin-like growth factor axis can contribute to failure of normal growth and development (Corkins, 2010).

B. Factors that interfere with growth in children with CKD or kidney failure include:
1. Protein-calorie malnutrition.
2. Acidosis.
3. Renal sodium wasting.
4. Renal bone disease.
5. Hypertension.
6. Corticosteroid treatment.
7. Tissue resistance to growth hormone.
8. Zinc deficiency.

C. Causes of protein-calorie malnutrition in children with CKD.
1. Anorexia and alterations in taste.
2. Catabolic uremic state.

a. Increased muscle protein breakdown.

b. Inhibition of protein synthesis.

3. Comorbidities such as chronic infection, vomiting, diarrhea, or constipation.

4. Loss of protein and amino acids in dialysate during hemodialysis or peritoneal dialysis.

5. Insulin resistance.

6. Personal food preference.

7. Limited financial resources.

II. Evaluation of nutrition and growth in pediatric patient.

A. Objective and subjective measures useful to determine how well the child is growing and developing.

B. One-time measures of height and weight indicate size at a point in time, but serial measurements are used to evaluate growth (KDOQI Guidelines for Nutrition [NKF, 2008]).

C. Dietary interview.

1. Includes parent or patient recall of usual intake for 24 hours, or for 3 days for better assessment of day-to-day variation.

2. Daily intake of calories, protein, sodium, potassium, phosphorus, fluid intake, and vitamin intake determined and compared to required needs.

3. History of other factors related to nutrition: nausea, vomiting, diarrhea, constipation, eating patterns, food preparation, economic resources, change in appetite or taste of food, swallowing difficulty, physical eating skills, and activity.

a. If the patient is less than 2 years old, evaluate monthly.

b. If the patient is older than 2 years, evaluate at least quarterly.

D. Anthropometric measurements.

1. The patient's measurements should be compared to the normal for age and gender (KDOQI Guidelines for Nutrition [NKF, 2008]).

2. Head circumference (FOC).

a. The FOC should be measured at each visit until 3 years of age.

b. In malnutrition, the FOC is last to be affected after weight and height.

c. A small FOC for age may reflect severe nutritional deficiency and growth retardation.

3. Length measurements in infants and toddlers should be obtained up to 36 months.

a. Plot monthly on World Health Organization (WHO) length growth charts.

b. Growth velocity (change in height per unit of time) can be calculated by the 2006 WHO Growth Standards. A negative change indicates poor growth.

4. Height measurements in children greater than 2 years, who are able to stand unassisted.

a. Plotted at least quarterly on the CDC height growth chart.

b. Should be within the 5th and 95th percentile for age.

c. In children with CKD, if height growth parallels but is less than the 5th percentile or falls off the curve, intervention is needed.

5. Weight should be assessed at each visit and plotted at least monthly on the growth chart.

a. A weight-for-length less than expected or below the 5th percentile for age may reflect nutritional deficiency.

b. The target weight should be estimated based on a euvolemic state, presence of edema, BP, lab values, and dietary evaluation.

c. Weight evaluations can be a challenge as weight gain is expected in a growing child.

6. Body Mass Index (BMI) for Height–Age percentile.

a. The BMI should be determined each time height and weight are measured.

b. The CDC defines underweight as BMI-for-age < 5th percentile, overweight as > 85th percentile, and obese as > 95th percentile.

E. Biochemical parameters.

1. Serum albumin.

a. The serum albumin level should be greater than 4.0 g/dL (KDOQI Guidelines for Nutrition, [NKF, 2008]).

b. It is affected by many factors, including:

(1) Loss in urine in children with nephrotic syndrome.

(2) Loss in dialysate, especially during peritoneal dialysis.

(3) Poor dietary intake.

(4) Can be depressed with systemic inflammation or volume-overload.

2. Serum bicarbonate.

a. Should be measured monthly.

b. The goal is to maintain the level greater than 22 mEq/L (KDOQI Guidelines for Nutrition [NKF, 2008]).

c. Uncorrected acidosis plays a significant role in growth retardation.

3. Bone disease parameters consist of monthly serum calcium, phosphorus, alkaline phosphatase, and quarterly intact PTH. Assessment of the PTH may need to be done more frequently if therapy is being adjusted to normalize the PTH.

4. Anemia parameters include a CBC monthly and

iron studies quarterly (see Anemia Management).
5. Urea kinetic modeling, including protein catabolic rate (PCR) (KDOQI Guidelines for Nutrition [NKF, 2008]).
   a. Can be normalized to a patient's weight (nPCR). First calculate the urea generation rate (G):

   G (mg/min)= {C2 x V2)- (C1 x V1)} / t
   where:
   C2= predialysis blood urea nitrogen (BUN) (mg/dL)
   C1= postdialysis BUN
   V2= predialysis total body water (dL; V2= 5.8 dL/ kg x predialysis weight in kg)
   V1= postdialysis total body water (dL; V1= 5.8 dL x postdialysis weight in kg)
   t= time (minutes) from end of the dialysis treatment to the beginning of the next treatment

   b. Then, using a modified Borah equation, nPCR is calculated:

   nPCR (g/kg/d)= 5.43 x est G/V1+ 0.17
   where:
   V1= postdialysis total body water
       (L; V1= 0.58 x postdialysis weight in kg)

   c. Must be measured monthly in patients on dialysis.
6. Bioelectrical impedance analysis (BIA)
   a. Allows estimation of body fluid compartment volumes, which can be used to make inferences about body composition.
   b. Can be influenced by fluid status, fat mass, or lean mass.
7. Sodium and water balance is monitored via monthly sodium levels and assessment of fluid balance with each visit.

F. Medications with nutritional implications.
   1. Should be evaluated monthly in patients on dialysis.
   2. Should include:
      a. Phosphate binders and calcitriol.
      b. Diuretics.
      c. Other vitamins.

G. Comorbidities that may affect the child's nutritional intake should be evaluated with each occurrence.

H. Psychologic or social factors that may affect nutritional intake should be evaluated frequently.

III. Dietary prescription for children.

A. Calories.
   1. 100% of estimated energy requirement (EER) is recommended starting point for pediatric patients with CKD stages 3 to 5. Further adjustment is based on weight gain or weight loss (KDOQI Guidelines for Nutrition [NKF, 2008]).
   2. Institute of Medicine (IOM) recommends 45% to 65% of energy from carbohydrates and 30% to 40% from fat.
   3. Calories from dialysate glucose in patients on peritoneal dialysis must be considered in initial prescription and may increase the total calorie intake by about 7 to 10 kcal/kg.
   4. Adjust calorie intake upward or downward according to the child's intake and nutritional assessment.

B. Protein.
   1. Maintain dietary protein intake: (KDOQI Guidelines for Nutrition [NKF, 2008]).
      a. CKD Stage 3: 100% to 140% of the daily recommended intake (DRI) for ideal body weight.
      b. CKD Stage 4–5: 100% to 120% of the DRI for ideal body weight.
   2. Patients on chronic hemodialysis may require 0.1 g/kg/day more than the DRI to account for dialytic losses.
   3. Patients on chronic peritoneal dialysis may require 0.2 g to 0.3 g/kg/day more than the DRI.
   4. If unable to consume adequate amounts of protein to meet the DRI, protein modulars or concentrated formula may be used.
   5. Inflammation or recent infection can contribute to protein catabolism and be considered when making recommendations on protein needs.

C. Vitamins.
   1. Vitamin supplementation should be based on assessment of dietary intake and identified deficiency.
   2. Consider supplementation of water-soluble vitamins to children on dialysis if measured blood vitamin levels are low, clinical evidence of deficiency is present, or the dietary intake alone does not meet or exceed 100% of the daily recommended intake.

D. Lipid management.
   1. Hyperlipidemia often occurs as CKD progresses; characterized by hypertriglyceridemia, elevated levels of very low-density lipoproteins (VLDL), low-density lipoproteins (LDL), and total cholesterol.
   2. In a malnourished child, additional restrictions maybe overwhelming and can further reduce caloric intake. Dietary intervention is not recommended for malnourished children with CKD. However, in nonmalnourished children with CKD, increase fiber, heart-healthy fat, and limit sugar intake (KDOQI Guidelines for Nutrition [NKF, 2008]).

IV. Special concerns for nutrition in children.

A. Infants.
   1. Feedings should be breastmilk or whey-based, low renal solute load formula.
   2. Poor nutrition at this age may adversely affect cognitive development.
   3. Gastrointestinal reflux is common in this age group and can impair feedings.
   4. Solid foods should be introduced on a normal schedule, but may be refused by infants with CKD stage 5 on dialysis who have anorexia.

B. It may be difficult to meet the protein needs because of a preference for carbohydrates in children. Protein modulars may be needed.

C. Adolescents.
   1. Dietary preferences may interfere with adherence to the diet.
   2. The desire for peer group acceptance may adversely affect adherence to sodium and fluid restricted diets.

D. Specific disease-related nutritional recommendations in children.
   1. Children with congenitally obstructed or dysplastic kidneys.
      a. May have polyuria, renal sodium wasting, and intravascular volume depletion without supplemental sodium and water intake.
      b. May have significant acidosis from tubular injury, but only mild to moderate CKD.
      c. Cow's milk should be avoided because of the high sodium and phosphate load.
   2. Children with acquired glomerulonephritis often require sodium restriction.
   3. Children treated with steroids.
      a. Monitor for hyperlipidemia.
      b. Advise of the steroid-induced appetite stimulus and potential to consume excessive calories and become obese.
   4. Children with nephrotic syndrome (NS) and severe edema.
      a. Evaluate for malabsorption and subsequent malnutrition.
      b. Sodium restriction is required.
      c. Monitor for hyperlipidemia and consider drug treatment if the NS is chronic and unremitting.
   5. Children with tubular defects.
      a. Associated with severe polyuria and renal solute loss.
      b. May benefit from high volume feedings and replacement of renal salt and mineral losses.

E. Supplemental nutrition.
   1. Consider when a child does not have normal height velocity.
   2. Consider when a child does not consume the DRI for protein and calories.
   3. Consider oral supplements, especially designed for kidney failure, that:
      a. Provide increased protein and calories.
      b. Do not provide increased electrolytes and phosphorus.
   4. Enteral tube feedings can be initiated if oral intake does not meet the nutritional needs of the child.
   5. Use intermittent bolus or continuous feeding to meet protein and caloric needs.
      a. Deliver feedings via nasogastric (NG) tube if short-term feeding is needed. Tolerated best by infants and small children.
      b. Common issues with NG tubes.
         (1) Often medications are also given through the NG tube and due to inadequate flushing after administration, the NG tube may clog and require frequent replacement.
         (2) Monitor for gastric reflux and emesis, aspiration, sinusitis, chronic irritation including oropharyngitis and esophagitis, and patient or parental anxiety.
      c. Deliver via gastrostomy tube (GT) if long-term feeding is needed.
         (1) The gastrostomy tube may be concealed beneath the clothes, especially if a gastrostomy button is used.
         (2) Monitor for gastric reflux and emesis, gastric leakage, exit-site irritation or infection, intestinal obstruction, gastrocutaneous fistula, peritoneal dialysate leak, and peritonitis.
   6. A trial of intradialytic parenteral nutrition (IDPN) is suggested for malnourished children (BMI for height-age < 5th percentile) receiving maintenance HD who are unable to meet their nutritional requirements through oral or tube feeding (KDOQI Guidelines for Nutrition [NKF, 2008]).

V. Growth patterns and issues in children.

A. Infancy.
   1. Nutrition is the most important determinant of growth.
   2. Growth rate in the first year is higher than at any other time of life.
   3. The potential for growth loss and recovery is greatest, so prevention and treatment during this stage is critical.

B. Childhood.
1. Growth hormone and insulin-like growth factors as well as caloric intake are important determinants of growth in this age group.
2. The potential for growth loss and recovery is great, so prevention and treatment during this stage is also critical.

C. Treatment and associated issues related to growth patterns.
1. CKD stages 3 and 4 is associated with poor height and weight growth.
2. Hemodialysis is associated with poor height and weight growth.
3. PD is associated with:
   a. Exaggerated losses of substances relevant for growth, especially amino acids and proteins.
   b. Marked insulin resistance related to peritoneal glucose uptake.
   c. Increased obesity related to the absorption of glucose from the dialysate in addition to high caloric intake.
   d. Feeling of satiety induced by large fill volumes.
4. Transplantation requiring chronic steroid therapy is associated with poor height growth and increased incidence of obesity.

D. Optimizing growth in children.
1. Optimize dialysis adequacy.
2. Control renal osteodystrophy.
3. Control acid-base balance.
4. Replace renal-wasting of sodium and fluid.
5. Insure adequate protein and energy intake.

E. Treatment with growth hormone (GH) to stimulate growth in children with CKD and kidney failure.
1. GH promotes anabolism and increased muscle mass.
2. It overcomes the relative resistance to growth hormone associated with CKD.
3. Indications.
   a. Height less than 2.0 standard deviations below the mean for chronologic age.
   b. Height velocity less than 2.0 standard deviations below the mean.
   c. Growth potential as documented by bone radiographs showing open epiphyses.
4. Pretreatment considerations.
   a. Correct protein-calorie malnutrition, acidosis, and hyperphosphatemia.
   b. Control hyperparathyroidism and renal osteodystrophy.
5. Treatment considerations.
   a. Identify target height, usually 50th percentile for chronologic age.
   b. Base dose on kg body weight and administer daily by subcutaneous route. (See minimizing

the trauma of repeated injections in the Anemia Management Section previously described.)
   c. Monitor for treatment adequacy as defined by increase in growth velocity every 3 months.
   d. Reasons to discontinue therapy.
      (1) No response in 12 months (growth velocity < 2 cm/year).
      (2) Target height achieved or final height reached, and epiphyses are closed.

Section K
Immunization Guidelines for Pediatric Patients with Kidney Disease

I. Overview.

A. Infants and children with CKD or kidney failure should receive all usual immunizations per the recommended childhood immunization schedule, except Hepatitis B vaccine, which should be given in an increased dose (Neu, 2012).

B. Pediatric kidney transplant patients and patients on immunosuppressive medications.
1. Require all usual immunizations with the following exception: avoid live vaccines, including measles/mumps/rubella (MMR), oral polio vaccine, and varicella vaccine.
2. Check MMR and varicella titers before transplantation and revaccinate if indicated (Danovitch, 2010).

II. Specific information.

A. Hepatitis B vaccine.
1. For effectiveness, the recommended dose is increased to 20 mcg for all pediatric patients with CKD, on dialysis, or with transplants. The dialysis formulation (40 mcg/mL) should be used (Neu, 2012).
2. Monitor yearly antibody titers and administer booster if titer less than 10 mIu/mL.

B. Influenza vaccine.
1. It should be given annually to pediatric patients on dialysis, pediatric transplant patients, and pediatric patients with CKD or nephrotic syndrome. These patients have increased susceptibility to the complications of influenza.
2. If less than 1 year old, administer split virus vaccine.
3. If less than 8 years old, administer two doses on first administration.

C. Pneumococcal vaccine.
1. It should be administered, especially to nephrotic patients because of their increased susceptibility to pneumococcal infection (Neu, 2012).
2. Pneumococcal 13-valent conjugate vaccine.
   a. Give at least 8 weeks prior to giving Pneumococcal polysaccharide vaccine (PPSV 23).
   b. Children under 6 years old will need two doses of Prevnar 13 at least 1 month apart.
   c. Children aged 6 to 18 years old will need one dose.
3. Pneumococcal polysaccharide vaccine (PPSV 23).
   a. Administer once if patient greater than 2 years old.
   b. Revaccinate after 3 to 5 years if patient is younger than 10 years old.
   c. Revaccinate after 6 years if patient is older than 10 years old.

D. The APRN's role in immunization management.
1. The APRN can lead a quality improvement project to increase vaccination rates in the dialysis unit.
2. Figure 5.2 is an example of an immunization protocol created by an APRN.

SECTION L
Emergency Care

I. Staff should be appropriately trained in Basic Life Support (BLS) and/or Pediatric Advanced Life Support (PALS). Appropriate equipment and supplies are suggested to be available for the child.

A. BLS equipment and supplies.
1. Oropharyngeal airways: infant, child, and adult (sizes 00 to 5).
2. Nasopharyngeal airways: sizes 18F–34F, or 4.5–8.5 mm.
3. Self-inflating resuscitation bag: child and adult size (child reservoir of 450 mL, adult reservoir 1000 mL).
4. Bag-valve-mask devices: infant, child, and adult sizes.
5. Oxygen masks: infant, child, and adult sizes.
6. Non-rebreathing masks: pediatric and adult sizes.
7. Suction catheters (6F–14F).
8. Bulb syringe.

B. PALS equipment and supplies.
1. Pediatric paddles for defibrillator (defibrillator should be able to deliver 5 to 360 joules).
2. Pediatric size monitoring electrodes.
3. Laryngoscope with straight blades 1 to 2, curved blades 2 to 4.

4. Endotracheal tube stylets: pediatric and adult sizes.
5. Endotracheal tubes: uncuffed sizes 2.5 to 6.0, cuffed sizes 6.0 to 8.0.
6. NG tubes: 8F to 16F.

II. Suggested medications to have available for pediatric cardiopulmonary resuscitation and their dosages.

A. Epinepherine (1:1000) for bradycardia or asystole: 0.1 mg/kg/dose IV or by endotracheal tube.

B. $NaHCO_3$ (1 mEq/mL): 1 mEq/kg/dose IV.

C. Atropine sulfate (0.1 mg/mL): 0.02 mg/kg/dose IV
1. Minimum dose: 0.1 mg.
2. Maximum single dose infants and children: 0.5 mg, adolescents 1.0 mg.

D. Calcium chloride (100 mg/mL, 10%): 20 mg/kg/dose IV.

E. Lidocaine (20 mg/mL): 1 mg/kg/dose.

III. Individual patient medication worksheets in the record for easy and accurate reference in an emergency.

A. Precalculated by physician or pharmacist with physician review.

B. Include patient name, weight, body surface area; endotracheal tube size; emergency medication doses in mg and in mL.

C. Update at least every 6 to 12 months to reflect changes in actual weight and height.

SECTION M
Atraumatic Care

I. Atraumatic care is defined as the provision of therapeutic care in settings, by personnel, and through the use of interventions that eliminate or minimize the psychological and physical distress experienced by children and their families in the healthcare systems (Wong, 1989).

II. Potential physical stresses.

A. Pain and discomfort (injections, needle punctures, dressing changes, and other invasive procedures such as a VCUG).

Immunization Protocol for Dialysis Unit

I. Introduction

To reduce the risk of morbidity and mortality from vaccine-preventable disease, physicians who care for potential transplant recipients should monitor the immunization status of their patients and keep abreast of changes in the recommended immunization guidelines (Chow & Golan, 2009). Because patients with end-organ disease, such as end-stage renal disease, have reduced immune responses to many vaccines, vaccination should be performed as early as possible during the course of these diseases. Furthermore, it is particularly important for live vaccines to be updated during the pretransplant assessment because such vaccines are contraindicated once a patient is maintained on immunosuppression (Chow & Golan, 2009).

II. Previous Immunization Records

All new patients to Texas Children's Hospital Dialysis Unit should bring a copy of their current immunization records within 1 month of starting dialysis. These records may be requested from:
– Pediatrician/Primary Care Provider
– Health Department
– School

III. Laboratory data to be collected with initial blood work

- Varicella titer level
- Hepatitis Panel (Including Hep A, B, C antigens/antibodies)

IV. Laboratory Results

– If positive Hepatitis B, dialysis machines should be isolated and not used on other patients.
– If positive Hepatitis results, lab tests should be repeated to determine if results are accurate.
– If positive Hepatitis C, order "Hepatitis C Quantitative RNA PCR."

Vaccine	Titer levels	Dosing/Schedule	Monitoring
Hepatitis B	Give booster if antibody < 10	Dialysis patients receive formulation of 40 mcg/mL. Dose = 20 mcg/mL IM if < 18 y/o.	Obtain titer on admission and yearly thereafter.
Hepatitis A	If antibody negative	Give 0.5 mL IM. If no previous history of Hep A vaccine, give booster in 6 months	
Varicella	Give vaccine if IgG < 1.10	Give 0.5 mL SQ	
Meningococcal	N/A	Give 0.5 mL IM at age 11–12 and booster at age 16. See CDC guidelines (attached) for catch-up schedule.	
Prevnar 13 Pneumococcal	N/A	Give 0.5 mL IM at least 8 weeks prior to giving PPSV 23. Children under 6 years old will need 2 doses of Prevnar 13 at least 1 month apart. Children ages 6–18 will need 1 dose.	
Pneumovax (PPSV 23)	N/A	Give 0.5 mL IM to all patients 8 weeks after completing the PCV 13 series.	
PPD	N/A	0.1 mL intradermally. Read test 48–72 hrs after placement.	PPD test on admission and yearly thereafter.

V. Patients needing immunizations

After the previous vaccine records and titer levels are reviewed, the Nurse Practitioner or rounding Physician should contact the primary Nephrologist to provide an update on needed vaccines. This should be done to determine if the patient has any contraindications to receiving the vaccine. All new patients should be current on their immunizations within 6 months of starting dialysis.

_____   _____

Medical Director of Dialysis   Date
Texas Children's Hospital

Figure 5.2. Immunization protocol for dialysis unit.

B. Immobility (tethered to dialysis equipment).

C. Sleep deprivation (nighttime therapy).

D. Inability to eat or drink (the dietary restrictions of CKD/ kidney failure).

E. Changes in elimination habits (constipation due to decreased oral fluid intake).

III. Potential psychological stresses.

A. Separation from family (from either child and/or parent's point of view).

B. Lack of privacy (open chronic dialysis environment).

C. Inability to communicate (developmental barriers, language barriers).

D. Inadequate knowledge and understanding of the situation.

E. Severity of illness.

F. Parental behavior (expression of concern).

G. Child behavior (appearing more ill).

IV. Potential environmental stresses.

A. Unfamiliar surroundings or crowding.

B. Unfamiliar noises (dialysis equipment sounds; telephones; monitoring; human sounds such as talking, crying, moaning, or retching).

C. Unfamiliar people (healthcare professionals – larger volumes in teaching institutions, patients, and visitors).

D. Unfamiliar and unpleasant smells (rubbing alcohol, adhesive remover, body odors, disinfectants).

E. Exam lights.

F. Activity related to other patients.

G. Sense of urgency or lack of concern among staff.

H. Inappropriate comments.

V. Principles of atraumatic care (see Table 5.12).

A. Prevent or minimize physical stresses.
1. Reduce intrusive and painful procedures.
   a. Painful injections: use the smallest gauge needle (ultrafine) for intradermal or subcutaneous injections; use topical anesthesia (i.e., EMLA®); use buffered lidocaine; use intravenous route when it is a viable alternative (e.g., ESAs during chronic hemodialysis).
   b. Fistula needle placement: prepare site with topical anesthetic; use buffered lidocaine;

buttonhole technique; self-cannulation.
2. Avoid or reduce other kinds of physical distress.
   a. Restraints: consider absolute need, and alternatives, such as therapeutic hugging for procedures (e.g., child sitting in parent's lap instead of being held down); minimize personnel involved when physical immobilization is necessary and focus on immobilizing just the child's joints.
   b. Sleeplessness: cluster care to provide 1-hour to 1.5-hour sleep cycles or naps (particularly around blood pressure monitoring).
   c. Smells: eliminate when possible (e.g., food preparation near dialysis treatment area, perfumes, disinfectants).
   d. Noise: minimize equipment noise; offer emotionally soothing alternative (e.g., age-appropriate music).
   e. Skin trauma: avoid tape when possible.
      (1) Tape is needed for securing fistula needles to prevent dislodgement, and ANNA recommends using the chevron taping technique.
      (2) Use surgical netting for securing peritoneal catheters.
      (3) Use skin barriers.
      (4) Use hydro-gel electrodes.
3. Control pain.
   a. Assess frequently using multidimensional approach and document findings.
   b. Use nonpharmacologic interventions as an adjunct to pharmacologic interventions.
4. Prevent or minimize parent/child separation.
   a. Promote family-centered care which fully recognizes the role that families play in ensuring the health and well-being of infants, children, adolescents, and family members of all ages.
      (1) Family and professional partnerships (e.g., families involved in program planning, family advisory councils).
      (2) Child and family participation in care (e.g., patient educational materials designed with families).
      (3) Child and family support (e.g., teaching professionals how to do procedures with families present).
   b. Use the same core group of nurses and technicians with the registered nursing staff managing the care.
   c. Consider parents' and children's preferences to be or not to be together.
      (1) Offer children and parents an informed choice if they choose or not choose to be together.
      (2) Prepare children and parents for the experience if they choose to be together.

Table 5.12

Developmental Age-Appropriate Care: Preparation and Education/Activity

Developmental Age	Nursing Interventions
0–12 months (infant)	➤ Support parent(s) ability to calm/comfort infant by providing parent(s) with adequate information and preparation to reduce their own anxiety. ➤ Provide opportunities for the parent(s) to hold the infant.
12–24 months (toddler)	➤ Support parent(s) ability to calm/comfort toddler by providing parent(s) with adequate information and preparation to reduce their own anxiety. ➤ Encourage parent(s) to involve toddler in developmentally appropriate scheduled activities. ➤ Whenever safe and possible, allow toddler to handle items used in his/her care (e.g., blood pressure cuff, face mask). ➤ Offer suggestions to parent(s) about helpful distractions during procedures. If parent(s) are unavailable, offer comfort and/or distraction as appropriate. ➤ Stoop to the child's eye level (face-to-face) and speak softly/calmly.
2–3 years (toddler)	➤ Support parent(s) ability to calm/comfort toddler by providing parent(s) with adequate information and preparation to reduce their own anxiety. ➤ Encourage parent(s) to use age-appropriate activity areas* when available. ➤ Actively involve child in treatment. Whenever safe, allow child to handle/examine equipment used in treatments and procedures. ➤ Provide comfort and/or distraction during tests and procedures. Preparation should begin immediately preceding the event. ➤ Give the child simple explanations of tests and procedures, using the sensory approach (i.e., what child will see, hear, taste, feel). ➤ Provide choices whenever possible (e.g., examine eyes or ears first). ➤ Stoop to the child's eye level (face-to-face) and speak softly/calmly.
3–5 years (preschooler)	➤ Actively involve child in treatment. ➤ Whenever safe, allow child to handle and explore medical equipment prior to use (e.g., peritoneal dialysis catheter). ➤ Provide comfort and/or distraction during and after tests/procedures. ➤ Use interventions that preserve the child's concept of body integrity (e.g., child-friendly Band-Aids for venipuncture sites). ➤ Give the child short, simple explanations of tests and procedures using the sensory approach (i.e., what child will see, hear, taste, feel). Ask for feedback. ➤ Preparation should be done far enough in advance for child to process information, but not too far in advance so that child has time to fantasize – preferably a few hours before the test or procedure. ➤ Encourage child to participate in age-appropriate activities. ➤ Provide choices whenever possible (e.g., exam which ear first). ➤ Stoop to (or sit at) the child's eye level (face-to-face) and speak softly/calmly.
6–9 years (school-age)	➤ Be honest. ➤ Encourage choices among options if possible (e.g., IV in right or left hand for the peritoneal dialysis patient receiving IV medication therapy). ➤ Whenever safe, allow child to handle and explore medical equipment before use. ➤ Provide comfort and/or distraction during and after tests or procedures. ➤ Give the child developmentally appropriate explanations of tests and procedures using the sensory approach (i.e., what child will see, hear, taste, feel). Ask for feedback. ➤ Preparation should be done far enough in advance for child to process information, but not too far in advance so that child has time to fantasize. ➤ Encourage child to participate in age-appropriate activities. ➤ Provide choices whenever possible (e.g., which limb for venipuncture).
9–12 years (preteen)	➤ Provide honest and accurate information about potential tests/procedures/treatments/etc. Ask for feedback about what the preteen understands. ➤ Provide developmentally appropriate explanations using the sensory approach (i.e., what the patient will see, hear, feel, etc.). ➤ Provide comfort and/or distraction as needed during procedures that may be uncomfortable or painful. ➤ Encourage participation in decision making whenever possible. ➤ Be clear about what expectations are in terms of learning/self-care/adherence. ➤ Preparation should be done far enough in advance for child to process information. ➤ Provide choices whenever possible (e.g., choices that lead to having some control, such as you or I applying tape).
13–18 years (adolescent)	➤ Provide rationale for treatment. Get feedback regarding adolescent's understanding of tests/procedures/disease process and treatment plans. ➤ Encourage adolescents to take responsibility for aspects of self-care. Provide positive reinforcement for successes. ➤ It is important to prepare adolescent for what he/she will see, hear, feel, taste, smell, and be expected to do.

*activity areas can include a playroom, playground, garden, library, school room, and/or teen room.
(Algrananti, 1998)

(3) Help parents support the child during the procedure. For example, be near the child's face to touch and use supportive, nonjudgmental language (e.g., "You are so brave"; "I am here with you").

B. Partner with a child-life specialist, whose discipline is devoted to translating medical issues into language, teaching methods, and coping skills appropriate for developmental age.

C. Employ arts and health interventions to facilitate understanding.

D. Reduce fear of the unknown.
  1. Educate about the hospital or clinic environment, kidney disease, and treatments; use doll models.
  2. Make the environment less threatening (e.g., identify safe areas where no procedures are performed; prominently display children's art).
  3. Allow the child to keep a familiar article (e.g., a toy or blanket or item belonging to an absent parent) during a short, unavoidable separation from family members.

E. Promote a sense of control.
  1. Respect and elicit the family's knowledge about the child and health condition(s).
  2. Promote parent-professional partnerships.

F. Provide opportunities for control.
  1. Age-appropriate participation in care.
  2. Maintain consistent and normalized daily schedule, including educational activities.

SECTION N
Special Considerations for Pediatric Programs

I. Quality of life program.

A. Assessment of Health-Related Quality of Life in Pediatric Patients.
  1. Now mandated at least once per year by the United States Centers for Medicaid and Medicare Services.
  2. PedsQLTM 3.0 (disease specific) and PedsQLTM 4.0 (generic scales for physical, emotional, social, and school functioning) have been validated in pediatric patients (Neul et al., 2013).
  3. Forms to be completed by both patient and the parent proxy.

B. How to communicate results with patient, family, and team members.
  1. Interventions.

2. Life Options/rehabilitation program (http://lifeoptions.org).

C. Facility and network support.
  1. One or more school teachers dedicated to working with patients in the pediatric dialysis unit.
  2. A standard review of school performance (e.g., grades, test scores) and patient's Individualized Education Program (IEP) or 504 plan.
  3. Summer camp opportunities for patients on maintenance dialysis.
  4. Renal Support Network, http://www.rsnhope.org
  5. American Kidney Fund, http://www.kidneyfund.org
  6. National Kidney Foundation, https://www.kidney.org

D. Transition to adult care.
  1. Actual transfer should be individualized for each patient; usually occurs between 18 to 21 years of age (Watson & Warady, 2011).
  2. Transfer may be least desirable during the stage of mid-adolescence (normally ages 14 to 17 years), when a teenager is at the height of risk-taking behavior, peer conformity, poor future orientation, and parental conflict (Bell, 2007).

E. Early preparation should begin by discussing transition expectations with the family at the time of diagnosis and annually thereafter. The formal transition process should begin between the ages of 10 and 14 and should be individualized according to the adolescent's neurocognitive and developmental status (Bell et al., 2008).

F. Transition preparation.
  1. A written transition plan needs to be established with the patient and family well in advance.
  2. Includes understanding of and ability to describe the underlying cause of the kidney failure. Initial education may have been focused toward the primary caregiver.
  3. Includes mastery of self-care skills, including:
    a. Knowing names and doses of medications.
    b. Taking medications accurately.
    c. Calling for own medication refills.
    d. Arranging clinic visits.
    e. Self-monitoring for signs and symptoms of kidney disease.
  4. For a patient on dialysis, arrange to make a visit to the adult facility, when a trusted nurse, social worker, or child life specialist can accompany the patient.
  5. For patients with kidney transplants, awareness of the long and short-term impacts of their medical condition on their overall health and other aspects of life (e.g., pregnancy, genetic counseling, cancer screenings, infection prevention, etc.).

References

Akcan-Arikan, A., Zappitelli1, M., Loftis, L.L., Washburn, K.K., Jefferson, L.S., & Goldstein, S.L. (2007). Modified RIFLE criteria in critically ill children with acute kidney injury. *Kidney International, 71*(10), 1028-1035.

Avner, E.D., Harmon, W.E., Niaudet, P., & Yoshikawa, N. (Eds.). (2009). *Pediatric nephrology* (6th ed.). Philadelphia: Springer.

Barbour, T., Johnson, S., Cohney, S., & Hughes, P. (2012). Thrombotic microangiopathy and associated renal disorders. *Nephrology Dialysis Transplantation, 27*(7), 2673-2685.

Bell, L. (2007). Adolescent dialysis patient transition to adult care: a cross-sectional survey. *Pediatric Nephrology, 22*(5), 720-726.

Bell, L.E., Bartosh, S.M., Davis, C.L., Dobbels, F., Al-Uzri, A., Lotstein, D., Reiss, J., & Dharnidharka, V.R. Adolescent transition to adult care in solid organ transplantation: A consensus conference report. *American Journal of Transplantation, 8*(11), 2230–2242.

Berry, S.G. (1980). Urine sediment examination. *Annals of Internal Medicine, 93*(6), 940-940.

Blowey, D.L. (2012). Update on the pharmacologic treatment of hypertension in pediatrics. *The Journal of Clinical Hypertension (Greenwich), 14*(6), 383-387.

Chase, J.P., Austin, P., Hoebeke, P., & McKenna, P. (2010). The management of dysfunctional voiding in children: A report from the Standardization Committee of the International Children's Continence Society. *The Journal of Urology, 183*(4), 1296-1302.

Cheung, C.K., & Khwaja, A. (2008). Chylous ascites: an unusual complication of peritoneal dialysis. A case report and literature review. *Peritoneal Dialysis International, 28*(3), 229–231.

Cochat, P., & G. Rumsby, G. (2013). Primary hyperoxaluria. *The New England Journal of Medicine, 369*(7), 649-658.

Corkins, M.R. (2010). *Pediatric nutrition support core curriculum.* Silver Spring, MD: American Society for Parenteral and Enteral Nutrition.

Danovitch, G.M. (2010). *Handbook of kidney transplantation.* Philadelphia: Lippincott Williams & Wilkins.

Dell, K.M. (2011). The spectrum of polycystic kidney disease in children. *Advances in Chronic Kidney Disease, 18*(5), 339-347.

Graham, K.M., & Levy, J.B. (2009). Enuresis. *Pediatrics in Review, 30*(5),165-173.

Grossman, J.M., Gordon, R., Ranganath, V.K., Deal, C., Caplan, L., Chen, W., … Saag, K.G. (2010). American College of Rheumatology 2010 recommendations for the prevention and treatment of glucocorticoid-induced osteoporosis. *Arthritis Care & Research, 62*(11), 1515–1526

Hains, D.S., Bates, C.M., Ingraham, S., & Schwaderer, A.L. (2009). Management and etiology of the unilateral multicystic dysplastic kidney: A review. *Pediatric Nephrology, 24*(2), 233-241.

Hildebrandt, F., Attanasio, M., & Otto, E. (2009). Nephronophthisis: Disease mechanisms of a ciliopathy. *Journal of the American Society of Nephrology, 20*(1), 23-35.

International Society of Nephrology (ISN). (2012). Summary of recommendation statements. *Kidney International Supplements 2*(2), 8-12. doi:10.1038/kisup.2012.7

Kleta, R., Basoglu, C., & Kuwertz-Bröking, E. (2000). New treatment options for Bartter's syndrome. *New England Journal of Medicine, 343*(9), 661-662.

Koziell, A., & Grundy, R. (1999). Frasier and Denys-Drash syndromes: Different disorders or part of a spectrum? *Archives of Disease in Childhood, 81*(4), 365-369.

National Kidney Foundation (NKF). (2000). NKF-K/DOQI clinical practice guidelines for peritoneal dialysis adequacy: Update 2000. *American Journal of Kidney Diseases, 37*(1), S65-S136.

National Kidney Foundation (NKF). (2006). Clinical practice guidelines for hemodialysis adequacy: Update 2006. *American Journal of Kidney Diseases, 48*, S2–S90.

National Kidney Foundation (NKF). (2007). KDOQI clinical practice guideline and clinical practice recommendations for anemia in chronic kidney disease: 2007 update of hemoglobin target. *American Journal of Kidney Diseases, 50*(3), 471–530.

National Kidney Foundation (NKF). (2008). KDOQI clinical practice guideline for nutrition in children with CKD: 2008 update. *American Journal of Kidney Diseases, 53*(3 Suppl. 2), S11-104.

Neu, A.M. (2012). Immunizations in children with chronic kidney disease. *Pediatric Nephrology, 27*(8), 1257-1263.

Neul, S.K., Minard, C.G., Currier, H., & Goldstein, S.L. (2013). Health-related quality of life functioning over a 2-year period in children with end-stage renal disease. *Pediatric Nephrology, 28*(2), 285-293.

Nguyen, H.T., Herndon, C.D.A., Cooper, C., Gatti, J., Kirsch, A., Kokorowski, P., & Campbell, J.B. (2010). The Society for Fetal Urology consensus statement on the evaluation and management of antenatal hydronephrosis. *Journal of Pediatric Urology, 6*(3), 212-231.

Ohler, L., & Cupples, S. (2008). *Core curriculum for transplant nurses.* Philadelphia: Mosby.

Pham, P.T., Pham, P.C., Wilkinson, A.H., & Lew, S.Q. (2000). Renal abnormalities in sickle cell disease. *Kidney International, 57*(1), 1-8.

Roberts, K.B. (2011). Urinary tract infection: Clinical practice guideline for the diagnosis and management of the initial UTI in febrile infants and children 2 to 24 months. *Pediatrics, 128*(3), 595-610.

Rodriguez-Soriano, J. (1999). Bartter's syndrome comes of age. *Pediatrics, 103*(3), 663.

Salusky, I.B., & Goodman, W.G. (2001). Adynamic Renal Osteodystrophy: Is there a problem? *Journal of the American Society of Nephrology, 12*(9), 1978-1985.

Sorof, J., & Daniels, S. (2002). Obesity hypertension in children: A problem of epidemic proportions. *Hypertension, 40*(4), 441-447.

Stevens, P.E., & Levin, A. (2013). Evaluation and management of chronic kidney disease: Synopsis of the kidney disease: Improving global outcomes 2012 clinical practice guideline. *Annals of Internal Medicine, 158*(11), 825-830.

Trnka, P. (2013). Henoch-Schönlein purpura in children. *Journal of Paediatrics and Child Health, 49*(12), 995-1003. doi:10.1111/jpc.12403

Warady, B.A., Bakkaloglu, S., Newland, J., Cantwell, M., Verrina, E., Neu, A., & Schaefer, F. (2012). Consensus guidelines for the prevention and treatment of catheter-related infections and peritonitis in pediatric patients receiving peritoneal dialysis: 2012 update. *Peritoneal Dialysis International, 32*(Suppl. 2), S32-86.

Warady, B.A., Schaefer, F., Fine, R.N., & Alexander, S.R. (2004). *Pediatric Dialysis.* Netherlands: Springer.

Watson, A.R., & Warady, B.A. (2011). Transition from pediatric to adult-centered care. *Dialysis & Transplantation, 40*(4), 156–158.

Wyatt, R.J., & Julian, B.A. (2013). IgA nephropathy. *New England Journal of Medicine, 368*(25), 2402-2414.

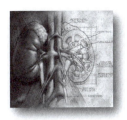

SELF-ASSESSMENT QUESTIONS FOR MODULE 6

These questions apply to all chapters in Module 6 and can be used for self-testing. They are not considered part of the official CNE process.

Chapter 1

1. The specific scope of practice for each APRN is governed by the
    a. Renal Physicians Association.
    b Center for Medicare and Medicaid Services.
    c. individual state (e g., Alabama, Alaska).
    d. American Nurses Association.

2. A major recommendation of the Institute of Medicine Report, "The Future of Nursing: Leading Change, Advancing Health" related to APRN practice is
    a. implement universal standards to control practice.
    b. remove barriers related to scope of practice.
    c. devise common contracts for practice as an APRN.
    d. reimburse APRNs based on level of independence in practice.

3. Hospice referrals can be made
    a. only by a physician.
    b. by anyone.
    c. only by a physician/APRN/PA.
    d. only by a certified palliative care provider.

4. One approach to geriatric renal palliative care categorizes older adults into phenotypes including all of the following EXCEPT
    a. healthy/usual.
    b. frail.
    c. vulnerable.
    d. healthy/unusual.

5. Predictors of increased risk of early mortality include all of the following EXCEPT
    a. older age.
    b. intellect.
    c. peripheral vascular disease.
    d. decreased albumin.

6. For chronic management of neuropathic pain, the following is recommended:
    a. acetaminophen (Tylenol).
    b. nonsteroidal antiinflammatory drugs (NSAIDs).
    c. meperidine (Demerol®).
    d. gabapentin (Neurontin®).

Chapter 2

7. The CKD predictive model that provides the most useful information in older adults and in persons with GFR 45–74 mL/min/1.73 m² is
    a. MDRD.
    b. CKD-EPI.
    c. CKD-EPI creatinine-cystatin C equation.
    d. CKD-EPI cystatin C equation.

8. A patient factor that can increase susceptibility to chronic kidney disease includes
    a. history of anemia.
    b. extreme exercise.
    c. low income.
    d. BMI < 25.

9. What is the goal for transferrin saturation for patients with CKD?
    a. > 20%.
    b. > 30%.
    c. > 40%.
    d. > 50%.

Mr. Y. is a 66-year-old Caucasian male with eGFR 45 mL/min, BP 154/98 in clinic, home BP log showed BP ranges from 126/78 to 142/86, urine albumin to creatinine ratio < 30 mg/g. His current medication regimen is HCTZ 25 mg daily, amlodipine 10 mg daily, lisinopril 5 mg daily.

10. What would be the next best step in management of this patient's blood pressure?
    a. Recheck creatinine and electrolytes and increase Lisinopril to 10 mg daily.
    b. Stop HCTZ and replace with furosemide 20 mg bid.
    c. Make no changes in regimen.
    d. Obtain 24-hour BP monitor to verify BP trends at home before adjusting regimen.

11. When should you discontinue the use of an ACE inhibitor?
    a. If serum creatinine elevates greater than 50%.
    b. When proteinuria has decreased by 40–50%.
    c. When BP gets less than 130/80.
    d. If serum potassium is 4.8.

12. What class of antihypertensive is used with proteinuria and chronic kidney disease?
    a. Angiotensin receptor blockers (ARBs).
    b. Dihydropyridine calcium channel blockers.
    c. Beta blockers.
    d. Vasodilators.

13. When should vitamin D levels be first measured?
    a. At the first visit.
    b. CKD stage 4.
    c. CKD stage 3.
    d. CKD stage 5.

14. Patients diagnosed with chronic kidney disease are at increased risk for acute kidney injury.
    a. True.
    b. False.

15. Which class of medications should be avoided or discontinued once diagnosed with chronic kidney disease?
    a. Antibiotics.
    b. NSAIDs.
    c. Antihistamines.
    d. None of the above.

16. What guidelines are followed once chronic kidney disease is diagnosed?
    a. American Society of Nephrology.
    b. American Nephrology Nurses' Association.
    c. Renal Physicians Association.
    d. Kidney Disease Improving Global Outcomes.

17. How can CKD patients and families prepare psychosocially for kidney replacement therapy?
    a. Encourage participation in multidisciplinary educational offerings.
    b. Acknowledge fear, anxiety, and sense of loss.
    c. Focus on positives and provide constant encouragement and hope.
    d. All of the above.

Chapter 3

18. The APRN on a transplant team performs the following functions during the pretransplant phase:
    a. Obtains history and physical, reviews diagnostic studies, reviews risk factors for sensitization, and reviews infectious disease history.
    b. Obtains history and physical, reviews diagnostic studies, reviews financial status, and reviews risk factors for sensitization.
    c. Obtains history and physical, reviews diagnostic studies, conducts dietary screen, and reviews risk factors for sensitization.
    d. Obtains history and physical, reviews diagnostic studies, reviews infectious disease history, and conducts psychosocial assessment.

19. Which of the following patients would receive induction therapy?
    a. Individuals with a high PRA, individuals of African-American ethnicity, younger individuals, and individuals with blood type B.
    b. Individuals with a high PRA, individuals of Caucasian ethnicity, younger individuals, and individuals who have had a prior transplant.
    c. Individuals with a high PRA, individuals of African-American ethnicity, younger individuals, and individuals who have had a prior transplant.
    d. Individuals with a low PRA, individuals of African-American ethnicity, younger individuals, and individuals who have had a prior transplant.

20. Which immunosuppressive medication causes posttransplant diabetes?
    a. Prednisone.
    b. Mycophenolate mofiteil.
    c. Prograf.
    d. Both a and c.

21. Which of the following drugs has 50% removal by dialysis?
    a. Hydralazine.
    b. Carvedilol.
    c. Lisinopril.
    d. Amlodipine.

22. Which of the following should be evaluated when dosing vitamin D analogs?
    a. Intact parathyroid hormone results only.
    b. Intact parathyroid hormone and corrected serum calcium results.
    c. Intact parathyroid hormone and uncorrected serum calcium results.
    d. Intact parathyroid hormone, corrected serum calcium, and serum phosphorus results.

23. After access placement, avoidance of compression includes which of the following:
    a. No IVs or blood draws to access arm.
    b. No blood pressures to access arm.
    c. Avoid carrying heavy items draped over the access arm.
    d. All the above.

24. During the 2-week postop evaluation of the dialysis access, which of the following is true?
    a. The thrill should be continuous and strongest at the arterial anastomosis.
    b. To differentiate bruising/ecchymosis from infection, bruising/ecchymosis is nonblanchable.
    c. It is common to have tingling and numbness to access hand.
    d. Both a and b.

25. Referral for malfunctioning dialysis access should occur when
    a. there is a vessel spasm during dialysis.
    b. the BP is low and has decreased blood flow through access.
    c. there are persistent changes in access surveillance parameters.
    d. there is an infiltration during dialysis.

26. Lack of needle site rotation is the only cause of aneurysms/pseudoaneurysms.
    a. True.
    b. False.

27. Use of duplex ultrasound can assist in determining cause of slow to mature fistula.
    a. True.
    b. False.

28. If the patient on icodextrin was diabetic, what would you mention about his glucometer?
    a. Just make sure to check blood sugar twice daily, no special cautions.
    b. Maltose is a metabolite of icodextrin and can lead to falsely low blood sugars if the glucometer strips use GDH-PDQ.
    c. Maltose can lead to falsely high blood sugar readings if the glucometer or strips use GDH-PDQ as testing reagent.
    d. The maltose in the icodextrin can lead to early corrosion of the glucometer.

29. Your patient is a 56-year-old female with diabetes, hypertensive, and a normal BMI. She has been on PD and now has very little residual kidney function. Her routine test for adequacy shows a significant decrease. Her regimen is 8 hours of APD overnight, fill volumes 2 liters, and a 1-liter day dwell. How can you help her?
    a. Increase her total overnight time only.
    b. Just increase her fill volumes.
    c. Just increase her day dwell volume.
    d. Use a prescription modeling program.

30. Mr. S. is in the unit with cloudy effluent and abdominal pain. He is treated empirically for peritonitis per unit protocol. Culture results show *Staphylococcus epidermidis*. He is discouraged because he had the same infection 3 weeks ago. How would you categorize this present infection?
    a. Relapsing peritonitis.
    b. Recurrent peritonitis.
    c. Reinfection.
    d. New infection.

31. To satisfy all documentation, recordkeeping, and reporting requirements, the CMS Conditions for Coverage requires patients to agree to report to the ESRD facility providing support services all data information at least every
    a. 30 days.
    b. 45 days.
    c. 60 days
    d. 90 days.

32. Greg is approaching chronic kidney failure and is relocating to be a home hemodialysis patient in your center. He was started on the hepatitis B vaccine series prior to his transfer. All but one of the following statements is true regarding the hepatitis B vaccine. Which one is NOT TRUE?
    a. Hemodialysis patients are less likely to have protective levels of antibody after vaccination with standard dose vaccine.
    b. Patients on in-center hemodialysis require the same dose as patients on home hemodialysis.
    c. Vaccination is not recommended because he will be dialyzing at home.
    d. Patients vaccinated before starting dialysis have shown higher sero protective rates and antibody titers.

Chapter 4

33. Which of the following findings would you expect in the urine of a patient with rhabdomyolysis?
    a. Nonacidic.
    b. Pigmented brown granular casts.
    c. Urinary sodium concentration < 20 mEq/L.
    d. FENA < 1%.

34. According to the KIDGO guidelines, AKI Stage 2 is characterized by
    a. serum creatinine 1.5 to 1.9 times baseline.
    b. serum creatinine 2.0 to 2.9 times baseline.
    c. urine output < 0.5mL/kg/h for 6–12 hours.
    d. urine output < 0.3mL/kg/h for ≥24 hours.

35. The typical finding in urine osmolality when comparing prerenal to intrarenal AKI is
    a. in prerenal AKI the osmolality is low.
    b. in prerenal AKI the osmolality is high.
    c. in intrarenal AKI the osmolality is high.
    d. there is no difference in the osmolality.

36. In a patient with AKI who is going to start hemodialysis, it is important to consider the level of azotemia. If severe, azotemia will require
    a. that the patient be connected to cardiac monitoring.
    b. minimal ultrafiltration during the 4-hour treatment.
    c. a lower blood flow rate using a high efficiency dialyzer.
    d. reducing the urea to no more than 30%.

37. In a patient who has a vascular access and becomes hyperkalemic, it is more effective and less problematic to
    a. treat with Kayexalate®.
    b. administer dextrose and insulin.
    c. provide a dialysis treatment.
    d. give bicarb and calcium.

38. Samuel L. has a spot urine protein-to-creatinine ratio of 3.7 grams of protein. Which statement is true?
    a. He has a normal urine protein.
    b. He has nephrotic range proteinuria.
    c. This proteinuria could be only due to his diabetes and needs no further workup.
    d. Blood pressure control with ACE-inhibitors will have no effect on his degree of proteinuria.

39. Evaluation of acute kidney injury includes
    1. physical assessment and history.
    2. urinalysis.
    3. review of chart for precipitating events.
    4. medication review.
    5. assessment of eGFR and the degree of change.
    6. radiologic evaluation of kidneys/bladder.
        a. 2, 5, and 6.
        b. 1 and 2.
        c. 1, 3, and 5.
        d. All of the above.

40. Diabetic ketoacidosis is characterized by a triad of symptoms, including
    a. hyperglycemia, metabolic acidosis, and ketosis.
    b. hypoglycemia, metabolic acidosis, and ketosis.
    c. hyperglycemia, metabolic alkalosis, and ketosis.
    d. hypoglycemia, metabolic alkalosis, and ketosis.

41. The preferred vascular access for acute hemodialysis/CRRT is
    a. an AV fistula.
    b. an AV graft.
    c. a noncuffed catheter.
    d. a cuffed catheter.

42. The percentage of kidney function is in flux at all times.
    a. True.
    b. False.

Chapter 5

43. Jody Garza is a 12-year-old female with CKD stage 5 starting hemodialysis (HD) in-center 4 days a week. Her risk for anemia includes
    a. extracorporeal blood loss and menorrhagia.
    b. delayed bone age and mineral bone disease.

c. frequent blood draws and access via arteriovenous fistula.
d. increased transferrin saturation and increased ferritin.

44. Sam, a 2-year-old male with CKD stage 5 on peritoneal dialysis (PD), is seen in the clinic for a PD catheter exit-site infection. Cultures are obtained and are positive for methicillin-susceptible *S. aureus*. Based on the International Society for Peritoneal Dialysis (ISPD), the recommended treatment for this PD catheter exit-site infection is antibiotics given
    a. intravenously.
    b. orally.
    c. intraperitoneally.
    d. intramuscularly.

45. Renal tubular acidosis (RTA) can only be the result of an inherited autosomal dominant gene.
    a. True.
    b. False.

46. Johnny has been referred to your clinic from his primary care provider for proteinuria and hematuria on a routine urinalysis. Mother reports he has progressive hearing loss and has been referred to an ophthalmologist for decreased visual acuity. Based on his symptoms, you suspect
    a. atypical hemolytic uremic syndrome.
    b. Jeune syndrome.
    c. Alport's syndrome.
    d. Henoch-Schönlein purpura.

47. The nurse practitioner is reviewing immunization records for a new patient in the hemodialysis unit undergoing evaluation for a living related kidney transplant from her mother. Of the following vaccines which is the most important to have prior to transplant?
    a. Tetanus, diphtheria, pertussis (TdaP).
    b. Human papillomavirus (HPV).
    c. Varicella (VZV).
    d. Hepatitis A (Hep A).

48. When doing education for a patient initiating growth hormone, the mother asks, "How will my child's growth be monitored?" The nurse practitioner's best response is
    a. Growth velocity will be evaluated every 3 months.
    b. Records will be kept of how often he outgrows his clothes.
    c. Bone scans will be performed every 6 months.
    d. The level of GH will be monitored quarterly.

49. You are consulted to see a 3-year-old female who presented to the emergency department with complaints of lower extremity edema and hypertension at her primary care provider's office. Her lab results were significant for the following: albumin 2 g/dL, K 3.5 mmol/L, triglycerides 300 mg/dL, and urinalysis with 4+ protein. Based on these lab results, the APRN suspects
    a. nephrotic syndrome.
    b. systemic lupus erythematosus.
    c. renal dysplasia.
    d. chronic glomerulonephritis.

50. As early as CKD stage 1, a child can experience
    a. metabolic acidosis.
    b. hyperkalemia.
    c. anemia.
    d. a and b.

Answer Key

Chapter 1
1. c
2. b
3. b
4. d
5. b
6. d

Chapter 2
7. c
8. c
9. a
10. d
11. a
12. a
13. c
14. a
15. b
16. d
17. d

Chapter 3
18. a
19. c
20. d
21. c
22. d
23. d
24. d
25. c
26. b
27. a

28. c
29. d
30. a
31. a
32. c

Chapter 4
33. b
34. b
35. b
36. d
37. c
38. b
39. d
40. a
41. c
42. a

Chapter 5
43. a
44. b
45. b
46. c
47. a
48. a
49. a
50. d

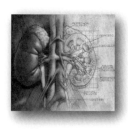

INDEX FOR MODULE 6

Page numbers followed by **f** indicate figures.
Page numbers followed by **t** indicate tables